Frailty and Sarcopenia in Cirrhosis

Puneeta Tandon • Aldo J. Montano-Loza
Editors

Frailty and Sarcopenia in Cirrhosis

The Basics, the Challenges, and the Future

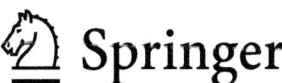 Springer

Editors
Puneeta Tandon
Division of Gastroenterology and Liver Unit
University of Alberta
Edmonton
AB
Canada

Aldo J. Montano-Loza
Division of Gastroenterology and Liver Unit
University of Alberta
Edmonton
AB
Canada

ISBN 978-3-030-26225-9   ISBN 978-3-030-26226-6   (eBook)
https://doi.org/10.1007/978-3-030-26226-6

This Springer imprint is published by the registered company Springer Nature Switzerland AG
The registered company address is: Gewerbestrasse 11, 6330 Cham, Switzerland

Preface

Frailty and sarcopenia have long been recognized as essential elements for prognostication in the aging population. In the recent past, an ever-increasing number of studies have explored the prevalence, pathogenesis, and robust prognostic relevance in patients with cirrhosis. This rising tide of data has already resulted in a change in how we describe our patients, the terms frailty and sarcopenia now permeating our vocabulary.

As an emerging area of study in cirrhosis, some important questions have been answered, but many questions remain. How can frailty and sarcopenia be measured? How do they behave over time? What are the changes in muscle cellular and molecular biology that result in atrophy and weakness? How should the information about a patient's frailty or sarcopenia be used to guide rehabilitation? Should a diagnosis of frailty or sarcopenia change whether patients are considered for liver transplant?

Recognizing the importance of these questions, it is our distinct pleasure to bring together the efforts of an international team of experts and share with you a practical review of "the basics, the challenges, and the future" of frailty and sarcopenia in patients with cirrhosis.

Chapters 1, 2, 3, 4, 5, 6, and 7 introduce the basics of the definitions and diagnosis of each of these entities in research and in the clinical setting, their pathogenesis and prognostic implications, and practical approaches to nutrition and exercise-based therapy. Chapters 8, 9, 10, 11, 12, 13, and 14 focus on the challenges. How do gender, age, and ethnicity alter body composition? Is muscle mass assessment alone enough? How can we assess muscle quality, and what impact does it have on prognosis? Do these entities change with time? Do they improve after liver transplant? Chapters 15, 16, 17, and 18 discuss future considerations including practical bedside measures, upcoming pharmacological therapies, the concept of expanding our thinking to multidimensional frailty, and a research wish list.

We are extremely grateful to our panel of distinguished contributors, experts in the field, from Australia, Europe, and North and South America. We also extend a special thanks to the Springer publishing team who helped to bring these ideas to reality.

It has been a pleasure to be a part of the frailty and sarcopenia evolution in cirrhosis. The contributions of the authors of this book and many others across the world will undoubtedly see the journey continue, questions get answered, and more interrogations arise. With an impact on both quantity and quality of life, frailty and sarcopenia assessment and management will very soon be interwoven as an indispensable part of our daily clinical practice.

Edmonton, AB, Canada   Puneeta Tandon, MD, FRCP(C), MSc(Epi)
                                                          Aldo J. Montano-Loza, MD, PhD, FAASLD, FACG

Contents

Contributors

Pranab Barman Division of Gastroenterology and Hepatology, Duke University Hospital, Durham, NC, USA

Kirsten Elizabeth Bell Department of Kinesiology, University of Waterloo, Waterloo, ON, Canada

Chantal Bémeur Département de nutrition, Université de Montréal, and Hepato-Neuro Lab, CRCHUM, Montreal, QC, Canada

Rahima A. Bhanji Division of Gastroenterology and Liver Unit, Department of Medicine, University of Alberta, Edmonton, AB, Canada

Stefan Buettner Department of Surgery, Erasmus MC University Medical Center, Rotterdam, The Netherlands

Elizabeth J. Carey Division of Gastroenterology and Hepatology, Mayo Clinic, Phoenix, AZ, USA

Hui-Wei Chen Division of Gastroenterology Hepatology and Nutrition, University of Pittsburgh, Pittsburgh, PA, USA

Daria D'Ambrosio Gastroenterology and Hepatology Unit, Department of Translational and Precision Medicine, Sapienza University of Rome, Rome, Italy

Srinivasan Dasarathy Department of Gastroenterology, Hepatology, Cleveland Clinic, Cleveland, OH, USA

Ilana Roitman Disi Division of Anesthesia, Faculty of Medicine Foundation of the University of Sao Paulo, Cancer Institute of Sao Paulo, Sao Paulo, SP, Brazil

Andres Duarte-Rojo Division of Gastroenterology Hepatology and Nutrition, University of Pittsburgh, Pittsburgh, PA, USA

Center for Liver Diseases and Thomas E. Starzl Transplantation Institute, University of Pittsburgh Medical Center, Pittsburgh, PA, USA

Michael A. Dunn Center for Liver Diseases, Thomas E. Starzl Transplantation Institute, Pittsburgh, PA, USA

Pittsburgh Liver Research Center, University of Pittsburgh, Pittsburgh, PA, USA

Maryam Ebadi Department of Medicine, Division of Gastroenterology and Liver Unit, University of Alberta, Edmonton, AB, Canada

Nicoletta Fabrini Gastroenterology and Hepatology Unit, Department of Translational and Precision Medicine, Sapienza University of Rome, Rome, Italy

Maria Cristina Gonzalez Catholic University of Pelotas, Pelotas, RS, Brazil

Penelope Hey Department of Gastroenterology and Hepatology, Austin Health, Melbourne, VIC, Australia

The University of Melbourne, Melbourne, VIC, Australia

Jan N. M. IJzermans Department of Surgery, Erasmus MC University Medical Center, Rotterdam, The Netherlands

Kathleen P. Ismond Division of Gastroenterology, Department of Medicine, Faculty of Medicine and Dentistry, University of Alberta, Edmonton, AB, Canada

Matthew R. Kappus Division of Gastroenterology and Hepatology, Duke University Hospital, Durham, NC, USA

Barbara Lattanzi Gastroenterology and Hepatology Unit, Department of Translational and Precision Medicine, Sapienza University of Rome, Rome, Italy

Alice Liguori Gastroenterology and Hepatology Unit, Department of Translational and Precision Medicine, Sapienza University of Rome, Rome, Italy

Manuela Merli Gastroenterology and Hepatology Unit, Department of Translational and Precision Medicine, Sapienza University of Rome, Rome, Italy

Aldo J. Montano-Loza Division of Gastroenterology and Liver Unit, Department of Medicine, University of Alberta, Edmonton, AB, Canada

Marina Mourtzakis Department of Kinesiology, University of Waterloo, Waterloo, ON, Canada

Graeme M. Purdy Department of Physical Therapy, Faculty of Rehabilitation Medicine, University of Alberta, Edmonton, AB, Canada

Kenneth J. Riess Department of Physical Therapy, Faculty of Rehabilitation Medicine, University of Alberta, Edmonton, AB, Canada

School of Health and Life Sciences, Northern Alberta Institute of Technology, Edmonton, AB, Canada

Darryl B. Rolfson Division of Geriatric Medicine, Department of Medicine, University of Alberta, Edmonton, AB, Canada

Christopher F. Rose Département de médecine, Université de Montréal, and Hepato-Neuro Lab, CRCHUM, Montreal, QC, Canada

Marie Sinclair Department of Gastroenterology and Hepatology, Austin Health, Melbourne, VIC, Australia

The University of Melbourne, Melbourne, VIC, Australia

Christopher J. Sonnenday, MD, MHS Department of Surgery, University of Michigan, Ann Arbor, MI, USA

Guido Stirnimann Division of Gastroenterology & Liver Unit, University of Alberta Hospital, Edmonton, AB, Canada

Department of Visceral Surgery and Medicine, University Hospital Inselspital and University of Bern, Bern, Switzerland

Puneeta Tandon Division of Gastroenterology and Liver Unit, Department of Medicine, Faculty of Medicine and Dentistry, University of Alberta, Edmonton, AB, Canada

Department of Medicine, Cirrhosis Care Clinic, University of Alberta, Edmonton, AB, Canada

Elliot B. Tapper Division of Gastroenterology and Hepatology, University of Michigan, Ann Arbor, MI, USA

Gastroenterology Section, VA Ann Arbor Healthcare System, Ann Arbor, MI, USA

Jeroen L. A. van Vugt Department of Surgery, Erasmus MC University Medical Center, Rotterdam, The Netherlands

Jingjie Xiao Department of Agricultural, Food and Nutritional Science, University of Alberta, Edmonton, AB, Canada

Division of Palliative Care Medicine, Department of Oncology, University of Alberta, Edmonton, AB, Canada

Covenant Health Palliative Institute, Edmonton, AB, Canada

Part I
The Basics

Chapter 1
Definition and Diagnosis of Sarcopenia in the Research and Clinical Settings

Aldo J. Montano-Loza and Maryam Ebadi

Sarcopenia or muscle wasting is a common feature in patients with cirrhosis. Currently, it is well established that this complication is known to be a significant risk factor for overall mortality, mortality on the liver transplantation (LT) wait list, postoperative complication, and even post-LT death.

It is important to distinguish that sarcopenia is not the same as frailty. While sarcopenia is one of the main components of frailty, the latter is a syndrome characterized by decreased physiologic reserve and increased vulnerability to health stressors that predisposes patients to adverse health outcomes.

Muscle mass decreases with aging, with a loss of approximately 1% per year up to age 70, which increases later to 1.5% per year. However, the annual rate of muscle loss is twofold faster in patients with cirrhosis, and losses greater than 3% per year increase the risk of mortality, independent of the severity of liver disease [1].

In some cases, severe sarcopenia can be identified on clinical routine examination; however, early stages of muscle loss may not be visually evident, and the presence of ascites and obesity might make sarcopenia recognition difficult. As a result, objective, reproducible, and validated measures of muscle loss are essential. In addition, quantification of muscle mass provides objective data, which might be relevant for central decisions, such as candidacy for LT.

Sarcopenia refers to loss of muscle mass and function according to the European Working Group on Sarcopenia in Older People (EWGSOP). However, majority of studies of sarcopenia in patients with liver disease focus on the measurement of muscle mass alone. This might be related to the fact that function studies such as handgrip have not shown to correlate with CT muscle assessment in patients with cirrhosis [2]. In addition, muscle function can be affected by acute illness, particularly complicating inpatient assessment, whereas muscle mass is a more stable and

A. J. Montano-Loza (✉) · M. Ebadi
Department of Medicine, Division of Gastroenterology and Liver Unit, University of Alberta, Edmonton, AB, Canada
e-mail: montanol@ualberta.ca

© Springer Nature Switzerland AG 2020
P. Tandon, A. J. Montano-Loza (eds.), *Frailty and Sarcopenia in Cirrhosis*,
https://doi.org/10.1007/978-3-030-26226-6_1

objective parameter that is insensitive to acute changes in cognition or global physical function.

Sarcopenia provides an objective measurement of physical fitness that is applicable even to patients who cannot participate in bedside measures of frailty or for whom estimates of performance status may not reflect their overall health status.

In this chapter, we summarize the evidence from the medical literature to address definition of sarcopenia in patients with cirrhosis in the clinical and research setting.

Definition of Sarcopenia

Sarcopenia is a term which was first adopted by Rosenberg in 1989 in the geriatric literature [3]. Sarcopenia was initially defined as an age-related loss of skeletal muscle, generally described as lean appendicular mass (normalized to height squared) greater than two standard deviations below that typical for healthy young adults [4]. The term sarcopenia has since been expanded to reflect low muscle mass leading to negative effects on physical performance and clinical outcomes across a broad range of disease states.

The new International Statistical Classification of Diseases and Related Health Problems, 10th revision (ICD-10-CM) (M62.84), code for sarcopenia represents a significant recognition as a disease [5]. Great heterogeneity in the metric used to define sarcopenia exists among published study cohorts [6]. Furthermore, studies have varied in their use of a standard definition of sarcopenia defined by threshold values, versus evaluating sarcopenia by percentile among a specific population. The specific definition used for determining sarcopenia is obviously linked to the method of measurement, as not all metrics apply or have been validated across modalities.

Modalities to Evaluate Muscle Mass in Patients with Cirrhosis

Multiple modalities exist for muscle mass quantification, including indirect and direct techniques such as anthropometry, bioelectrical impedance analysis (BIA), dual-energy X-ray absorptiometry (DEXA), ultrasound (US), magnetic resonance imaging (MRI), and computed tomography (CT) (Table 1.1).

Choosing an appropriate assessment technique for clinical practice versus research depends on various features such as cost, accuracy, accessibility, and feasibility of the technique in the population of interest. While all methods may be applicable in the general population, many are not appropriate or accurate in cirrhosis. Mid-arm muscle circumference measurement, a form of anthropometry, requires specialized training and has a low reproducibility.

DEXA which has become the standard of care modality for measuring bone mineral density, may also be used to measure appendicular skeletal muscle mass.

Table 1.1 Modalities evaluating sarcopenia in cirrhosis

	Advantages	Disadvantages
Sarcopenia tools for the clinical setting		
Mid-arm muscle circumference (MAMC)	Cheap, noninvasive, wide availability	Low reproducibility, measurements are affected by subcutaneous adipose tissue loss, requires specialized training
Bioelectrical impedance analysis (BIA)	Noninvasive, quick, simple, inexpensive	Fluid retention, diuretic use, liquid and food intake before the test, and physical activity alter the results
Dual-energy X-ray absorptiometry (DEXA)	Noninvasive, inexpensive, wide availability, consistent results, and little radiation exposure	Influenced by lower limb edema
Sarcopenia tools for the research setting		
Ultrasound (thigh muscle thickness)	Noninvasive, simple, reliable, inexpensive without radiation exposure, independent of edema	Unidentified reproducibility
CT/ MRI	Quick, precise, independent of ascites or edema, capability to quantify muscle and adipose tissue quality and quantity	Expensive, radiation exposure in longitudinal CT images

DEXA-estimated appendicular skeletal muscle mass, which is adjusted to body size, has been adopted by consensus groups (International Working Groups on Sarcopenia and the EWGSOP) to define criteria for the determination of sarcopenia [7]. However, these criteria have not been validated in larger data sets and diverse populations, and since it is a projection-based rather than cross-sectional modality, DEXA inherently suffers from challenges related to tissue overlap. In addition, the fluid shifts common to patients with decompensated cirrhosis reduce the accuracy of DEXA and BIA.

In contrast, US is a promising modality that deserves additional study as it is inexpensive, noninvasive, and free of radiation exposure, has applicability in a variety of practice settings, and can provide results independent of fluid retention [8]. However, more studies are needed before it can be recommended in clinical practice.

Cross-sectional imaging is a routine part of LT assessment in most centers to evaluate the vascular and biliary anatomy for surgical planning and as screening for hepatocellular carcinoma (HCC). The existence of routine cross-sectional imaging in patients evaluated for LT has provided an opportunity for assessment of muscle mass in patients with cirrhosis without the need for additional testing. Indeed, the majority of studies on sarcopenia in LT have used CT imaging.

MRI is also commonly used in LT patients and provides an additional opportunity to assess body composition. While preliminary reports suggest that CT and MRI-based imaging yield equivalent results [9], validity across both techniques needs to be established. Sensitivity and specificity of techniques for capturing longitudinal changes are inevitable criteria for predicting patients' long-term outcomes.

Muscle area on cross-sectional CT images can be assessed by using the Hounsfield units from −29 to +150. Measurements can be obtained in a semiauto-mated way with the help of the software SliceOmatic (TomoVision, Montreal, Quebec, Canada). Besides SliceOmatic, other software has been used to determine the SMI (FatSeg, OsiriX, ImageJ).

Overall, CT image analysis can be used for opportunistic body composition assessment, and therefore, inclusion of cross-sectional imaging as part of LT assess-ment should be considered in the future to develop and validate consistent criteria for sarcopenia.

While individual investigators have made these techniques relatively high throughput in a research setting, an efficient clinical tool or process for measuring muscle mass in clinical practice has not been developed. "Single-slice" or abbrevi-ated CT is a technique with obvious appeal, as it is based upon the modality with the most use in published research studies and is widely available [10]. While caution regarding radiation exposure is appropriate in general, the dose involved in such limited CT scans is miniscule compared with other medical imaging modalities (e.g., equivalent to a standard chest X-ray). Furthermore, such limited scans can be done without the need for intravenous contrast exposure. Importantly, since CT is often performed in these patients for other reasons, these images may already be available for analysis in a large proportion of patients. However, automation of mea-surement of muscle mass such that a diagnosis of sarcopenia could be readily made has not been established. Nevertheless, this modality is likely to be the most appli-cable to clinical practice, as it requires little additional work for the clinician, is not of undue burden to patients, and minimizes operator error in measurement. Similar research efforts have been attempted using single-slice MRI, which eliminates the concern of radiation exposure although may be logistically and financially more costly [11].

Determination of Sarcopenia in Patients with Cirrhosis

In the past decade, a blast of research on sarcopenia in cirrhosis has emerged. This information has significantly advanced our knowledge; however, the field is cur-rently hampered by heterogeneous definitions, measurements, and study design. A main factor confounding the current literature is the use of different cutoffs to define sarcopenia in cirrhosis.

Englesbe et al. first reported sarcopenia using the cross-sectional area of the total psoas area (TPA) on CT imaging. Using the lowest quartile to define sarcopenia, an association between TPA and post-LT mortality was found [12]. Subsequent studies evaluating patients assessed for LT used CT cutoffs for sarcopenia associated with higher mortality risk derived from skeletal muscle index (SMI) in cancer patients [13]. CT-measured SMI, calculated as total muscle area at the third lumbar vertebra (L3) normalized to height squared, is a strong surrogate of whole body muscle mass [10] and can be applied as a reliable marker of whole body muscularity. Among

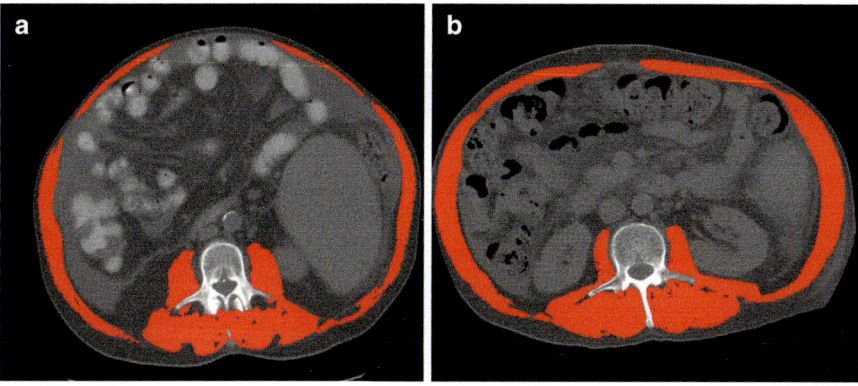

Fig. 1.1 Total muscle area quantification at the level of third lumbar vertebra using abdominal CT images from two male patients with cirrhosis. (**a**) and (**b**), respectively, present a patient who had low SMI (39 cm^2/m^2) and high SMI (54 cm^2/m^2)

patients with cirrhosis, CT-measured SMI at L3 has been the most well-validated tool to define sarcopenia and correlates strongly with survival. To create standardized cutoff points for sarcopenia in cirrhosis, Carey et al. recently defined sarcopenia as SMI <50 cm^2/m^2 in male and <39 cm^2/m^2 in female patients with cirrhosis, listed for LT based on the data from North America centers, part of the Fitness, Life Enhancement, and Exercise in Liver Transplantation (FLEXIT) Consortium [14]. Defined in this way, sarcopenia was delineated based on sex-specific SMI values associated with mortality independent of age and MELD score [14]. To date, this is the only North American study to define sarcopenia using the data derived from a diverse population of patients with cirrhosis awaiting LT. Figure 1.1 highlights the total skeletal muscle quantification at L3 from two male patients.

Apart from total SMI at L3, various psoas muscle measurements including cross-sectional area [12, 15], index [16], and thickness [17] have been applied to predict mortality risk in patients with cirrhosis. However, it has been recently reported that psoas muscle index has limited performance for identifying patients with higher waitlist mortality risk in cirrhosis as compared to SMI [18].

Discrepancies in sarcopenia prevalence between studies likely result from divergent criteria for defining sarcopenia (values below 5th percentile of age- and sex-matched normal population or optimal cut points for the mortality discriminations), outcome of interest, and study population (Table 1.2). In the past, cut points derived from other populations, such as patients with cancer, have been applied, and these may not be appropriate for patients with cirrhosis. The use of different imaging software between studies does not appear to be a significant concern, as excellent agreement has been observed between various software programs when compared directly for quantification of abdominal skeletal muscle cross-sectional area [19].

Sarcopenia in cirrhosis has classically been associated with increased mortality in both genders; however, emerging evidence suggests male sex as a predisposing factor for sarcopenia and increased mortality in cirrhosis [20]. This emphasizes the

Table 1.2 Summary of studies investigating sarcopenia diagnosis in cirrhosis

Author/year	Study population	Sarcopenia assessment	Sarcopenia cutoff	Criteria for cutoff
Merli et al. 2010 [30]	150 patients with cirrhosis hospitalized to a tertiary care	Mid-arm muscle circumference (MAMC)	NA	MAMC below the 5th percentile of age- and sex-matched normal population
Englesbe et al. 2010 [12]	163 LT recipients	CT-measured psoas muscle	TPA <1420 mm² at the level of the fourth lumbar vertebra (L4)	Lowest TPA quartile
Montano-Loza et al. 2012 [13]	112 patients with cirrhosis evaluated for LT	CT at the level of the third lumbar vertebrae	L3 SMI ≤38.5 cm²/m² for women and ≤52.4 cm²/m² for men	Mortality-associated SMI cutoffs in cancer [31]
Krell et al. 2013 [28]	207 LT recipients	CT-measured psoas muscle	TPA <1499 mm² for men and <954 mm² for women	Lowest TPA tertile
DiMartini et al. 2013 [25]	338 LT recipients	CT at the level of the third lumbar vertebrae	L3 SMI ≤38.5 cm²/m² for women and ≤52.4 cm²/m² for men	Mortality-associated SMI cutoffs in cancer [31]
Masuda et al. 2014 [27]	204 patients undergoing LT	CT-measured psoas muscle	PMA <800 cm² for men and <380 cm² for women	PMA below the 5th percentile for each sex
Durand et al. 2014 [17]	562 patients listed for LT	CT-measured psoas muscle	Transversal psoas muscle thickness [TPMT/height (mm/m)] at the level of the umbilicus ≤16.8 mm/m	Optimal cutoffs of TPMT/height to discriminate waiting list mortality
Hara et al. 2016 [32]	161 patients with cirrhosis	Bioelectrical impedance analysis (BIA)- measured upper limb skeletal muscle mass (kg)	1.2 kg/m² for women and 1.7 kg/m² for men	Values less than −1 standard deviation from the mean values in the control group (diabetic patients)
Carey et al. 2017 [14]	396 patients listed for LT	CT at the level of the third lumbar vertebrae	SMI <39 cm²/m² for women and <50 cm²/m² for men	Optimal cutoffs of SMI to discriminate waiting list mortality
Golse et al. 2017 [15]	256 LT recipients	CT-measured psoas muscle	PMA <1561 mm² for men and <1464 mm² for women	Optimal cutoffs of PMA to discriminate 1-year post-LT mortality

Table 1.2 (continued)

Author/year	Study population	Sarcopenia assessment	Sarcopenia cutoff	Criteria for cutoff
Tandon et al. 2016 [8]	159 patients evaluated for LT	CT at the level of the third lumbar vertebrae	L3 SMI $\leq$38.5 cm^2/m^2 for women and $\leq$52.4 cm^2/m^2 for men	Mortality-associated SMI cutoffs in cancer [31]
Belarmino et al. 2018 [33]	144 male patients with cirrhosis	Appendicular skeletal muscle index (ASMI) with dual-energy X-ray absorptiometry (DEXA)	DEXA-ASMI $\leq$7 kg/m^2	Lowest tertiles of the DXA-ASMI
Van Vugt et al. 2018 [29]	224 patients listed for LT	CT at the level of the third lumbar vertebrae	L3 SMI <44.1 for men and <37.9 for women	Lowest sex-specific quartile of SMI
Praktiknjo et al. 2018 [34]		Magnetic resonance imaging (MRI)	Fat-free muscle area <2895 mm^2 for women and Fat-free muscle area <3197 mm^2 for men	Optimal cutoffs to discriminate 3-year survival

importance of survival analysis stratification by sex rather than simply adjusting for sex. The prevalence of sarcopenia within each BMI category is another consideration when building a consensus definition to incorporate into clinical practice. Lastly, divergent study outcomes, such as overall mortality in evaluated patients, waitlist mortality in listed patients, post-LT mortality in patients undergoing LT, and short-term versus long-term outcomes, confound the comparison between studies and development of generalized definitions.

Although a detailed definition of sarcopenia in cirrhosis for use in clinical practice is lacking, low muscle mass is a main indicator of adverse outcomes in this population, including poor quality of life [21], hepatic decompensation (ascites, hepatic encephalopathy, and variceal bleeding) [22], mortality in patients with cirrhosis evaluated for LT [17, 22–25], longer hospital and intensive care unit stay [26, 27], higher incidence of infection following LT [26, 28], and higher overall healthcare cost [29]

In summary, at the current time, it is clear that sarcopenia is an important predictor of poor clinical outcomes in cirrhosis. SMI measured by CT constitutes the best studied technique for measuring sarcopenia in patients with cirrhosis. Cutoff values for sarcopenia, defined as SMI <50 cm^2/m^2 in male and <39 cm^2/m^2 in female patients, constitute the validated definition for sarcopenia in patients with cirrhosis. Many questions remain, including more practical and accessible modalities for measuring muscle mass with the optimal cutoff values for sarcopenia, the ideal timing and frequency of muscle mass assessment, and how to best incorporate the concept of sarcopenia into clinical decision-making. A detailed definition of sarcopenia should be established for use in clinical practice with consideration of age, gender, and ethnicity. Standardized tools, validation between techniques, and functional deterioration are important considerations for sarcopenia prognosis.

References

1. Hanai T, Shiraki M, Ohnishi S, Miyazaki T, Ideta T, Kochi T, et al. Rapid skeletal muscle wasting predicts worse survival in patients with liver cirrhosis. Hepatol Res. 2016;46(8):743–51. https://doi.org/10.1111/hepr.12616.
2. Giusto M, Lattanzi B, Albanese C, Galtieri A, Farcomeni A, Giannelli V, et al. Sarcopenia in liver cirrhosis: the role of computed tomography scan for the assessment of muscle mass compared with dual-energy X-ray absorptiometry and anthropometry. Eur J Gastroenterol Hepatol. 2015;27(3):328–34. https://doi.org/10.1097/MEG.0000000000000274.
3. Rosenberg IH. Summary comments. Am J Clin Nutr. 1989;50(5):1231–3. https://doi.org/10.1093/ajcn/50.5.1231.
4. Baumgartner RN, Koehler KM, Gallagher D, Romero L, Heymsfield SB, Ross RR, et al. Epidemiology of sarcopenia among the elderly in New Mexico. Am J Epidemiol. 1998;147(8):755–63.
5. Anker SD, Morley JE, von Haehling S. Welcome to the ICD-10 code for sarcopenia. J Cachexia Sarcopenia Muscle. 2016;7(5):512–4. https://doi.org/10.1002/jcsm.12147.
6. Fielding RA, Vellas B, Evans WJ, Bhasin S, Morley JE, Newman AB, et al. Sarcopenia: an undiagnosed condition in older adults. Current consensus definition: prevalence, etiology, and consequences. International working group on sarcopenia. J Am Med Dir Assoc. 2011;12(4):249–56. https://doi.org/10.1016/j.jamda.2011.01.003.
7. Cruz-Jentoft AJ, Baeyens JP, Bauer JM, Boirie Y, Cederholm T, Landi F, et al. Sarcopenia: European consensus on definition and diagnosis: report of the European working group on sarcopenia in older people. Age Ageing. 2010;39(4):412–23. https://doi.org/10.1093/ageing/afq034.
8. Tandon P, Low G, Mourtzakis M, Zenith L, Myers RP, Abraldes JG, et al. A model to identify sarcopenia in patients with cirrhosis. Clin Gastroenterol Hepatol. 2016;14(10):1473–80 e3. https://doi.org/10.1016/j.cgh.2016.04.040.
9. Tandon P, Mourtzakis M, Low G, Zenith L, Ney M, Carbonneau M, et al. Comparing the variability between measurements for sarcopenia using magnetic resonance imaging and computed tomography imaging. Am J Transplant. 2016;16(9):2766–7. https://doi.org/10.1111/ajt.13832.
10. Shen W, Punyanitya M, Wang Z, Gallagher D, St-Onge MP, Albu J, et al. Total body skeletal muscle and adipose tissue volumes: estimation from a single abdominal cross-sectional image. J Appl Physiol. 2004;97(6):2333–8. https://doi.org/10.1152/japplphysiol.00744.2004.
11. Schweitzer M. Stages of technical efficacy: journal of magnetic resonance imaging style. J Magn Reson Imaging. 2016;44(4):781–2. https://doi.org/10.1002/jmri.25417.
12. Englesbe MJ, Patel SP, He K, Lynch RJ, Schaubel DE, Harbaugh C, et al. Sarcopenia and mortality after liver transplantation. J Am Coll Surg. 2010;211(2):271–8. https://doi.org/10.1016/j.jamcollsurg.2010.03.039.
13. Montano-Loza AJ, Meza-Junco J, Prado CM, Lieffers JR, Baracos VE, Bain VG, et al. Muscle wasting is associated with mortality in patients with cirrhosis. Clin Gastroenterol Hepatol. 2012;10(2):166–73, 73 e1. https://doi.org/10.1016/j.cgh.2011.08.028.
14. Carey EJ, Lai JC, Wang CW, Dasarathy S, Lobach I, Montano-Loza AJ, et al. A multicenter study to define sarcopenia in patients with end-stage liver disease. Liver Transpl. 2017;23(5):625–33. https://doi.org/10.1002/lt.24750.
15. Golse N, Bucur PO, Ciacio O, Pittau G, Sa Cunha A, Adam R, et al. A new definition of sarcopenia in patients with cirrhosis undergoing liver transplantation. Liver Transpl. 2017;23(2):143–54. https://doi.org/10.1002/lt.24671.
16. Izumi T, Watanabe J, Tohyama T, Takada Y. Impact of psoas muscle index on short-term outcome after living donor liver transplantation. Turk J Gastroenterol. 2016;27(4):382–8. https://doi.org/10.5152/tjg.2016.16201.

17. Durand F, Buyse S, Francoz C, Laouenan C, Bruno O, Belghiti J, et al. Prognostic value of muscle atrophy in cirrhosis using psoas muscle thickness on computed tomography. J Hepatol. 2014;60(6):1151–7. https://doi.org/10.1016/j.jhep.2014.02.026.
18. Ebadi M, Wang CW, Lai JC, Dasarathy S, Kappus MR, Dunn MA, et al. Poor performance of psoas muscle index for identification of patients with higher waitlist mortality risk in cirrhosis. J Cachexia Sarcopenia Muscle. 2018;9(6):1053–62. https://doi.org/10.1002/jcsm.12349.
19. van Vugt JL, Levolger S, Gharbharan A, Koek M, Niessen WJ, Burger JW, et al. A comparative study of software programmes for cross-sectional skeletal muscle and adipose tissue measurements on abdominal computed tomography scans of rectal cancer patients. J Cachexia Sarcopenia Muscle. 2017;8(2):285–97. https://doi.org/10.1002/jcsm.12158.
20. Ebadi M, Tandon P, Moctezuma-Velazquez C, Ghosh S, Baracos VE, Mazurak VC, et al. Low subcutaneous adiposity associates with higher mortality in female patients with cirrhosis. J Hepatol. 2018;69(3):608–16. https://doi.org/10.1016/j.jhep.2018.04.015.
21. Norman K, Kirchner H, Lochs H, Pirlich M. Malnutrition affects quality of life in gastroenterology patients. World J Gastroenterol. 2006;12(21):3380–5.
22. Alvares-da-Silva MR, Reverbel da Silveira T. Comparison between handgrip strength, subjective global assessment, and prognostic nutritional index in assessing malnutrition and predicting clinical outcome in cirrhotic outpatients. Nutrition. 2005;21(2):113–7. https://doi.org/10.1016/j.nut.2004.02.002.
23. van Vugt JL, Levolger S, de Bruin RW, van Rosmalen J, Metselaar HJ, JN IJ. Systematic review and meta-analysis of the impact of computed tomography-assessed skeletal muscle mass on outcome in patients awaiting or undergoing liver transplantation. Am J Transplant. 2016;16(8):2277–92. https://doi.org/10.1111/ajt.13732.
24. Montano-Loza AJ, Duarte-Rojo A, Meza-Junco J, Baracos VE, Sawyer MB, Pang JX, et al. Inclusion of sarcopenia within MELD (MELD-sarcopenia) and the prediction of mortality in patients with cirrhosis. Clin Transl Gastroenterol. 2015;6:e102. https://doi.org/10.1038/ctg.2015.31.
25. DiMartini A, Cruz RJ Jr, Dew MA, Myaskovsky L, Goodpaster B, Fox K, et al. Muscle mass predicts outcomes following liver transplantation. Liver Transpl. 2013;19(11):1172–80. https://doi.org/10.1002/lt.23724.
26. Montano-Loza AJ, Meza-Junco J, Baracos VE, Prado CM, Ma M, Meeberg G, et al. Severe muscle depletion predicts postoperative length of stay but is not associated with survival after liver transplantation. Liver Transpl. 2014;20(6):640–8. https://doi.org/10.1002/lt.23863.
27. Masuda T, Shirabe K, Ikegami T, Harimoto N, Yoshizumi T, Soejima Y, et al. Sarcopenia is a prognostic factor in living donor liver transplantation. Liver Transpl. 2014;20(4):401–7. https://doi.org/10.1002/lt.23811.
28. Krell RW, Kaul DR, Martin AR, Englesbe MJ, Sonnenday CJ, Cai S, et al. Association between sarcopenia and the risk of serious infection among adults undergoing liver transplantation. Liver Transpl. 2013;19(12):1396–402. https://doi.org/10.1002/lt.23752.
29. van Vugt JLA, Buettner S, Alferink LJM, Bossche N, de Bruin RWF, Darwish Murad S, et al. Low skeletal muscle mass is associated with increased hospital costs in patients with cirrhosis listed for liver transplantation-a retrospective study. Transpl Int. 2018;31(2):165–74. https://doi.org/10.1111/tri.13048.
30. Merli M, Lucidi C, Giannelli V, Giusto M, Riggio O, Falcone M, et al. Cirrhotic patients are at risk for health care-associated bacterial infections. Clin Gastroenterol Hepatol. 2010;8(11):979–85. https://doi.org/10.1016/j.cgh.2010.06.024.
31. Prado CM, Lieffers JR, McCargar LJ, Reiman T, Sawyer MB, Martin L, et al. Prevalence and clinical implications of sarcopenic obesity in patients with solid tumours of the respiratory and gastrointestinal tracts: a population-based study. Lancet Oncol. 2008;9(7):629–35. https://doi.org/10.1016/S1470-2045(08)70153-0.
32. Hara N, Iwasa M, Sugimoto R, Mifuji-Moroka R, Yoshikawa K, Terasaka E, et al. Sarcopenia and Sarcopenic obesity are prognostic factors for overall survival in patients with cirrhosis. Intern Med. 2016;55(8):863–70. https://doi.org/10.2169/internalmedicine.55.5676.

33. Belarmino G, Gonzalez MC, Sala P, Torrinhas RS, Andraus W, D'Albuquerque LAC, et al. Diagnosing sarcopenia in male patients with cirrhosis by dual-energy X-ray absorptiometry estimates of appendicular skeletal muscle mass. JPEN J Parenter Enteral Nutr. 2018;42(1):24–36. https://doi.org/10.1177/0148607117701400.
34. Praktiknjo M, Book M, Luetkens J, Pohlmann A, Meyer C, Thomas D, et al. Fat-free muscle mass in magnetic resonance imaging predicts acute-on-chronic liver failure and survival in decompensated cirrhosis. Hepatology. 2018;67(3):1014–26. https://doi.org/10.1002/hep.29602.

Chapter 2
The Definition and Diagnosis of Frailty in the Research and Clinical Settings

Hui-Wei Chen and Andres Duarte-Rojo

Frailty is defined as physiologic decline and reduced physiological reserve that leads to increased vulnerability to health stressors with subsequent physical dependency and multiple adverse outcomes including death [1]. Sarcopenia, an anatomical loss of skeletal muscle mass and function, is not synonymous with frailty, but it often accompanies frailty. The concept of frailty was initially described in the geriatric literature as it is prevalent in advanced age populations; however, it is also ubiquitous in patients with chronic medical conditions.

It is important to recognize that frailty is a disorder of physical function that occurs on a continuum, which ranges from mild deconditioning that affects leisure activity (also known as "pre-frail") to end-stage disease with failure to thrive (Fig. 2.1). In the elderly, it has been shown that pre-frail patients have similar negative outcomes as frail patients but in lesser degree and that the former are more likely to be able to regain the "robust" state when compared to the latter [2, 3]. This fact makes early identification of pre-frail state valuable in order to timely intervene and prevent progression or to serve as a model for frailty reversibility efforts.

While frailty and sarcopenia are major healthcare concerns for older adults, they are also very prevalent in people with chronic medical diseases such as chronic liver disease, chronic kidney disease, and cancer, which accelerate the progression of physical dysfunction and muscle atrophy regardless of age. Due to these conditions' robust association with adverse outcomes, frailty and sarcopenia have attracted

H.-W. Chen
Division of Gastroenterology Hepatology and Nutrition, University of Pittsburgh, Pittsburgh, PA, USA

A. Duarte-Rojo (✉)
Division of Gastroenterology Hepatology and Nutrition, University of Pittsburgh, Pittsburgh, PA, USA

Center for Liver Diseases and Thomas E. Starzl Transplantation Institute, University of Pittsburgh Medical Center, Pittsburgh, PA, USA
e-mail: duarterojoa@upmc.edu

© Springer Nature Switzerland AG 2020
P. Tandon, A. J. Montano-Loza (eds.), *Frailty and Sarcopenia in Cirrhosis*,
https://doi.org/10.1007/978-3-030-26226-6_2

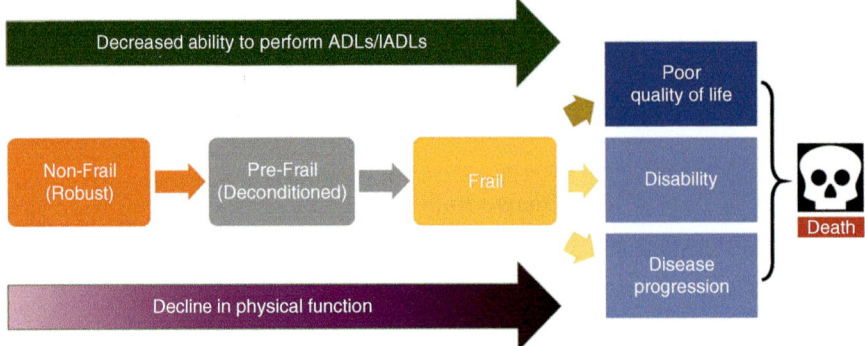

Fig. 2.1 The continuum of physical function disorders, its drivers, and ultimate consequences. Frailty occurs on a spectrum ranging from mild deconditioning to failure to thrive. As patients with cirrhosis begin to have decreased ability to perform ADLs and/or IADLs along with declining physical performance, they gradually become frailer with declining quality of life, worsening disability, and disease progression. Ultimately, significant physical deterioration or frailty leads to various adverse outcomes, such as unplanned hospitalization and death

growing interest in cirrhosis and liver transplantation. From available studies, it is known that development of frailty in patients with cirrhosis leads to increased incidence of hepatic decompensation, recurrent/prolonged hospitalizations, posttransplantation complications, and mortality [1, 4–6]. It has also been validated repeatedly that frailty alone is an independent risk factor for waitlist removal and death while on the transplant waitlist, regardless of the standard prognostic tools such as the Model for End-Stage Liver Disease (MELD) and Child-Turcotte-Pugh (CTP) scores [7–9]. Despite it being a growing field, there is currently no clinical practice guideline to provide directions to the clinician in assessing and diagnosing frailty.

Measurement of Frailty

There are many frailty assessment tools that have been developed to identify at-risk patients. Some of these incorporate mostly subjective components. Activities of daily living (ADL) and instrumental activities of daily living (IADL) are questionnaire-based tools that allow clinicians to assess patient's difficulty with performing daily self-care activities and activities that allow an individual to live independently, respectively [10, 11]. The Karnofsky Performance Scale (KPS) and Clinical Frailty Scale (CFS) incorporate both the ADL and IDAL in addition to limitations one may experience with chronic diseases as well as cognitive decline. These scales (KPS and CFS) attempt to better categorize patients into different frailty groups by assigning the degree of frailty with numerical scores [4, 12]. The Braden Scale, a traditional tool used to risk-stratify for pressure ulcers based on physical exam and assessment of six criteria, has also been used as a standardized measure of frailty [8]. While these questionnaires are easily attainable and have been associated with adverse outcomes, they rely heavily on the self-reported information and judgment from the personnel administering the test. Moreover, when self-reported physical activity was compared with objective data collected by a physical activity tracker, it was noticed that patients overrepresented their activities disclosing mildly limited to normal physical function when in fact their physical activity was very limited [13]. Thus, as in many other self-reported scenarios, there is a tendency for magnifying the actual physical accomplishments potentially resulting in a high rate of false negatives (overestimates functionality) and precluding the usefulness of these scales as accurate screening methods.

Based on a comprehensive review of frailty measurement tools in the geriatric literature, the Fried Frailty Phenotype (FFP) is the most commonly cited frailty diagnostic tool [14]. The FFP criteria were devised based on observation of physical declines and weakness in the geriatric population, whom are most vulnerable to adverse outcomes. This assessment tool encompasses five characteristics: weight loss, exhaustion, weakness, slow walking speed, and decreased physical activity. It divides patients into three different groups based on the number of characteristics that an individual has fulfilled: frail, when one fulfills three or more of the five criteria; pre-frail, when having one or two of these characteristics; and robust, when one does not have any characteristics [15]. While the FFP has been validated in multiple studies [14–17], its utility in assessing for frailty in patients with end-stage liver disease is more limited [4, 5, 7]. The reason being that the characteristics included in FFP are part of the symptoms and/or can be affected by the clinical manifestations commonly seen in patient with cirrhosis, which would lead to inaccurate assessment of frailty. As we know, fluid overload and ascites are very common manifestations of patients with cirrhosis, and its presence makes it difficult to accurately assess patient's true weight. Moreover, exhaustion and weakness are subjective symptoms frequently reported in cirrhosis, and they are further aggravated in patients with hepatic encephalopathy. Because of the aforementioned confounding factors, FFP is unable to accurately assess frailty in patients with cirrhosis (underestimates functionality). As such, it is currently understood that assessment of frailty in the setting of cirrhosis or advanced liver disease must rely mainly on objective physical function characteristics.

In addition to the FFP criteria, there are other objective frailty measurement tools which have been employed to capture frailty in patients with cirrhosis. Grip strength and gait speed test (GST) are popular simple physical function tests to screen for frailty, and decline in either has been shown to be an independent risk factor for hospitalizations in patients with different chronic diseases [6, 18–20]. More comprehensive testing that is performance-based such as the Short Physical Performance Battery (SPPB) including repeated chair stands, balance testing, and 4-meter walk is also commonly used and has been predictive of disability, hospitalization, and mortality [7, 21]. A novel frailty assessment for patients with cirrhosis, termed the Liver Frailty Index (LFI), was devised after using available assessment frailty tools with subsequent modeling of different combinations. It was found that the combination of three simple tests – grip strength, chair stands, and balance – was able to best

Table 2.1 Operational characteristics of tests used to evaluate frailty in patients with cirrhosis

	FFP	SPPB	LFI	GST	6MWT	CPET
Includes subjective data	Yes	No	No	No	No	No
Clinical accessibility	Moderate	Easy	Moderate	Easy	Moderate	Poor
Changes over time	N/A	Yes	Yes	Yes	Yes	Yes
Changes post-intervention	N/A	N/A	N/A	N/A	Yes	Yes
Changes pre- to posttransplant	N/A	N/A	Yes	N/A	Yes	Yes

FFP Fried Frailty Phenotype, *SPPB* Short Physical Performance Battery, *LFI* Liver Frailty Index, *GST* gait speed test, *6MWT* 6-minute walk test, *CPET* cardiopulmonary exercise testing

predict frailty in patients with cirrhosis [22]. Moreover, the predictive usefulness of LFI was independent of the degree of liver dysfunction, and it presumably outperformed both FFP and SPPB. LFI is also reproducible and practical, and although it has shown responsiveness to change over time, no data on improvement following an intervention has been published to date.

With so many assessment tools that are at a clinician's disposal to use in clinic, it remains uncertain which test(s) should be incorporated into our clinical practice. Clinical accuracy, reproducibility, and practicality are essential values that the clinical frailty testing should have. These tools should also have an independent predictive value for outcomes from known disease-related prognostic variables including MELD score and CPT score [23]. Current data does not support the use of a screening test followed by a confirmatory test, and rather using any of the tests showed in Table 2.1 to diagnose frailty is encouraged. Although there are no head-to-head comparisons on the accuracy of these tests, LFI is the one most rigorously validated as a result of large multidisciplinary and multicenter research efforts.

Clinical Relevance of Frailty

As mentioned previously, it is now recognized that frailty is a poor prognostic factor associated with increased morbidity and mortality in patients with chronic liver diseases (Table 2.2). It is found that cirrhotic patients with increasing frailty are associated with increased unplanned hospitalizations or death from cirrhosis-related complications regardless of the severity of the liver disease based on MELD scores [4–7].

Tandon et al. had shown that liver-related complications accounted for 85% of all the unplanned hospitalizations – the three most common causes being hepatic encephalopathy, volume overload/acute kidney injury, and infection. Furthermore, 57% of the frail patients stratified by CFS were admitted to the hospital or died within 6 months as compared with 24% of the non-frail patients. It was found that for every one-point increase in the CFS, the odds for an unplanned hospitalization or death within 6 months was 1.9 and independent from other prognostic factors. What was striking about the study is that unplanned hospitalization occurred in almost one-third of the 300 patients over 6 months despite a mean MELD score of

Table 2.2 Prospective studies evaluating frailty assessed with performance-based tools and its relationship with clinical outcomes

1st author (year)	Study duration	Characteristics	Study group(s)	Tool assessment	Outcomes
Lai et al. [7] (2014)	12 months	Median MELD 15 CTP-A 9% CTP-B 61% CTP-C 30% $n = 294$	Stratified by frailty (FFP ≥3): Frail ($n = 51$) Not frail ($n = 243$)	FFP, SPPB, ADL, and IADL	Frail patients had significantly more death/delisting compared to non-frail patients (22% vs. 10%) Frailty patients had increased mortality independent of the severity of the liver disease Each 1-unit increase in the FFP was associated with 45% increased risk of waitlist mortality Each 1-unit decrease in the SPPB was associated with 19% increased risk of waitlist mortality Patients with MELD <18 and frail phenotype have higher waitlist mortality than those with non-frail patients and MELD <18 or MELD ≥18
Tandon et al. [4] (2016)	6 months	MELD 12 ± 4.8 CTP-A 39% CTP-B 43% CTP-B 18% $n = 300$	Stratified by frailty (CFS >4): Frail ($n = 54$) Not frail ($n = 246$)	CFS, FFP, and SPPB	Liver-related reasons accounted for 85% of the unplanned hospitalization Approximately one-third of the study cohort had unplanned hospitalization despite mean MELD of 12 Frail patients had significantly more unplanned hospitalization than non-frail patients (57% vs. 24%)
Dunn et al. [6] (2016)	12 months	MELD 14.7 ± 5.8 $n = 373$	Cirrhotic patients on waitlist, in evaluation or declined	Gait speed Grip strength	Cirrhotic patient experienced 2.14 hospital days/100 days (7.81 days/year) Each 0.1 m/s gait speed decrease was associated with 22% greater hospital days Grip strength showed similar association as gait speed, however, not statistically significant
Lai et al. [27] (2018)	12 months	Median MELD 15 (pretransplant) Median MELD 20 (at transplant) $n = 214$	Stratified by frailty: "Robust" – LFI <3.2 ($n = 53$) "Pre-frail" – 3.2 ≤LFI <4.5 ($n = 62$) "Frail" – ≥4.5 ($n = 44$)	LFI	Majority of patient experienced worsening of frailty status at 3 months with incremental improvement at 12 months compared to the pretransplant state Pretransplant LFI was a potent predictor of posttransplant robustness Patients who were frail pretransplant had significantly higher transplant length of stay and hospitalized days within 3 months of transplant compared to non-frail patients

Abbreviations: *MELD* Model for End-Stage Liver Disease, *CTP* Child-Turcotte-Pugh score, *CFS* Clinical Frailty Scale, *ADL* activities of daily living, *IADL* instrumental activities of daily living, *FFP* Fried Frailty Phenotype, *SPPB* Short Physical Performance Battery, *LFI* Liver Frailty Index

12 suggesting that MELD score alone is an inadequate measure for mortality and morbidity in patients with cirrhosis [4].

Furthermore, Dunn et al. demonstrated that GST, a surrogate measurement of frailty, is an independent and potentially modifiable risk factor for adverse outcomes such as hospitalization due to complications associated with cirrhosis and waitlist removal. Interestingly, it was found that every 0.1 m/s decrease in gait speed was associated with a 22% increase in days of hospitalization, independently of MELD score. Grip strength was also evaluated as a potential marker for frailty, and while it showed similar trend as gait speed, it did not reach significance with the same outcomes. The fact that such a minimal change in GST would lead to an otherwise enormous negative outcome suggests that more studies need to be done to identify and intervene potentially modifiable risk factors to reverse frailty (or prefrailty) [6].

In a landmark study, Lai et al. showed that frailty predicts waitlist mortality in patients awaiting liver transplant independently of the severity of their liver disease based on MELD score. It demonstrated that frail patients assessed by FFP had significantly more death/delisting compared to non-frail patients (22% vs. 10%). Interestingly, it was also found that patients deemed frail with MELD <18 experienced higher waitlist mortality/delisting than patients who were not frail regardless of their MELD scores, suggesting that frailty plays an essential prognostic role in predicting mortality and/or delisting in patients with cirrhosis [7]. This again demonstrates that MELD score alone is likely to underestimate the mortality risk in this population.

Given that frailty assessment in cirrhosis is being limited to physical function and performance, tests more traditionally used to assess cardiorespiratory endurance or aerobic fitness, such as the 6-minute walk test (6MWT) and the cardiopulmonary exercise testing (CPET), have been linked to frailty as well [23]. As such, by providing sound information on heart, lungs, vascular, and skeletal muscle functions during a bout of exercise, the 6MWT and CPET yield an accurate estimate of overall physical function as well. Carey et al. initially described that patients with cirrhosis not able to achieve 250 meters or more had a higher mortality while on the transplant waitlist, independently of MELD score and other variables [24]. Although the authors confirmed their results in a subsequent larger study, the predictive value of 6MWT was not as meaningful per multivariable analysis [25]. A systematic review including 7 studies with 1107 patients identified both the peak exercise oxygen uptake (peak VO_2) and anaerobic threshold from CPET were associated with either pre- or posttransplant mortality and secondarily with shorter intensive care unit and total hospital stay [26]. Notably, both 6MWT and CPET have shown improvement following exercise in patients with cirrhosis, making them attractive to monitor change in response to interventions aiming to treat frailty. Although CPET is a more sophisticated test, it has remained limited to the research arena given its impracticality and lack of third-payer coverage.

Frailty is thus useful in prognosticating mortality and hospitalization in all cirrhotic patients, as well as waitlist removal for those on the transplant waitlist. Not surprisingly, a study including posttransplant follow-up has shown that patients with higher pretransplant frailty scores (i.e., LFI) have decreased odds of becoming robust 1 year after undergoing liver transplantation [27]. This study highlights the need to identify at-risk groups (e.g., pre-frail) and intervene prior to development of frailty in order to decrease mortality, morbidity, and independence of patients both before and following liver transplantation.

Potential Application in Healthcare

In spite of the absence of robust evidence in the published literature, it is widely accepted that frailty in cirrhosis must be a reversible condition [9]. As the dynamic syndrome that it encompasses, frailty should be viewed as a spectrum including pre-frail or deconditioned stages, where patients are at risk of progressing to a frail condition with increased risk for experiencing adverse outcomes. Moreover, within each stage it must be understood that patients with more severe physical dysfunction bear greater risk, and thus appropriate diagnosis and stratification are necessary in order to facilitate interventions to transition patients toward lower levels of physical dysfunction. In this regard, frailty tests using a continuous scale that is easy to interpret (e.g., SPPB, LFI, GST, 6MWT) would be particularly important in order to better monitor improvement or deterioration (Table 2.3). Although future research will need to define what the clinically relevant changes are in either direction (i.e., improvement or deterioration), such model of care might benefit a larger proportion of patients by having a complementary evaluation on the response to interventions and physical resilience, rather than a unique and static frailty assessment. It is likely that an isolated assessment, by providing an incomplete picture of physical function, would result in precipitated decisions severely affecting a patient's prognosis (e.g., removal from liver transplant list).

While most frailty studies were performed in the outpatient setting [4–7], there is a paucity of data in the inpatient setting. Tapper et al. showed that measuring frailty via ADL, the Braden Scale and Morse fall risk scores on patients upon admission to a liver unit significantly predicted 90-day mortality [8]. Although these results are promising, none of the frailty tools used in this study objectively assessed

Table 2.3 Frailty assessment tools with their respective cutoffs in patients with cirrhosis

	Non-frail	Pre-frail	Frail
FFP	0	1–2	≥3
SPPB	≥10		<10
LFI	<3.2	3.3–4.4	≥4.5
GST	>0.8 m/s	≤0.8 m/s	
6MWT	>250 m	<250 m	
CPET	>60%	<60%	

FFP Fried Frailty Phenotype, *SPPB* Short Physical Performance Battery, *LFI* Liver Frailty Index, *GST* gait speed test, *6MWT* 6-minute walk test, *CPET* cardiopulmonary exercise testing physical function and therefore are not compatible with the tests validated in the outpatient setting. Ideally, the same test used as outpatient should be used during hospitalizations in order to facilitate continuity in monitoring. However, given the lack of validated data on performance-based testing during hospitalization, such tests should be considered exclusively for research purposes and within the context of the particular acute setting (e.g., weigh its limited clinical relevance in patients with overt hepatic encephalopathy or severe fluid overload).

Although not formally studied, reversal of frailty following liver transplantation in some but not all transplanted patients supposes that liver failure is the main driver in some, whereas in others frailty is likely facilitated by comorbidities or nonclinical circumstances. As such, when pondering frailty in the decision to proceed with liver transplantation, the clinician needs to estimate whether frailty is potentially reversible with liver transplantation or not (hepatic-driven vs. non-hepatic-driven and acute vs. chronic). In the absence of more extensive literature, addressing frailty reversibility, having a documented response to prior physical interventions, and knowing how resilient patient and caregiver are can help predict reversibility.

Impact of Frailty on Healthcare Systems

In addition to the clinical consequences, the compromised function associated with frailty has a major impact on the healthcare system. The unplanned hospitalizations have a particularly heavy burden on physical dysfunction, leading to worsened prognosis while exponentially increasing healthcare costs [5]. The cost has been estimated at upward of $25,000 per admission, with 30-day readmission rates estimated to be as high as 37% [6, 28–30]. It was also shown that, when compared to patients with a normal GST (1 m/s), those with a GST of 0.5 m/s and 0.25 m/s had a three- to sixfold increase in estimated yearly hospital stay with costs in excess of $60,000 to $135,000, respectively [6]. Furthermore, studies have shown that frail and pre-frail patients incur significantly more healthcare cost when compared to their non-frail counterparts after controlling for age, comorbidity, and general sociodemographic characteristics [31]. Hence, the need to identify individuals at high risk of hepatic decompensation and hospitalization can have important patient and healthcare system benefits [32].

Proposed Model of Care

Despite the growing recognition of the need to identify frailty in patients with cirrhosis, we lack a standardized protocol to assess frailty in the clinical setting. This is likely related to (1) lack awareness of existing research and available tests, (2) limited clinical time to assess and intervene on physical function, and (3) missing institutional support due to the fact that frailty evaluations and interventions are not reimbursable (or even not available). In Fig. 2.2 we propose a model to integrate

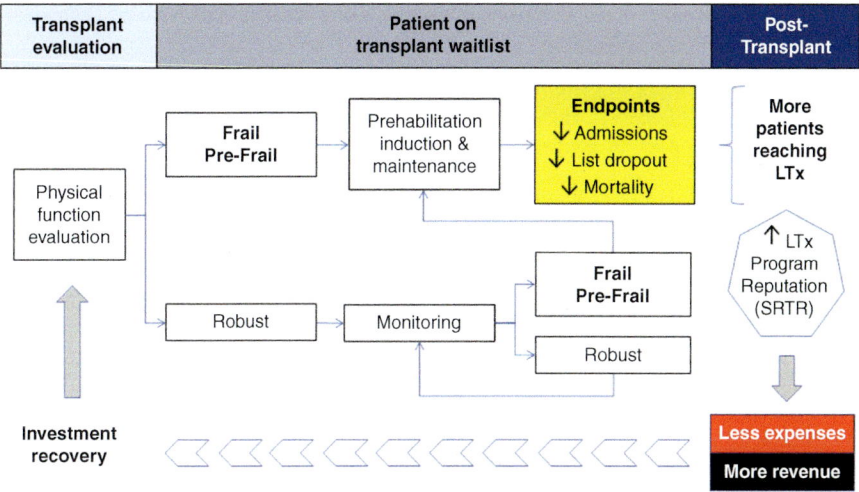

Fig. 2.2 Conceptualization of a model of care integrating a frailty assessment as part of liver transplantation. The incorporation of a certified exercise professional into the liver transplant staff can facilitate routine evaluations of frailty using tests that objectively examine physical function. Testing should allow recognition of the three stages of physical function and should be used serially (i.e., every 4 to 12 weeks) to monitor deterioration or improvement. Prehabilitation interventions to counteract physical deterioration should then be implemented for frail and pre-frail patients. With such intervention patients responding to treatment should have less admissions to hospital, be able to remain on the waitlist, and reach liver transplantation. Improved clinical outcomes would translate into reputational and economic benefits for the transplant program allowing recovery of financial investment

frailty assessments as part of routine clinical practice. Although this model mostly applies to waitlisted patients for liver transplantation, similar models can be generated for non-transplant candidates with cirrhosis. Importantly, the test(s) chosen to investigate frailty should be performance-based (i.e., objectively evaluating physical function), easily administered by any personnel, and provide reproducible results with a robust association with clinically relevant outcomes such as mortality, transplant waitlist removal, unplanned hospitalizations, or falls. Eventually, the assessment should be incorporated into the electronic medical record in order to allow clinicians to track changes in physical function overtime and take clinical decisions accordingly.

References

1. Morley JE, Vella B, van Kan GA, Anker SD, et al. Frailty consensus: a call to action. J Am Med Dir Assoc. 2013;14:392–7.
2. Crow R, Lohman M, Titus A, et al. Mortality risk along the frailty spectrum: data from the national health and nutrition examination survey 1999 to 2004. J Am Geriatr Soc. 2018;66(3):496–502.

3. Gill TM, Gahbauer EA, Allore HG, et al. Transitions between frailty states among community-living older persons. Arch Intern Med. 2006;166:418–23.
4. Tandon P, Tangri N, Thomas L, et al. A rapid bedside screen to predict hospitalization in cirrhosis. Am J of Gastroenterol. 2016;111:1749–67.
5. Sinclair M, Poltavskiy E, Dodge J, Lai J. Frailty is independently associated in increased hospitalization days in patients on the liver transplant waitlist. World J Gastroenterol. 2017;23(5):899–905.
6. Dunn M, Josbeno D, Tevar A, et al. Frailty as tested by gait speed is an independent risk factor for cirrhosis complications that required hospitalization. Am J Gastroenterol. 2016;111:1768–75.
7. Lai JC, Feng S, Terrault NA, et al. Frailty predicts waitlist mortality in liver transplant candidates. Am J Transplant. 2014;14:1870–9.
8. Tapper EB, Finkelstein D, Mittleman MA, et al. Standard assessments of frailty are validated predictors of mortality in hospitalized patients with cirrhosis. Hepatology. 2015;62:584–90.
9. Lai JC, Dodge JL, Sen S, et al. Functional decline in patients with cirrhosis awaiting liver transplantation: results from the functional assessment in liver transplantation FrAILTY study. Hepatology. 2016;63:574–80.
10. Katz S, Ford AB, Moskowitz RW, et al. Studies of illness in the aged. The index of ADL: a standardize measure of biological and psychological function. JAMA. 1963;15:914–9.
11. Lawton MP, Brody EM. Assessment of older people: self-maintaining and instrumental activities of daily living. Gerontologist. 1969;9:179–86.
12. Dolgin NH, Marins PN, Movahedi B, et al. Functional status predicts postoperative mortality after liver transplantation. Clin Transpl. 2016;30(11):1403–10.
13. Dunn M, Josbeno D, Schmotzer A, et al. The gap between clinically assessed physical performance and objective physical activity in liver transplant candidates. Liver Transpl. 2016;22:1324–32.
14. Buta BJ, Walston JD, Godino JG, et al. Frailty assessment instruments: systematic characterization of the uses and contexts of highly-cited instruments. Ageing Res Rev. 2016;26:53.
15. Fried LP, Tangen CM, Walston J, et al. Frailty in older adults: evidence for a phenotype. J Gerontol A Biol Sci Med Sci. 2001;56:M146.
16. Makary MA, Segev DL, Pronovost PJ, et al. Frailty as a predictor of surgical outcomes in older patients. J Am Coll Surg. 2010;210:901.
17. Rothman MD, Leo-Summers L, Gill TM. Prognostic significance of potential frailty criteria. J Am Geriatr Soc. 2008;56:2211.
18. Kutner NG, Zhang R, Huang Y, et al. Gait speed and mortality, hospitalization, and functional status change among hemodialysis patients: a US renal data system special study. Am J Kidney Dis. 2015;66:297–304.
19. Kon SS, Jones SE, Schofield SJ, et al. Gait speed and readmission following hospitalization for acute exacerbation of COOPD: a prospective study. Thorax. 2015;70:1131–7.
20. Garcia-Pena C, Farcia-Fabela LC, Gutierrez-Robledo LM, et al. Handgrip strength predicts functional decline at discharge in hospitalized male elderly a hospital cohort study. PLoS One. 2013;8(7):e69849.
21. Volpato S, Cavalieri M, Sioulis F, et al. Predictive value of the short physical performance battery following hospitalization in older patients. J Gerontol A Biol Sci Med Sci. 2011;66:89–96.
22. Lai JC, Covinsky K, Dodge J, et al. Development of a novel frailty index to predict mortality in patients with end-stage liver disease. Hepatology. 2017;66(2):564–74.
23. Tandon P, Ismond K, Riess K, et al. Exercise in cirrhosis: translating evidence and experience to practice. J Hepatol. 2018;69(5):1164–77.
24. Carey E, Steidley E, Aqel B, et al. Six-minute walk distance predicts mortality in liver transplant candidates. Liver Transpl. 2010;16:1373–8.
25. Yadav A, Chang YH, Carpenter S, et al. Relationship between sarcopenia, six-minute walk distance and health-related quality of life in liver transplant candidates. Clin Transpl. 2015;29:134–41.

26. Ney M, Haykowsky MJ, Vanermeer B, et al. Systematic review: pre- and post-operative prognostic value of cardiopulmonary exercise testing in liver transplant candidates. Aliment Pharmacol Ther. 2016;44(8):796–806.
27. Lai JC, Segev D, McCulloch C, et al. Physical frailty after liver transplantation. Am J Transplant. 2018;18:1986–94.
28. Volk ML, Tocco RS, Bazick J, et al. Hospital readmissions among patients with decompensated cirrhosis. Am J Gastroenterol. 2012;107:47–52.
29. Berman K, Tandra S, Forssell K, et al. Incidence and predictors of 30-day readmission among patients hospitalized for advanced liver disease. Clin Gastroenterol Hepatol. 2011;9:254–9.
30. Bini EJ, Weinshel EH, Generoso R, et al. Impact of gastroenterology consultation on the outcomes of patients admitted to the hospital with decompensated cirrhosis. Hepatology. 2001;34:1089–95.
31. Bock JO, Konig HH, Brenner H. Association of frailty with health care costs – results of the ESTHER cohort study. BMC Health Service Research. 2016;16:128.
32. Kim WR. The burden of hepatitis C in the United States. Hepatology. 2002;36:S30–4.

Chapter 3
Deciphering the Cirrhotic Patient's Present Status: The Overlap Between Physical Frailty, Disability, and Sarcopenia

Elliot B. Tapper

Introduction

"It is often difficult to decide whether a trial of [chemotherapy] is indicated."

"The decision should be based on a review of the patient's history and an evaluation of his present status, so that an estimate can be made of the probable therapeutic effect of the agent in a particular situation." – Dr. David Karnofsky [1]

Transplant, like many therapies, possesses a therapeutic window. In much the same way that Karnofsky described the performance status as a decision aid to define the therapeutic window for chemotherapy, clinicians often turn to factors beyond the Model for End-Stage Liver Disease (MELD) in order to classify patients who are and are not likely to benefit from transplantation. Among the known "non-MELD" indicators, frailty, disability, and sarcopenia are the concepts. As predictors, they are closely associated with adverse events including hospitalization, transplant delisting, and death [2]. Each is captured using different measures. Frailty, a syndrome of decreased physiologic reserve, is best captured through demonstrations of physical function (e.g., chair stands, handgrip, balance); disability, or limited activity, is typically captured by patient report (e.g., activities of daily living [ADLs]). Sarcopenia or loss of muscle bulk can be quantified using multiple imaging modalities, anthropometrics, and bioimpedance. However, despite the differences in how each concept is measured, they share common roots. Taken together, each factor provides helpful information for clinicians seeking an enhanced understanding of the patient's present status with an eye toward that which can (or cannot) be rehabilitated.

In this chapter we review the derivation and application of these concepts in the context of cirrhosis care with a focus on their shared pathogenesis.

E. B. Tapper (✉)
Division of Gastroenterology and Hepatology, University of Michigan, Ann Arbor, MI, USA

Gastroenterology Section, VA Ann Arbor Healthcare System, Ann Arbor, MI, USA
e-mail: ctapper@umich.edu

© Springer Nature Switzerland AG 2020   25
P. Tandon, A. J. Montano-Loza (eds.), *Frailty and Sarcopenia in Cirrhosis*,
https://doi.org/10.1007/978-3-030-26226-6_3

A Conceptual Model

Sarcopenia, frailty, and disability are often present simultaneously; however, they may have developed disynchronously. A patient who can perform their ADLs but falls routinely and therefore walks very slowly may be frail. Whereas the disabled patient is generally physically frail, this is not necessarily true for patients limited primarily by cognitive dysfunction. Understanding the differences underpinning one's path to a given present status are essential to understand the prognosis and benefits of interventions. As reflected in Fig. 3.1, the specific expression of a patient's poor "present status" varies according to multiple factors including the duration of illness, severity of disease, comorbidities, and socioeconomics.

First, a patient with a rapid decline in health such as acute-on-chronic liver failure due to alcoholic hepatitis or hepatitis B flare may present as disabled and frail but with preserved muscle bulk. Conversely, a patient with nonalcoholic steatohepatitis (NASH)-related cirrhosis who has had refractory ascites for multiple years may present with preserved ability, mild or absent frailty, and severe sarcopenia. Relatedly, the patient's present status is fundamentally a snapshot of a dynamic health status. It varies with the fluctuations of encephalopathy and ascites and changes drastically in response to treatment (e.g., alcohol abstinence, treatment of ascites/hepatic encephalopathy [HE]) and illness (e.g., infection, falls, hospitalization).

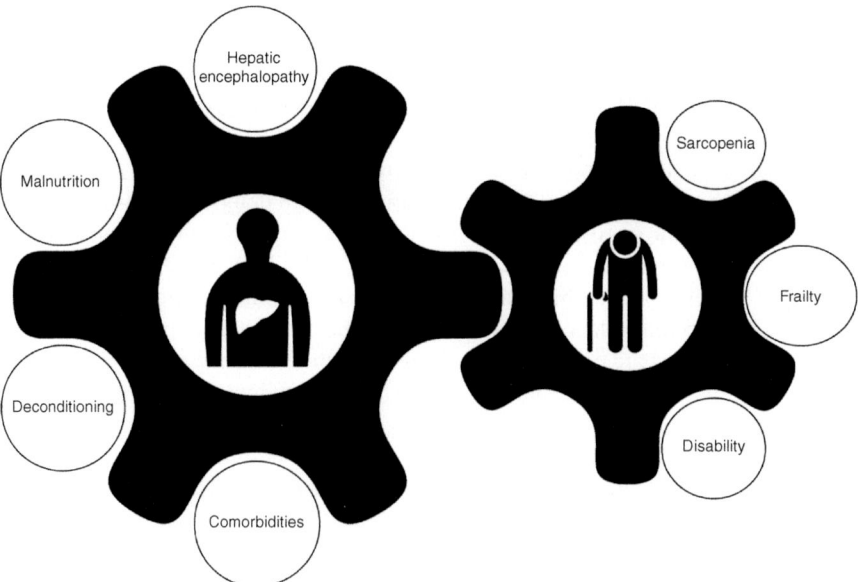

Fig. 3.1 Underlying forces that shape the patient's present status. Patients with cirrhosis have a unique physiology. How these factors manifest in the general assessment of a patient's present status varies from person to person

Second, and relatedly, the severity of liver disease is a key driver of poor present status. Above all, the presence of HE is a central governing factor in the patient's clinical phenotype. HE is disabling and interferes with cognitive function, balance, and coordination [3], confounding the assessment of frailty [2]. Hyperammonemia is myotoxic and causes sarcopenia [4]. Ascites limits physical function, diminishes appetite, and causes excess caloric burning.

Third, extrahepatic comorbidities further define the patient's status commensurate with their severity and the organs effected. Fourth, socioeconomic status reflects employment categories such as manual labor that may be associated with strength that could remain disproportionate to global muscle loss. It also speaks to food security and food choices which impact nutritional status.

Methodological Considerations

Sarcopenia

Sarcopenia is common in patients with cirrhosis and is associated with worse outcomes before and after liver transplantation [5–7]. The mechanism for the sarcopenia's association with mortality in patients with cirrhosis is unclear but appears most closely linked to an increased risk of infections [7]. However, the current epidemiology and associations with sarcopenia are confounded in important ways. Accurate estimates of sarcopenia's prevalence in patients with cirrhosis are complicated by multiple factors. First, studies of sarcopenia have employed highly heterogeneous methodologies ranging from the area examined (e.g., ultrasound, bioimpedance, total psoas area, psoas at L3, psoas at L4; adjusted for height using the skeletal muscle index). Second, the prevalence of sarcopenia varies with severity of liver disease as captured by Child classification or MELD score, factors which are heterogeneously distributed in cohorts that examine the clinical impact of sarcopenia. Third, there are few prospective validations of sarcopenia as a biomarker for risk in patients with cirrhosis. Sarcopenia is therefore determined from tests that have been ordered for other reasons. Although it is unclear, the reasons for the scan in which sarcopenia was disclosed may impact the risk of sarcopenia. At the same time many patients may not be candidates for the modality chosen. For example, chronic kidney disease is associated with sarcopenia as well [8]. However, many CT (computed tomography) scans are performed only in patients with either preserved renal function (given the risks of iodinated contrast) or those who are undergoing hemodialysis. Similarly, patients with abdominal symptoms, perhaps leading to anorexia and malnutrition, may be more likely to receive a CT from which sarcopenia can be measured.

Frailty

The value and clinical impact of frailty in patients with cirrhosis is largely derived from studies of the outpatient transplant-waitlisted population [2, 9–13]. This population is likely markedly different from and may not generalized to patients who are compensated, newly decompensated, actively encephalopathic, critically ill, or undergoing an evaluation as an inpatient. In contrast to sarcopenia, however, frailty measures (e.g., 6-minute walk distance, handgrip, chair stands) are not routine components of the clinical evaluation. Accordingly, although the clinical context in which the frailty measure is obtained shapes the characteristics of the included cohort, studies of frailty are generally prospective allowing for accurate adjudication of future risks and outcomes.

Disability

Disability is evaluated subjectively by a trained observer or by patient report. Patient-reported ADL performance obtained by clinical nurses (or research assistants) has also been associated with a host of pretransplant outcomes including death, delisting, discharge to a nursing facility, and 30-day readmission after discharge [13–15]. The prototypical assessment of disability, the Karnofsky Performance Scale (KPS), has been extensively validated in patients with cirrhosis. The KPS is both a scale from 0 (death) to 100 (perfect health). It has demonstrated enhanced risk prediction in evaluating the survival hospitalized patients with decompensated cirrhosis [16, 17], waitlist mortality [18], and posttransplant survival [18–20]. Disability can be obtained in most clinical contexts and can also be evaluated retrospectively where it is recorded as part of clinical care [15]. Although it can be performed widely, it can be affected by acute changes in the patient's present status and may need adjustment, for example, for the presence of overt HE or infections [15, 17].

Practical Applications

Malnutrition

Given the overlap of sarcopenia, frailty, and disability, interventions to forestall their associated complications share common features. Foremost among these is malnutrition. Poor nutritional status can lead to sarcopenia and functional outcomes such as frailty or disability. Unsurprisingly, protein-energy malnutrition is associated with mortality in patients with cirrhosis [21, 22]. Furthermore, many patients who are objectively frail may not be able to reliably prepare adequate nutrition. In order to address malnutrition, a suite of interventions are needed.

The European Society for Parenteral and Enteral Nutrition recommends 35–40 kcal/kg/day and 1.2–1.5 g/kg ideal body weight/day of protein in patients with liver disease [23, 24]. A convenient rule of thumb to calculate protein needs adjusting for the conversion from actual to ideal body weight is to use 1 g/kg. This is particularly important for patients with HE who benefit from nutritional supplementation and high-protein diets [25, 26]. Protein restriction is categorically not recommended as it can lead to sarcopenia. Branched-chain amino acids can be supplemented safely for this purpose as well, although availability is limited and the data are not conclusive [27, 28].

The timing of nutritional administration seems to influence overall nourishment in cirrhosis. Owing to poor hepatic glycogen reserve as well as increased catabolic drive, sleeping itself – overnight fasting – may cause a decline in nutritional status by inducing catabolism and proteolysis [29, 30]. In a randomized controlled trial, 103 patients with cirrhosis received either isocaloric daytime or nighttime supplementary nutrition (710 kcal/day) [30]. The group receiving nighttime nutritional supplementation had significant increases in total body protein.

Patients with cirrhosis may also present with deficiencies in micronutrients that could impact the interpretation of frailty and disability. Particularly in the case of alcohol-related liver disease, zinc deficiency is often present [31]. Zinc deficiency may be associated with HE which, as above, could confound the interpretation of frailty [32]. Vitamin D deficiency is also common. Vitamin D deficiency is independently associated with falls and vitamin D deficiency-related osteoporosis is associated with fractures, both of which increase the risk of disability [33].

Deconditioning

Disability, frailty, and sarcopenia may all be sensitive to change from increased physical activity. It is easy to recommend exercise, but specific considerations should be addressed first [34]. We recommend beginning with 10-minute sessions once to twice daily and slowly increased the workload as tolerated. Subjects should note an increased heart rate and respiration or breathing rate, without experiencing anginal symptoms and allowing for unencumbered speech while exercising. While most non-disabled patients with cirrhosis can accomplish brisk walking, for those at high risk of falls or limited mobility, other approaches are needed. Consultation with physical therapy is often helpful. Beyond that, we refer patients to the videos produced by Go4Life, an exercise and physical activity campaign from the National Institute on Aging (https://go4life.nia.nih.gov/workout-videos/).

Hepatic Encephalopathy

As above, a patient with cirrhosis can be frail for many reasons. When present, HE plays an important, potentially primary role in the frailty phenotype. Hyperammonemia, one of the sources of HE, causes muscle catabolism which leads to sarcopenia [4, 35]. HE is associated with anorexia, exacerbating malnutrition and sarcopenia [36]. Similarly, HE leads to falls which can cause a fear of activity, increasing deconditioning. Above all, HE leads to hospitalization which worsens physical decline. We recently studied a large prospective cohort of patients assessed for frailty at the time of transplant evaluation [2]. We found that HE appears to be an important determinant of both the frailty phenotype and adverse health outcomes associated with frailty. It is not clear whether treatment of HE, including early identification of covert HE, would forestall or improve physical function. Further research is needed, but it is also justified. Basic science supports that ammonia-lowering interventions may reduce muscle proteolysis [4]. In patients, treatment of HE improves coordination in a driving simulator [37]. Trials are needed, however, to show whether HE-directed therapy improves sarcopenia, frailty, and disability in patients.

Conclusion

It is increasingly recognized that non-MELD factors such as disability, frailty, and sarcopenia are important predictors of meaningful outcomes for patients with cirrhosis. Although each concept is measured in different ways, they share a common biology. Understanding the overlap between these measures informs practice in important ways. Underlying each factor is malnutrition, deconditioning, and HE. Interventions to forestall or improve disability, frailty, or sarcopenia will require a deliberate, multimodal approach to address each of their drivers.

Disclosure

1. Elliot Tapper is the guarantor of this article.
2. Funding: Elliot Tapper receives funding from the National Institutes of Health through the Michigan Institute for Clinical and Health Research (KL2TR002241).

References

1. Karnofsky DA, Abelmann WH, Craver LF, Burchenal JH. The use of the nitrogen mustards in the palliative treatment of carcinoma. With particular reference to bronchogenic carcinoma. Cancer. 1948;1(4):634–56.
2. Tapper EB, Konerman M, Murphy S, Sonnenday CJ. Hepatic encephalopathy impacts the predictive value of the Fried Frailty Index. Am J Transplant. 2018;18:2566.
3. Bajaj JS, Thacker LR, Heuman DM, Sterling RK, Stravitz RT, Sanyal AJ, et al. Cognitive performance as a predictor of hepatic encephalopathy in pretransplant patients with cirrhosis receiving psychoactive medications: a prospective study. Liver Transpl. 2012;18(10):1179–87.
4. Kumar A, Davuluri G, Engelen MP, Ten Have GA, Prayson R, Deutz NE, et al. Ammonia lowering reverses sarcopenia of cirrhosis by restoring skeletal muscle proteostasis. Hepatology. 2017;65(6):2045–58.

5. van Vugt J, Levolger S, de Bruin R, van Rosmalen J, Metselaar H, IJzermans J. Systematic review and meta-analysis of the impact of computed tomography–assessed skeletal muscle mass on outcome in patients awaiting or undergoing liver transplantation. Am J Transplant. 2016;16(8):2277–92.

6. Cruz-Jentoft AJ, Baeyens JP, Bauer JM, Boirie Y, Cederholm T, Landi F, et al. Sarcopenia: European consensus on definition and diagnosis: Report of the European Working Group on Sarcopenia in Older People. Age Ageing. 2010;39(4):412–23.

7. Montano-Loza AJ, Meza-Junco J, Prado CM, Lieffers JR, Baracos VE, Bain VG, et al. Muscle wasting is associated with mortality in patients with cirrhosis. Clin Gastroenterol Hepatol. 2012;10(2):166–73, 73 e1.

8. Pereira RA, Cordeiro AC, Avesani CM, Carrero JJ, Lindholm B, Amparo FC, et al. Sarcopenia in chronic kidney disease on conservative therapy: prevalence and association with mortality. Nephrology Dialysis Transplantation. 2015;30(10):1718–25.

9. Lai JC, Covinsky KE, Dodge JL, Boscardin WJ, Segev DL, Roberts JP, et al. Development of a novel frailty index to predict mortality in patients with end-stage liver disease. Hepatology. 2017;66(2):564–74.

10. Lai JC, Covinsky KE, Hayssen H, Lizaola B, Dodge JL, Roberts JP, et al. Clinician assessments of health status predict mortality in patients with end-stage liver disease awaiting liver transplantation. Liver Int. 2015;35(9):2167–73.

11. Lai JC, Covinsky KE, McCulloch CE, Feng S. The Liver Frailty Index improves mortality prediction of the subjective clinician assessment in patients with cirrhosis. Am J Gastroenterol. 2018;113(2):235.

12. Lai JC, Dodge JL, Sen S, Covinsky K, Feng S. Functional decline in patients with cirrhosis awaiting liver transplantation: results from the functional assessment in liver transplantation (FrAILT) study. Hepatology. 2016;63(2):574–80.

13. Lai JC, Feng S, Terrault N, Lizaola B, Hayssen H, Covinsky K. Frailty predicts waitlist mortality in liver transplant candidates. Am J Transplant. 2014;14(8):1870–9.

14. Samoylova ML, Covinsky KE, Haftek M, Kuo S, Roberts JP, Lai JC. Disability in patients with end-stage liver disease: results from the functional assessment in liver transplantation study. Liver Transpl. 2017;23(3):292–8.

15. Tapper EB, Finkelstein D, Mittleman MA, Piatkowski G, Lai M. Standard assessments of frailty are validated predictors of mortality in hospitalized patients with cirrhosis. Hepatology. 2015;62(2):584–90.

16. Orman ES, Ghabril M, Chalasani N. Poor performance status is associated with increased mortality in patients with cirrhosis. Clin Gastroenterol Hepatol. 2016;14(8):1189–95. e1.

17. Tandon P, Reddy KR, O'leary JG, Garcia-Tsao G, Abraldes JG, Wong F, et al. A Karnofsky performance status–based score predicts death after hospital discharge in patients with cirrhosis. Hepatology. 2017;65(1):217 24.

18. Thuluvath PJ, Thuluvath AJ, Savva Y. Karnofsky performance status before and after liver transplantation predicts graft and patient survival. J Hepatol. 2018;69:818.

19. Serper M, Bittermann T, Rossi M, Goldberg DS, Thomasson AM, Olthoff KM, et al. Functional status, healthcare utilization, and the costs of liver transplantation. Am J Transplant. 2018;18(5).1187–96.

20. Dolgin NH, Martins PN, Movahedi B, Lapane KL, Anderson FA, Bozorgzadeh A. Functional status predicts postoperative mortality after liver transplantation. Clin Transpl. 2016;30(11):1403–10.

21. Alberino F, Gatta A, Amodio P, Merkel C, Di Pascoli L, Boffo G, et al. Nutrition and survival in patients with liver cirrhosis. Nutrition (Burbank, Los Angeles County, Calif). 2001;17(6):445–50.

22. Merli M, Riggio O, Dally L. Does malnutrition affect survival in cirrhosis? PINC (Policentrica Italiana Nutrizione Cirrosi). Hepatology (Baltimore, Md). 1996;23(5):1041–6.

23. Plauth M, Cabre E, Riggio O, Assis-Camilo M, Pirlich M, Kondrup J, et al. ESPEN Guidelines on Enteral Nutrition: Liver disease. Clinical nutrition (Edinburgh, Scotland) 2006;25(2):285–94.

24. Plauth M, Merli M, Kondrup J, Weimann A, Ferenci P, Muller MJ. ESPEN guidelines for nutrition in liver disease and transplantation. Clinical nutrition (Edinburgh, Scotland). 1997;16(2):43–55.
25. O'Brien A, Williams R. Nutrition in end-stage liver disease: principles and practice. Gastroenterology. 2008;134(6):1729–40.
26. Amodio P, Bemeur C, Butterworth R, Cordoba J, Kato A, Montagnese S, et al. The nutritional management of hepatic encephalopathy in patients with cirrhosis: International Society for Hepatic Encephalopathy and Nitrogen Metabolism Consensus. Hepatology (Baltimore, Md). 2013;58(1):325–36.
27. Kawaguchi T, Izumi N, Charlton MR, Sata M. Branched-chain amino acids as pharmacological nutrients in chronic liver disease. Hepatology (Baltimore, Md). 2011;54(3):1063–70.
28. Les I, Doval E, Garcia-Martinez R, Planas M, Cardenas G, Gomez P, et al. Effects of branched-chain amino acids supplementation in patients with cirrhosis and a previous episode of hepatic encephalopathy: a randomized study. Am J Gastroenterol. 2011;106(6):1081–8.
29. Owen OE, Trapp VE, Reichard GA Jr, Mozzoli MA, Moctezuma J, Paul P, et al. Nature and quantity of fuels consumed in patients with alcoholic cirrhosis. J Clin Invest. 1983;72(5):1821–32.
30. Plank LD, Gane EJ, Peng S, Muthu C, Mathur S, Gillanders L, et al. Nocturnal nutritional supplementation improves total body protein status of patients with liver cirrhosis: a randomized 12-month trial. Hepatology (Baltimore, Md). 2008;48(2):557–66.
31. Sengupta S, Wroblewski K, Aronsohn A, Reau N, Reddy KG, Jensen D, et al. Screening for zinc deficiency in patients with cirrhosis: when should we start? Dig Dis Sci. 2015;60(10):3130–5.
32. Takuma Y, Nouso K, Makino Y, Hayashi M, Takahashi H. Clinical trial: oral zinc in hepatic encephalopathy. Aliment Pharmacol Ther. 2010;32(9):1080–90.
33. Murphy SL, Tapper EB, Blackwood J, Richardson JK. Why do individuals with cirrhosis fall? a mechanistic model for fall assessment, treatment, and research. Dig Dis Sci. 2018:1–8.
34. Tapper EB, Martinez-Macias R, Duarte-Rojo A. Is exercise beneficial and safe in patients with cirrhosis and portal hypertension? Current Hepatology Reports. 2018:1–9.
35. Tapper EB, Jiang ZG, Patwardhan VR, editors. Refining the ammonia hypothesis: a physiology-driven approach to the treatment of hepatic encephalopathy. Mayo Clinic Proceedings, vol. 90: Elsevier; 2015. p. 646.
36. Nabi E, Thacker LR, Wade JB, Sterling RK, Stravitz RT, Fuchs M, et al. Diagnosis of covert hepatic encephalopathy without specialized tests. Clin Gastroenterol Hepatol. 2014;12(8):1384–9. e2.
37. Bajaj JS, Heuman DM, Wade JB, Gibson DP, Saeian K, Wegelin JA, et al. Rifaximin improves driving simulator performance in a randomized trial of patients with minimal hepatic encephalopathy. Gastroenterology. 2011;140(2):478–87. e1.

Chapter 4
The Pathogenesis of Physical Frailty and Sarcopenia

Srinivasan Dasarathy

Introduction

Sarcopenia or skeletal muscle loss is one of the most frequent complications of cirrhosis that adversely affects survival and development of and response to other complications of cirrhosis, quality of life, and post-liver transplantation outcomes [1–4]. Increasingly, frailty, a compendium of clinical manifestations due to impaired contractile function, is associated with sarcopenia [4–6]. Despite the high clinical significance, there are limited therapeutic options and no consistently effective therapies to prevent or reverse sarcopenia because the mechanisms are poorly understood [2, 7, 8]. Nutritional interventions including supplementation have generally been ineffective because it is increasingly recognized that cirrhosis is a state of anabolic resistance, due to impaired response to physiological anabolic stimuli [9–12]. Mechanistic understanding of the causes of anabolic stimuli that will permit development of therapies targeting sarcopenia and contractile dysfunction requires direct studies on skeletal muscle from human and experimental models of liver disease. Skeletal muscle is the largest store of proteins in mammals and consists of both structural proteins that maintain muscle mass and contractile proteins that are responsible for locomotor function [13, 14]. Muscle mass is maintained principally by a balance between protein synthesis and protein breakdown or protein homeostasis (proteostasis) [14]. Since the skeletal muscle cells are terminally differentiated, in addition to protein homeostasis, satellite cells that are myogenically committed stem cells provide myonuclei for maintenance of muscle mass and nuclear accretion during recovery [15]. Even though there are extensive data on satellite cell biology,

Supported in part by: NIH RO1 GM119174; RO1 DK 113196; P50 AA024333; R21 AR 71046; U01AA026976; UO1 DK 061732 and Mikati Foundation.

S. Dasarathy (✉)
Department of Gastroenterology, Hepatology, Cleveland Clinic, Cleveland, OH, USA
e-mail: dasaras@ccf.org

© Springer Nature Switzerland AG 2020
P. Tandon, A. J. Montano-Loza (eds.), *Frailty and Sarcopenia in Cirrhosis*,
https://doi.org/10.1007/978-3-030-26226-6_4

33

there is very limited data on satellite cell dysfunction in sarcopenia of disease, and loss of satellite cells does not consistently result in muscle loss [15–17]. Therefore, it is believed that dysregulated proteostasis is a major cause of sarcopenia and impaired contractile function in liver disease [2]. The underlying mechanisms of dysregulated protein homeostasis include defects in availability of substrates for protein synthesis, primarily amino acids and adenosine triphosphate (ATP), the principal cellular energy carrier generated in mitochondria, molecular signaling components that regulate protein synthesis and protein breakdown, and ribosomal components and function where protein synthesis occurs [8, 14]. Mediators of the nutritional, molecular, biochemical, and hormonal abnormalities that result in dys-regulated protein homeostasis and organelle dysfunction in the skeletal muscle are being increasingly recognized and are potential therapeutic targets to reverse or prevent sarcopenia in patients with liver disease.

The main focus of this review will be on the pathogenesis of dysregulated skel-etal muscle protein homeostasis and their potential mediators in cirrhosis that result in sarcopenia.

Impact of Terminology and Definitions in Identifying Pathophysiology of Sarcopenia

The term malnutrition in cirrhosis has been used in the past to refer to a constella-tion of nutritional deficiencies in patients with liver disease that adversely affected clinical outcomes [1, 8, 18]. However, a careful evaluation of these studies has shown that the principal component of malnutrition that affects clinical outcomes is the phenotype of skeletal muscle loss with or without fat loss and bioenergetic dys-function [1, 19–23]. In contrast to the past when the phenotype of malnutrition consisted primarily of muscle loss with varying degrees of fat loss, the epidemic of obesity has made it difficult to clinically recognize malnutrition or sarcopenia in these patients [24–26]. Therefore, with the increasing availability of imaging tech-niques, muscle mass can be quantified with increasing precision and reiterates the previous studies that muscle loss is a critical predictor of clinical outcomes in patients with liver disease [8]. Multiple groups have reported criteria to define sar-copenia based on local population-based normative values [27–30]. This is critical because physiological studies have shown that major predictors of skeletal muscle mass depend on age, gender, and ethnicity, and normative values need to be defined based on these characteristics [26, 31, 32]. Since muscle loss occurs physiologically with aging after about 50 years of age, females have lower muscle mass, and age- and gender-specific values should be used to define sarcopenia [28, 31]. This is criti-cal because identifying the mechanisms of sarcopenia and developing therapies and measures of response to interventions require appropriate measures of muscle mass. Currently, CT-based measures of the skeletal muscle index at the level of the 3rd lumbar vertebra are used to define sarcopenia in liver disease at most centers using published cutoff values [8, 29]. Even though loss of muscle mass is generally accompanied by impaired muscle contractile function, the term sarcopenia specifically refers to loss of muscle mass, while the term contractile dysfunction and frailty are used to define the disordered functional consequences in these patients [33, 34]. There is increasing recognition of the interplay between loss of muscle mass and impaired contractile function [35], and there may be shared and independent underlying mechanisms that cause sarcopenia and frailty. Unlike sarcopenia that has a defined phenotype, frailty is a constellation of functional abnormalities making it difficult to identify the pathogenesis [6, 34, 36, 37]. Therefore, the mechanisms of sarcopenia and contractile dysfunction are most likely to provide insights into the underlying pathogenesis of frailty.

Models of Sarcopenia in Liver Disease and Relevance to Mechanistic Studies

Even though patients with cirrhosis and age-, gender-, and ethnicity-matched healthy controls would be the best groups to identify the mechanisms of sarcopenia, heterogeneity of disease severity, impact of the underlying etiology of liver disease on muscle mass, and the duration of liver disease affect the specific readouts making it difficult to compare data from different groups of patients [2]. Additionally, the need for muscle tissue at specific times to evaluate response to interventions over time are difficult in human cirrhosis due to the risk of bleeding and infection at biopsy sites. Dissecting the mechanisms of sarcopenia and impaired contractile function is difficult in humans, and hence mechanistic studies necessitate the use of preclinical models. Even though it is possible to generate genetic models of rats, mice and cellular studies are most frequently used to dissect the molecular pathways of disease pathogenesis using loss and gain of function studies. In humans, sarcopenia in cirrhosis is due to both the consequences of hepatocellular dysfunction and vascular perturbations including portosystemic shunting. Animal models have been generated that permit the dissection of the consequences of hepatocellular dysfunction and portosystemic shunting. The various models used to study the mechanisms of sarcopenia and contractile dysfunction with their advantages and limitations are shown in Table 4.1 [38–48].

Skeletal Muscle Proteostasis in Cirrhosis

Since skeletal muscle mass is regulated by a dynamic balance between protein synthesis and proteolysis, both metabolic and molecular alterations contribute to protein loss and ultimately sarcopenia. The metabolic regulation of protein synthesis and proteolysis depends on the underlying molecular regulatory pathways, and there is now increasing interest in identifying how metabolic perturbations are sensed by and alter the cellular molecular signaling pathways.

Table 4.1 Common models used to study the pathogenesis of sarcopenia in liver disease

Model	Advantage	Limitations
Human cirrhosis	Most relevant to disease diagnosis and therapy	Variability between subjects Differences in etiology of liver disease Duration of disease is not known Hepatocellular dysfunction and vascular consequences contribute to sarcopenia Mechanistic studies are difficult to perform
Portocaval anastomosis (only rat)	Hyperammonemia and low testosterone mimic perturbations in human cirrhosis Vascular consequences due to portocaval shunting on sarcopenia can be studied independent of the hepatocellular necroinflammatory responses of cirrhosis Duration of disease is known – time of surgery	No underlying cirrhosis Potential variability of shunt diameter No portal hypertension – the underlying causal factor for portocaval anastomosis
Bile duct ligation (rat or mouse)	Liver is cirrhotic Hyperammonemia Increased circulating bile salts Genetic manipulations allow molecular dissection	Model of secondary biliary cirrhosis (a rare human disease) Confounding effects of bile salts and hyperammonemia on muscle protein turnover and signaling perturbations Steatorrhea and fat malabsorption cause severe calorie deficiency that affects muscle mass Onset of disease not certain – cirrhosis develops at varying times
Toxin-induced liver fibrosis Carbon tetrachloride (phenobarbitone) Thioacetamide Dimethyl/ diethyl nitrosamine (rat or mouse)	Hepatic fibrosis Hyperammonemia Genetic manipulations allow molecular dissection	Variability in duration and severity of fibrosis with inconsistent cirrhosis Reversible fibrosis upon stopping toxin Direct toxin-induced muscle injury Hepatocellular carcinoma develops Inconsistent vascular consequences – portal hypertension and portocaval shunting
Alcohol feeding models Acute Acute on chronic Chronic (rat or mouse)	Alcoholic liver disease Endotoxemia Fibrosis can occur Genetic manipulations allow molecular dissection	Variable response to ethanol Natural aversion of rodents to ethanol Ethanol effects on gut and liver confound muscle responses Direct effects of ethanol on muscle signaling and protein kinetics
Myotubes (mouse/rat)	Specific mediators can be studied Subcellular organelle responses can be studied Genetic manipulations allow molecular dissection	In vitro system, cannot reproduce whole-body responses Physiological relevance needs to be established in in vivo studies

Whole-Body and Muscle Metabolism in Physiology and Disease

The skeletal muscle is the major protein store in the body and serves as a source for amino acids during times of stress or fasting. Protein synthesis and breakdown occur physiologically in the skeletal muscle depending on the metabolic state that includes the postprandial or the fed state and the postabsorptive or the fasted state [49]. Physiologically, during the postprandial state that generally lasts about 4–6 h after a meal, muscle protein synthesis is stimulated by diet-derived substrates including carbon sources for energy (glucose, fatty acid) and nitrogen for protein synthesis (amino acids) [50]. The skeletal muscle is a net importer of amino acids, and proteolysis is suppressed in the postprandial state [51, 52]. Dietary substrates, specifically glucose, are the major source of energy, and amino acids are primarily used for protein synthesis in the skeletal muscle [53–55]. In the postabsorptive or fasted phase, nonessential protein synthesis is inhibited with a basal protein balance maintained by influx and efflux of substrates from and into circulation. During fasting, proteolysis is activated, and the skeletal muscle becomes a net exporter of amino acids [56]. The physiological response with amino acid release during fasting is required for both synthesis of essential proteins like cytokines, immunoglobulins, and enzymes that are necessary even in the fasted state and as gluconeogenic substrates. During fasting there is a switch in substrate utilization for energy from glucose to fatty acids generated by lipolysis [50]. However, since glucose is still the preferred substrate for certain organs, gluconeogenesis is activated during fasting, and amino acids (from muscle proteolysis) serve as the primary gluconeogenic substrates [50, 57, 58]. When the next meal is ingested, proteolysis is suppressed, and protein synthesis is stimulated to restore the protein content lost during the fasting state. In healthy subjects, the alternating fed and fasting cycle of substrate utilization regulates the muscle protein content and mass with the protein lost during fasting being restored during feeding to maintain a stable muscle mass (Fig. 4.1) [49, 50].

Unlike the physiological postprandial (fed) state that lasts about 4–6 h after each meal, cirrhosis is a state of accelerated starvation [8, 50, 59]. Indirect calorimetry studies demonstrate a more rapid switch from a carbohydrate/glucose preference for energy (high respiratory quotient) to fatty acids as the major energy substrate with amino acid catabolism serving as gluconeogenic substrates (low respiratory quotient) [50, 57, 60]. In addition to the accelerated starvation physiology with proteolysis that occurs much earlier in cirrhosis after a meal than in controls, a significant proportion of patients with cirrhosis are hypermetabolic [61–63]. The underlying pathophysiology of hypermetabolism in cirrhosis is not clear but is associated with worse clinical outcomes [64, 65]. These data suggest that the duration of fasting, when proteolysis and muscle loss occur, lasts longer and the postprandial protein synthesis period is shorter in cirrhosis. In addition to the shorter duration of the postprandial phase and longer postabsorptive or fasting phase, cirrhosis is believed to be a state of anabolic resistance characterized by impaired responses to anabolic stimuli [7, 66, 67]. Therefore, the restoration of the muscle protein loss during the postprandial or fed state may not completely reverse the losses of the postabsorptive

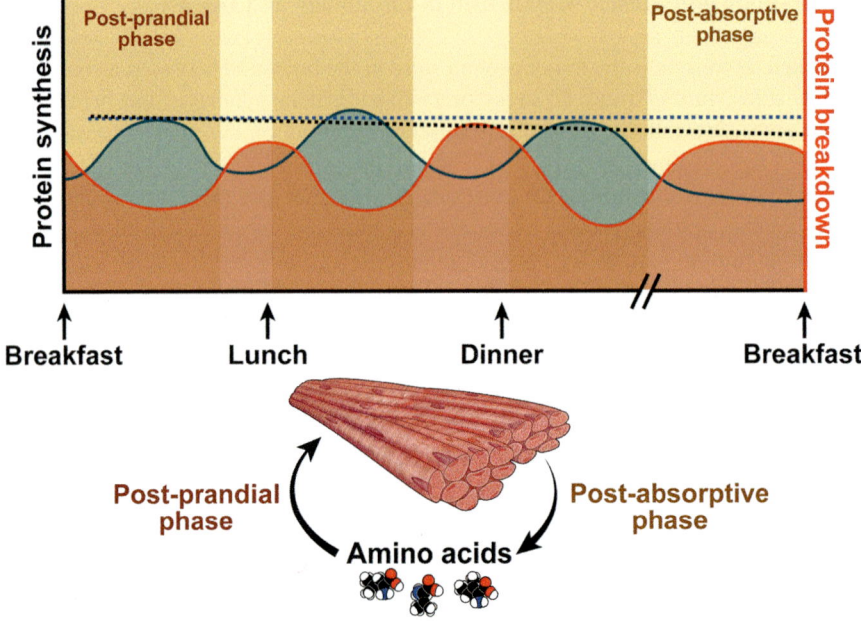

Fig. 4.1 Postprandial and postabsorptive protein homeostasis. Prior to a meal (fasted/postabsorptive phase), protein synthesis is decreased and protein breakdown is increased and following a meal (postprandial state) these changes are reversed. Since postprandial protein synthesis restores proteolysis-mediated loss of protein content, protein homeostasis is maintained (blue hatched line), while in cirrhosis, the duration of postabsorptive phase is extended due to accelerated starvation with dysregulated proteostasis and progressive loss of protein content and muscle mass

or fasting state resulting in a gradual but progressive muscle loss. Targeting the accelerated fasting in cirrhosis by frequent feeding and shortening the duration of the postabsorptive phase is a potential mechanistic therapeutic option to reverse and prevent worsening sarcopenia. The underlying mechanisms of these are currently under investigation, but cytokine and hormonal perturbations, including insulin resistance and endotoxemia, may contribute to these alterations.

Human Protein Kinetic Studies

A number of human studies have evaluated protein turnover with conflicting results. Increased, unaltered, and decreased rates of whole-body proteolysis and impaired protein synthesis have been reported using tracer kinetics [68–77]. This may be related to differences in etiology and severity of liver disease and duration of illness. A major limitation of these studies has been the lack of direct studies on the muscle since whole-body kinetics are influenced by organs besides the skeletal muscle. More recently, muscle protein synthesis measured using primed constant infusion and serial muscle biopsies before and following a single dose of branched chain amino acid supplementation showed similar rates of protein synthesis in cirrhosis and controls [78]. However, protein synthesis in the fasting state is currently not known.

Direct measures of muscle protein breakdown using tracer kinetics are challenging. 3-methyl histidine is formed by methylation of peptide-bound histidine in actin and myosin. After myofibrillar catabolism, 3-methyl histidine cannot be reutilized and is excreted in the urine. Studies using arteriovenous differences across the limb or urinary excretion of 3-methyl histidine used as measures of muscle protein breakdown also report conflicting results with increased, unaltered, or decreased muscle protein breakdown in cirrhosis [77, 79, 80].

Animal Studies

Decreased muscle mass with impaired muscle protein synthesis has been reported in the portocaval anastomosis rat and the bile duct-ligated rat [38, 81]. Direct measures of muscle protein breakdown in vivo are challenging. Instead, circulating amino acids and rate of appearance of specific metabolites have been used. There are no published data on direct measures of muscle protein breakdown using tracer kinetics in animals. Molecular measures of proteolysis have been used including altered ubiquitin proteasome pathway and autophagy [40, 41].

Cellular In Vitro Models

The best studied cellular system for a sarcopenic phenotype is the quantification of myotube size (diameter) in cellular cultures in response to potential mediators of muscle loss in cirrhosis [35, 40, 41, 46, 82–84]. These have been used to dissect the molecular and metabolic perturbations and have shown a reduction in protein synthesis, an increase in autophagy markers, and unaltered or decreased ubiquitin proteasome-mediated protein breakdown.

Molecular Perturbations in the Skeletal Muscle in Cirrhosis

In addition to direct studies in the skeletal muscle signaling pathways that regulate protein homeostasis, there is increasing interest in the regulation of these signaling perturbations in sarcopenia of liver disease [14, 59, 85]. Protein synthesis is regulated by two principal regulatory factors: myostatin, a transforming growth factor β superfamily member that inhibits protein synthesis, and locally generated insulin-like growth factor 1 (also known as mechanogrowth factor) that stimulates protein synthesis [2, 8, 40]. Canonical regulation of protein synthesis occurs via the Akt/mTORC1 that increases and the eukaryotic initiation factor 2α dependent regulatory pathway that inhibits protein synthesis [86]. A number of proteolytic pathways have been identified in the skeletal muscle and include the ubiquitin proteasome pathway, the lysosomal autophagy pathway, and the calcium-dependent calpain pathway of which there is robust literature in the former two proteolytic pathways in the muscle from models of liver disease [41, 45]. Perturbations in a number of upstream mediators including hyperammonemia, endotoxin, hormones, and nutrients cause dysregulation of these signaling pathways with impaired proteostasis and consequent sarcopenia [8, 14, 87, 88]. Understanding these perturbations is gaining increasing clinical interest because of the increasing availability of therapeutic options to restore proteostasis as a targeted approach to treat sarcopenia in liver disease.

Mediators of the Liver-Muscle Axis

Cirrhosis and other forms of liver disease with loss of muscle mass result in a number of biochemical, hormonal, cytokine, and metabolic perturbations that alter molecular signaling responses in the muscle culminating in dysregulated proteostasis and loss of muscle mass [7, 8]. Some of these have been studied directly in patients and models of cirrhosis, while others have been studied in non-hepatic disorders but are expected to result in activation of similar molecular perturbations. Of these, hyperammonemia is one of the best characterized mediators of the liver-muscle axis [89].

Physiologically, ammonia is a cytotoxic molecule generated mainly by gut bacterial metabolism as well as endogenous amino acid catabolism and purine breakdown during exercise in the skeletal muscle [90, 91]. Hepatocytes are the primary mechanism of ammonia disposal by the formation of urea, an energy requiring reaction [92]. In cirrhosis, ureagenesis is decreased due to hepatocellular dysfunction and portosystemic shunting with resultant hyperammonemia [93–95]. Even though hepatic encephalopathy is the best recognized adverse consequence of hyperammonemia [85], more recently the role of skeletal muscle in ammonia disposal and its consequences have been identified [96]. In a healthy subject, muscle is a net exporter of ammonia during fasting and exercise due to amino acid and purine catabolism with little clinical consequences because of normally functioning hepatocytes. In cirrhosis, multiple groups have reported an increased muscle uptake of ammonia [97, 98]; muscle ammonia uptake was generally believed to be a benign process. However, in the past decade, it is increasingly recognized that the skeletal muscle accumulates ammonia and functions as a metabolic partner to the liver [40, 41, 82]. Accumulation of ammonia in the skeletal muscle is not benign and initiates a series of metabolic, molecular, and organelle dysfunction with dysregulated protein homeostasis and potentially contributing to anabolic resistance [14, 40, 41]. Emerging data suggests that ammonia uptake by the transporter, RhBG, is increased by ammonia itself as well as causes of liver disease including ethanol [99].

Other potential mediators of the liver-muscle axis include endotoxemia with altered toll-like receptor signaling-mediated dysregulated protein homeostasis and muscle cell regeneration [87, 100], hormonal abnormalities including altered growth hormone secretion or resistance, and hypogonadism with decreased testosterone [101–103] and altered nutrient intake [104] and decreased physical activity [105]. This is however not a comprehensive list of potential mediators of the liver-muscle axis but includes those that have been evaluated in the development of sarcopenia. Other complications of cirrhosis including gastrointestinal bleeding, encephalopathy, ascites, renal dysfunction, and development of hepatocellular malignancy also aggravate the adverse consequences of the liver-muscle axis on skeletal muscle proteostasis, and their interaction with or contribution to the mediator (s) of the liver-muscle axis is not well characterized. Targeting the mediators of the liver-muscle axis is critical to reverse anabolic resistance, restore proteostasis, and improve muscle mass and function in cirrhosis.

Hormonal Perturbations in Cirrhosis

Male patients with cirrhosis and the PCA rat have lower circulating testosterone [106, 107]. Testosterone supplementation increases muscle mass in male patients with cirrhosis [103]. One of the potential mechanisms of testosterone is by a reduction in myostatin expression, but a more rapid aromatization of testosterone can accelerate its conversion to estradiol and impair beneficial responses [108]. Long-term safety of testosterone is also a concern, but given that testosterone or other aromatase resistant androgenic agents can inhibit muscle myostatin and protein synthesis, low androgens may be a potential mediator of decreased muscle protein synthesis in cirrhosis.

Growth hormone resistance or loss of the periodicity of growth hormone secretion has been reported in cirrhosis [102, 109, 110]. Growth hormone activates local insulin-like growth factor 1 and inhibits myostatin, and loss of growth hormone signaling may contribute to muscle loss [111].

Endotoxemia in Cirrhosis

Endotoxin is the lipopolysaccharide molecule in Gram-negative bacteria that is toxic to organisms primarily by the activation of host immune responses [112]. Low-grade sepsis and circulating endotoxemia have been reported in cirrhosis and patients with liver disease that can mediate muscle loss [87, 113, 114]. Endotoxin has been reported to impair protein synthesis by reduction in translational efficiency [12, 115]. The mechanistic basis of LPS-induced muscle loss is suggested to be mediated via a toll-like receptor (TLR)-4-dependent signaling with increased P65NFkB signaling, activation of inflammatory responses, and initiation of a cascade of molecular events that culminate in dysregulated proteostasis and muscle loss [100]. Even though overt sepsis may not be common, the low-grade

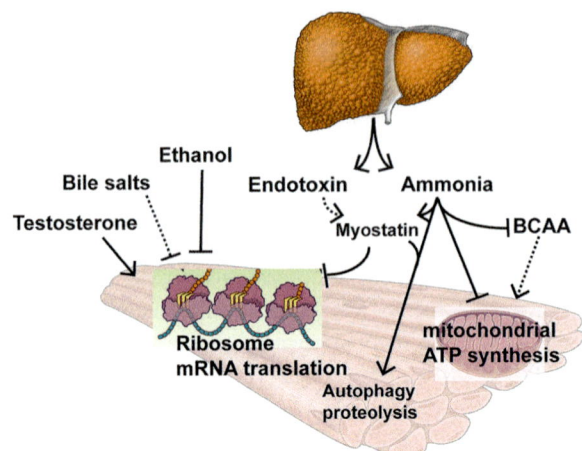

Fig. 4.2 Mediators of the liver-muscle axis. Hyperammonemia is a consistent abnormality and is one of the best characterized as a mediator of the liver-muscle axis. Other mediators include low-grade endotoxemia due to impaired gut barrier and decreased hepatic Kupffer cell function. Reduced testosterone and altered branched chain amino acids also contribute to impaired protein homeostasis by adverse impact on ribosomal function and translation of mRNA as well as increased protein breakdown via increased autophagy. Additionally, mitochondrial dysfunction also contributes to the bioenergetic deficiency and dysregulated proteostasis

endotoxemia due to a combination of increased gut permeability and impaired hepatic clearance of lipopolysaccharide has been referred to as metabolic endotoxemia [8]. Metabolic endotoxemia has been shown to impair muscle recovery responses and contribute to atrophy [116]. However, whether metabolic endotoxemia causes sarcopenia of cirrhosis and if the potential benefits of long-term antibiotics outweigh the risks are not known. Novel approaches to modulate TLR4 signaling and approaches to control metabolic endotoxemia are needed.

A schematic of these regulatory mediators is shown in (Fig. 4.2).

Signaling Pathways that Regulate Protein Homeostasis

Detailed reviews of translational regulation can be found elsewhere [86]. As mentioned earlier, skeletal muscle expression of myostatin is increased in cirrhosis and inhibits protein synthesis [40, 81]. Myostatin binds to activin IIB receptor, a type II TGFβ receptor, that upon ligand binding forms a heteromer complex with a type I receptor, activin-like kinases 4 and 5 [117]. The heterotetrameric receptor complex functions as a kinase for the Smad group of transcription factors which in turn inhibit the canonical Akt/mTORC1 pathway and consequent protein synthesis [118]. Details of myostatin signaling are beyond the scope of this work and can be reviewed elsewhere [117, 119, 120]. Insulin-like growth factor 1 is a known activator of the Akt/mTORC1 pathway to stimulate protein synthesis [120]. Protein synthesis is regulated primarily at the level of translational control when mRNA is translated to proteins in the ribosomes. The canonical translational regulation is mediated by mammalian target of rapamycin complex 1 (mTORC1) in the skeletal muscle [121]. Physiologically, mTORC1 is regulated by the upstream activator, protein kinase B/Akt, and inhibitor, AMP kinase, an energy sensor. Both Akt and AMPK phosphorylate tuberous sclerosis complex (TSC) 1 and 2 that either activates or inhibits mTORC1 kinase function depending on the sites of phosphorylation on the TSC protein [122]. Activated mTORC1 phosphorylates and activates downstream targets, P70S6 kinase and 4E binding protein 1. These two proteins are critical regulators of ribosomal translational initiation, the most energy requiring and critically regulated step in protein synthesis. mTORC1 causes translation of mRNA with a terminal oligopyrimidine tract at their 5′ end. The eukaryotic initiation factor-mediated translational control affects global translational control.

In brief, a number of eukaryotic initiation factors (eIF) are involved in translation initiation that involves binding of the 5′-methyl G cap structure on the mRNA to eIF4F, a cap binding protein complex [86]. The eIF4F-bound mRNA recruits the 43S initiation complex comprised of the 40S ribosomal subunit, a ternary complex containing an initiator tRNA molecule (eIF2.GTP.tRNA^{Met}) and the multisubunit initiation factor eIF3. The 43S initiation complex scans the 5′-untranslated region in a 5′ to 3′ direction [85, 123]. Recognition of the initiation codon results in a series of steps that result in commitment of the arrested ribosome to initiation mediated by eIF5 and eIF2-specific GTPase activating protein (GAP). Recognition of the AUG start codon and delivery of the initiator met-tRNA involve a GTP hydrolysis step which leaves the eIF2 complex in the inactive GDP-bound state. The translation initiation factor eIF2B regenerates an active ternary complex via its guanine nucleotide exchange (GEF) activity by recruiting a new initiator met-tRNA to the complex. The recycling of the ternary complex is necessary continuing translation initiation. During stress, eIF2 phosphorylation at its α-subunit (eIF2α) acts as an inhibitor of the eIF2B GEF activity and stalls recycling of the ternary complex with global inhibition of protein synthesis [124]. During cellular stress, a diverse group of eIF2α kinases are activated that phosphorylate Ser^{51} on eIF2α resulting in translational repression and decreased protein synthesis. Recovery from acute translational repression is mediated via dephosphorylation of eIF2α and selective translation of certain mRNA including ATF4 and CHOP to restore cellular homeostasis [125].

Hyperammonemic Stress Response

Responses to increased circulating ammonia and elevated muscle ammonia have been studied in human, animal, and cellular models [39, 40, 81–83, 126]. Hyperammonemia causes impaired protein synthesis by activation of the eIF2α kinase, general control non-derepressible 2 (GCN2), an amino acid deficiency sensor [46, 78, 83]. During cellular amino acid deficiency, uncharged tRNA concentrations increase that bind to the histidinyl tRNA-like binding site on GCN2 that results in its autophosphorylation and activation of the eIF2α kinase function with phosphorylation of the Ser[51] on eIF2α [127, 128]. Even though activation of GCN2 can occur due to any cellular amino acid deficiency, during hyperammonemia, activated *GCN2* is responsive to leucine supplementation in cellular systems despite no biochemical deficiency of leucine in myotubes [78, 83]. Instead, leucine is partitioned into the mitochondria to potentially serve as a substrate for mitochondrial ammonia disposal resulting in a potential compartmental deficiency in the cytosol [83, 119]. This cytosolic leucine deficiency results in impaired mTORC1 signaling and GCN2 activation, both of which can be reversed by high-dose leucine replacement. Unlike in the classical integrated stress response with initiation of adaptive responses, during hyperammonemia, expression of ATF4/CHOP or GADD34, the protein phosphatase 1 subunit required for dephosphorylation of eIF2α, is not increased. A partial recovery is mediated by an increased expression of a leucine exchanger, SLC7A5, and greater transport of leucine into the muscle, but this adaptive response is incomplete possibly because of reduced circulating branched chain amino acid concentrations [83].

More recently, ammonia withdrawal in myotubes and ammonia lowering therapy in the PCA rat showed an increase in muscle mass and muscle fiber diameter with partial reversal of an increased expression of myostatin, reduced protein synthesis, increased autophagy, impaired mTORC1 signaling, and increased eIF2α phosphorylation [46]. These data complement studies in the hyperammonemic models showing that ammonia is a mediator of the liver-muscle axis and impairs proteostasis.

Ammonia-Induced Skeletal Muscle Biochemical Perturbations and Organelle Dysfunction

Since ammonia is a chemical, its uptake by cellular systems is expected to result in biochemical responses. In cells other than hepatocytes, ammonia disposal is achieved by non-ureagenic metabolism. A major pathway that has been recognized in astrocytes and muscle cells is the initiation of cataplerosis or loss of critical tricarboxylic acid (TCA) cycle intermediate, α-ketoglutarate (αKG), to generate glutamate and subsequently glutamine [82, 129]. Glutamine is then exported into the circulation in exchange for leucine by the leucine exchanger, SLC7A5, referred to above in the HASR. Even though this reaction promotes ammonia disposal, it results in a reduction in mitochondrial intermediates that are expected to lower ATP synthesis. Consistently, in myotubes mitochondrial intermediates are lower, ATP content is reduced, and oxygen consumption is increased during hyperammonemia [82]. The reduction in ATP content contributes to lower protein synthesis since translation initiation is one of the most energy-requiring cellular processes [130]. Additionally, lower ATP content can also explain the reduced muscle contractile force reported in human cirrhosis, animal models, and hyperammonemic myotubes

[35]. In addition to a reduction in TCA cycle intermediates, skeletal muscle hyper-ammonemia impairs electron transport chain components, specifically complex 1, NADH oxidase [82]. The alteration in cellular redox ratio results in accumulation of NADH. Hyperammonemia also causes leak of electrons primarily from complex III with oxidative modification of cellular components. In addition to these altera-tions in mitochondrial intermediates, alternative pathways for ammonia disposal in the muscle include metabolic diversion of pyruvate away from oxidative metabo-lism to alanine and diversion of the malate aspartate pathway favoring aspartate. The combination of reduced TCA cycle intermediates with accumulation of NADH can also redirect pyruvate to lactate that can explain the elevated lactate in cirrhosis.

These metabolic perturbations can also result in molecular responses including reactive oxygen species-induced activation of autophagy and mitochondrial struc-tural defects that are areas of ongoing investigation.

A simplified schematic of these pathways is shown in (Fig. 4.3).

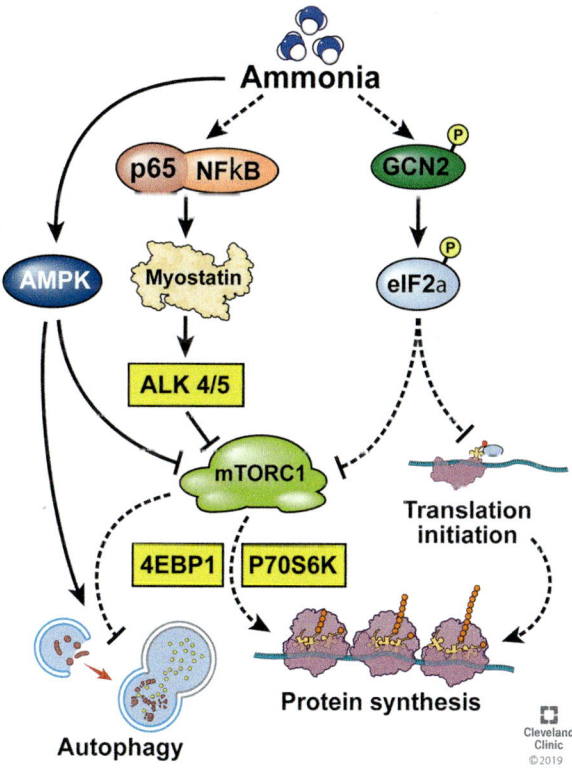

Fig. 4.3 Ammonia induced perturbations in signaling pathways that results in dysregulated proteostasis and sarcopenia. Hyperammonemia transcriptionally upregulates myostatin via a p65NFkB-mediated mechanism. Additionally, ammonia also activates amino acid deficiency sensor, GCN2, a eukaryotic initiation factor 2α kinase. Both myostatin and eIF2α impair mTORC1 signaling with reduced protein synthesis and increased autophagy

Pathogenesis of Skeletal Muscle Contractile Dysfunction and Frailty

A number of recent studies have shown that impaired skeletal muscle contractile function is also common in cirrhosis and accompanies sarcopenia or reduced muscle mass [35]. Whether impaired contractile function accompanies muscle loss and whether recovery of muscle mass is a necessary requirement for recovery of muscle contractile function is not clear. Frailty is a term that has been used to refer to a functional decline, due to muscle contractile dysfunction, and is accompanied by muscle loss [4, 6, 34, 36, 37, 131, 132]. Fatigue is another manifestation of skeletal muscle contractile dysfunction with reduced maximum contraction, impaired ability to sustain maximum contraction, and inability to perform repetitive activity all of which are also observed with frailty [35]. Both frailty and fatigue can be the result of loss of contractile proteins that occur with sarcopenia, impaired mitochondrial function with reduced ATP generation, and impaired function of contractile proteins due to posttranslational modifications including oxidative changes and nitration. Exercise in physiological states results in muscle ammonia generation due to a variety of factors including purine breakdown due to rapid breakdown of ATP to generate AMP that in turn is catabolized to inosine and finally ammonia release. Another potential mechanism of activity-induced muscle ammoniagenesis is the utilization of branched chain amino acids as a source of acetyl CoA for oxidation in the citric acid (TCA) cycle. Therefore, ammonia-induced perturbations in molecular and metabolic responses of exercise that decrease contractile function include hyperammonemia-mediated alterations in mitochondrial function and protein modifications. Even though changes in blood flow can affect muscle function, there are no data to support impaired muscle blood flow in cirrhosis [133, 134]. However, oxygen consumption by the muscle is impaired during hyperammonemia, and an increased lactate concentration can contribute to fatigue and impaired contractile function [82, 135, 136]. The term dysoxia has been used to refer to the impaired oxygen utilization despite adequate delivery [137, 138]. Dysoxia is a potential mechanism underlying muscle contractile dysfunction in cirrhosis as evidenced by impaired mitochondrial function during hyperammonemia [82]. During muscle contraction, increased utilization of oxygen occurs, but due to the hyperammonemia-induced mitochondrial dysfunction, contractility may be significantly impaired resulting in frailty. Since increased blood oxygen content cannot reverse dysoxia, strategies to restore mitochondrial homeostasis and reversing muscle contractile protein modifications are needed to improve fatigue and frailty. Whether the metabolic and molecular responses of regular activity in cirrhosis mimic the responses to active exercise in physiological states is not known. Finally, it is important to reiterate that precise definitions of the components of frailty and fatigue are necessary to dissect the pathogenic mechanisms.

Summary and Conclusions

Both hepatocellular dysfunction and vascular consequences due to portal hypertension and portosystemic shunting contribute to the metabolic, hormonal, and nutritional perturbations that alter skeletal muscle protein homeostasis and consequent sarcopenia and contractile dysfunction. Even though hyperammonemia is a consistent abnormality in cirrhosis and is a mediator of the liver-muscle axis, hormonal changes and metabolic endotoxemia are increasingly recognized to contribute to sarcopenia. Whether sarcopenia is a necessary component of frailty and if it is possible to reverse frailty are currently not known. However, hand grip strength, a measure of contractile dysfunction, is at least partially reversed following liver transplantation despite unaltered or further reduction in muscle mass which suggests that muscle strength does not necessarily correlate completely with muscle mass. Dissecting the metabolic perturbation, substrate preference, subcellular alterations, and molecular changes in the skeletal muscle will lay the foundation to develop targeted therapies to restore proteostasis, reverse muscle mass, and possibly improve frailty in cirrhosis.

References

1. Periyalwar P, Dasarathy S. Malnutrition in cirrhosis: contribution and consequences of sarcopenia on metabolic and clinical responses. Clin Liver Dis. 2012;16:95–131.
2. Dasarathy S. Consilience in sarcopenia of cirrhosis. J Cachexia Sarcopenia Muscle. 2012;3:225–37.
3. Ebadi M, Montano-Loza AJ. Insights on clinical relevance of sarcopenia in patients with cirrhosis and sepsis. Liver Int. 2018;38:786–8.
4. Ebadi M, Montano-Loza AJ. Sarcopenia and frailty in the prognosis of patients on the liver transplant waiting list. Liver Transpl. 2019;25:7–9.
5. Sinclair M, Poltavskiy E, Dodge JL, Lai JC. Frailty is independently associated with increased hospitalisation days in patients on the liver transplant waitlist. World J Gastroenterol. 2017;23:899–905.
6. Lai JC, Covinsky KE, McCulloch CE, Feng S. The liver frailty index improves mortality prediction of the subjective clinician assessment in patients with cirrhosis. Am J Gastroenterol. 2018;113:235–42.
7. Dasarathy S. Cause and management of muscle wasting in chronic liver disease. Curr Opin Gastroenterol. 2016;32:159–65.
8. Dasarathy S, Merli M. Sarcopenia from mechanism to diagnosis and treatment in liver disease. J Hepatol. 2016;65:1232–44.
9. Antar R, Wong P, Ghali P. A meta-analysis of nutritional supplementation for management of hospitalized alcoholic hepatitis. Can J Gastroenterol. 2012;26:463–7.
10. Koretz RL. The evidence for the use of nutritional support in liver disease. Curr Opin Gastroenterol. 2014;30:208–14.
11. Fialla AD, Israelsen M, Hamberg O, Krag A, Gluud LL. Nutritional therapy in cirrhosis or alcoholic hepatitis: a systematic review and meta-analysis. Liver Int. 2015;35:2072–8.
12. Ney M, Vandermeer B, van Zanten SJ, Ma MM, Gramlich L, Tandon P. Meta-analysis: oral or enteral nutritional supplementation in cirrhosis. Aliment Pharmacol Ther. 2013;37:672–9.

13. Anthony TG. Mechanisms of protein balance in skeletal muscle. Domest Anim Endocrinol. 2016;56(Suppl):S23–32.
14. Dasarathy S, Hatzoglou M. Hyperammonemia and proteostasis in cirrhosis. Curr Opin Clin Nutr Metab Care. 2018;21:30–6.
15. Sirabella D, De Angelis L, Berghella L. Sources for skeletal muscle repair: from satellite cells to reprogramming. J Cachexia Sarcopenia Muscle. 2013;4:125–36.
16. Fry CS, Lee JD, Mula J, Kirby TJ, Jackson JR, Liu F, et al. Inducible depletion of satellite cells in adult, sedentary mice impairs muscle regenerative capacity without affecting sarcopenia. Nat Med. 2015;21:76–80.
17. McCarthy JJ, Mula J, Miyazaki M, Erfani R, Garrison K, Farooqui AB, et al. Effective fiber hypertrophy in satellite cell-depleted skeletal muscle. Development. 2011;138:3657–66.
18. Tandon P, Raman M, Mourtzakis M, Merli M. A practical approach to nutritional screening and assessment in cirrhosis. Hepatology. 2017;65:1044–57.
19. Fiore P, Merli M, Andreoli A, De Lorenzo A, Masini A, Ciuffa L, et al. A comparison of skinfold anthropometry and dual-energy X-ray absorptiometry for the evaluation of body fat in cirrhotic patients. Clin Nutr. 1999;18:349–51.
20. Merli M, Riggio O, Dally L. Does malnutrition affect survival in cirrhosis? PINC (Policentrica Italiana Nutrizione Cirrosi). Hepatology. 1996;23:1041–6.
21. Romiti A, Merli M, Martorano M, Parrilli G, Martino F, Riggio O, et al. Malabsorption and nutritional abnormalities in patients with liver cirrhosis. Ital J Gastroenterol. 1990;22:118–23.
22. Merli M, Nicolini G, Angeloni S, Riggio O. Malnutrition is a risk factor in cirrhotic patients undergoing surgery. Nutrition. 2002;18:978–86.
23. Riggio O, Angeloni S, Ciuffa L, Nicolini G, Attili AF, Albanese C, et al. Malnutrition is not related to alterations in energy balance in patients with stable liver cirrhosis. Clin Nutr. 2003;22:553–9.
24. Schiavo L, Busetto L, Cesaretti M, Zelber-Sagi S, Deutsch L, Iannelli A. Nutritional issues in patients with obesity and cirrhosis. World J Gastroenterol. 2018;24:3330–46.
25. Eslamparast T, Montano-Loza AJ, Raman M, Tandon P. Sarcopenic obesity in cirrhosis-the confluence of 2 prognostic titans. Liver Int. 2018;38:1706–17.
26. Stenholm S, Harris TB, Rantanen T, Visser M, Kritchevsky SB, Ferrucci L. Sarcopenic obesity: definition, cause and consequences. Curr Opin Clin Nutr Metab Care. 2008;11:693–700.
27. Dasarathy J, Alkhouri N, Dasarathy S. Changes in body composition after transjugular intrahepatic portosystemic stent in cirrhosis: a critical review of literature. Liver Int. 2011;31:1250–8.
28. Tsien C, Garber A, Narayanan A, Shah SN, Barnes D, Eghtesad B, et al. Post-liver transplantation sarcopenia in cirrhosis: a prospective evaluation. J Gastroenterol Hepatol. 2014;29:1250–7.
29. Carey EJ, Lai JC, Wang CW, Dasarathy S, Lobach I, Montano-Loza AJ, et al. A multicenter study to define sarcopenia in patients with end-stage liver disease. Liver Transpl. 2017;23:625–33.
30. Ebadi M, Wang CW, Lai JC, Dasarathy S, Kappus MR, Dunn MA, et al. Poor performance of psoas muscle index for identification of patients with higher waitlist mortality risk in cirrhosis. J Cachexia Sarcopenia Muscle. 2018;9:1053–62.
31. Gallagher D, Visser M, De Meersman RE, Sepulveda D, Baumgartner RN, Pierson RN, et al. Appendicular skeletal muscle mass: effects of age, gender, and ethnicity. J Appl Physiol. (1985) 1997;83:229–39.
32. Heymsfield SB, Peterson CM, Thomas DM, Heo M, Schuna JM Jr. Why are there race/ethnic differences in adult body mass index-adiposity relationships? A quantitative critical review. Obes Rev. 2016;17:262–75.
33. Cesari M, Landi F, Vellas B, Bernabei R, Marzetti E. Sarcopenia and physical frailty: two sides of the same coin. Front Aging Neurosci. 2014;6:192.
34. Kok B, Tandon P. Frailty in patients with cirrhosis. Curr Treat Options Gastroenterol. 2018;16:215–25.

35. McDaniel J, Davuluri G, Hill EA, Moyer M, Runkana A, Prayson R, et al. Hyperammonemia results in reduced muscle function independent of muscle mass. Am J Physiol Gastrointest Liver Physiol. 2016;310:G163–70.
36. Lai JC, Covinsky KE, Dodge JL, Boscardin WJ, Segev DL, Roberts JP, et al. Development of a novel frailty index to predict mortality in patients with end-stage liver disease. Hepatology. 2017;66:564–74.
37. Lai JC, Volk ML, Strasburg D, Alexander N. Performance-based measures associate with frailty in patients with end-stage liver disease. Transplantation. 2016;100:2656–60.
38. Bosoi CR, Oliveira MM, Ochoa-Sanchez R, Tremblay M, Ten Have GA, Deutz NE, et al. The bile duct ligated rat: a relevant model to study muscle mass loss in cirrhosis. Metab Brain Dis. 2017;32:513–8.
39. Dasarathy S, Muc S, Hisamuddin K, Edmison JM, Dodig M, McCullough AJ, et al. Altered expression of genes regulating skeletal muscle mass in the portacaval anastomosis rat. Am J Physiol Gastrointest Liver Physiol. 2007;292:G1105–13.
40. Qiu J, Thapaliya S, Runkana A, Yang Y, Tsien C, Mohan ML, et al. Hyperammonemia in cirrhosis induces transcriptional regulation of myostatin by an NF-kappaB-mediated mechanism. Proc Natl Acad Sci U S A. 2013;110:18162–7.
41. Qiu J, Tsien C, Thapalaya S, Narayanan A, Weihl CC, Ching JK, et al. Hyperammonemia-mediated autophagy in skeletal muscle contributes to sarcopenia of cirrhosis. Am J Physiol Endocrinol Metab. 2012;303:E983–93.
42. Fortea JI, Fernandez-Mena C, Puerto M, Ripoll C, Almagro J, Banares J, et al. Comparison of two protocols of carbon tetrachloride-induced cirrhosis in Rats- improving yield and reproducibility. Sci Rep. 2018;8:9163.
43. Jimenez W, Claria J, Arroyo V, Rodes J. Carbon tetrachloride induced cirrhosis in rats: a useful tool for investigating the pathogenesis of ascites in chronic liver disease. J Gastroenterol Hepatol. 1992;7:90–7.
44. Munoz Torres E, Paz Bouza JI, Lopez Bravo A, Abad Hernandez MM, Carrascal ME. Experimental thioacetamide-induced cirrhosis of the liver. Histol Histopathol. 1991;6:95–100.
45. Thapaliya S, Runkana A, McMullen MR, Nagy LE, McDonald C, Naga Prasad SV, et al. Alcohol-induced autophagy contributes to loss in skeletal muscle mass. Autophagy. 2014;10:677–90.
46. Kumar A, Davuluri G, Silva RNE, Engelen M, Ten Have GAM, Prayson R, et al. Ammonia lowering reverses sarcopenia of cirrhosis by restoring skeletal muscle proteostasis. Hepatology. 2017;65:2045–58.
47. Lopez-Lirola A, Gonzalez-Reimers E, Martin Olivera R, Santolaria-Fernandez F, Galindo-Martin L, Abreu-Gonzalez P, et al. Protein deficiency and muscle damage in carbon tetrachloride induced liver cirrhosis. Food Chem Toxicol. 2003;41:1789–97.
48. Gayan-Ramirez G, van de Casteele M, Rollier H, Fevery J, Vanderhoydonc F, Verhoeven G, et al. Biliary cirrhosis induces type IIx/b fiber atrophy in rat diaphragm and skeletal muscle, and decreases IGF-I mRNA in the liver but not in muscle. J Hepatol. 1998;29:241–9.
49. Burd NA, Tang JE, Moore DR, Phillips SM. Exercise training and protein metabolism: influences of contraction, protein intake, and sex-based differences. J Appl Physiol. 1985) 2009;106:1692–701.
50. Tsien CD, McCullough AJ, Dasarathy S. Late evening snack: exploiting a period of anabolic opportunity in cirrhosis. J Gastroenterol Hepatol. 2012;27:430–41.
51. Mitchell WK, Wilkinson DJ, Phillips BE, Lund JN, Smith K, Atherton PJ. Human skeletal muscle protein metabolism responses to amino acid nutrition. Adv Nutr. 2016;7:828S–38S.
52. Atherton PJ, Smith K. Muscle protein synthesis in response to nutrition and exercise. J Physiol. 2012;590:1049–57.
53. Kiens B, Essen-Gustavsson B, Christensen NJ, Saltin B. Skeletal muscle substrate utilization during submaximal exercise in man: effect of endurance training. J Physiol. 1993;469:459–78.

54. Hoppeler H. Skeletal muscle substrate metabolism. Int J Obes Relat Metab Disord. 1999;23(Suppl 3):S7–10.
55. Westerterp KR. Food quotient, respiratory quotient, and energy balance. Am J Clin Nutr. 1993;57:759S–64S; discussion 764S–765S.
56. Pozefsky T, Tancredi RG, Moxley RT, Dupre J, Tobin JD. Effects of brief starvation on muscle amino acid metabolism in nonobese man. J Clin Invest. 1976;57:444–9.
57. Glass C, Hipskind P, Tsien C, Malin SK, Kasumov T, Shah SN, et al. Sarcopenia and a physiologically low respiratory quotient in patients with cirrhosis: a prospective controlled study. J Appl Physiol. 1985) 2013;114:559–65.
58. Romijn JA, Endert E, Sauerwein HP. Glucose and fat metabolism during short-term starvation in cirrhosis. Gastroenterology. 1991;100:731–7.
59. Dasarathy J, McCullough AJ, Dasarathy S. Sarcopenia in alcoholic liver disease: clinical and molecular advances. Alcohol Clin Exp Res. 2017;41:1419–31.
60. Plank LD, Gane EJ, Peng S, Muthu C, Mathur S, Gillanders L, et al. Nocturnal nutritional supplementation improves total body protein status of patients with liver cirrhosis: a randomized 12-month trial. Hepatology. 2008;48:557–66.
61. Muller MJ, Bottcher J, Selberg O. Energy expenditure and substrate metabolism in liver cirrhosis. Int J Obes Relat Metab Disord. 1993;17(Suppl 3):S102–6; discussion S115.
62. Muller MJ, Lautz HU, Plogmann B, Burger M, Korber J, Schmidt FW. Energy expenditure and substrate oxidation in patients with cirrhosis: the impact of cause, clinical staging and nutritional state. Hepatology. 1992;15:782–94.
63. Muller MJ, Bottcher J, Selberg O, Weselmann S, Boker KH, Schwarze M, et al. Hypermetabolism in clinically stable patients with liver cirrhosis. Am J Clin Nutr. 1999;69:1194–201.
64. Muller MJ, Boker KH, Selberg O. Are patients with liver cirrhosis hypermetabolic? Clin Nutr. 1994;13:131–44.
65. Peng S, Plank LD, McCall JL, Gillanders LK, McIlroy K, Gane EJ. Body composition, muscle function, and energy expenditure in patients with liver cirrhosis: a comprehensive study. Am J Clin Nutr. 2007;85:1257–66.
66. Morton RW, Traylor DA, Weijs PJM, Phillips SM. Defining anabolic resistance: implications for delivery of clinical care nutrition. Curr Opin Crit Care. 2018;24:124–30.
67. Rennie MJ, Wilkes EA. Maintenance of the musculoskeletal mass by control of protein turnover: the concept of anabolic resistance and its relevance to the transplant recipient. Ann Transplant. 2005;10:31–4.
68. Tessari P, Inchiostro S, Barazzoni R, Zanetti M, Orlando R, Biolo G, et al. Fasting and postprandial phenylalanine and leucine kinetics in liver cirrhosis. Am J Phys. 1994;267:E140–9.
69. Tessari P, Barazzoni R, Kiwanuka E, Davanzo G, De Pergola G, Orlando R, et al. Impairment of albumin and whole body postprandial protein synthesis in compensated liver cirrhosis. Am J Physiol Endocrinol Metab. 2002;282:E304–11.
70. Tessari P, Biolo G, Inchiostro S, Orlando R, Vettore M, Sergi G. Leucine and phenylalanine kinetics in compensated liver cirrhosis: effects of insulin. Gastroenterology. 1993;104:1712–21.
71. Tessari P, Kiwanuka E, Vettore M, Barazzoni R, Zanetti M, Cecchet D, et al. Phenylalanine and tyrosine kinetics in compensated liver cirrhosis: effects of meal ingestion. Am J Physiol Gastrointest Liver Physiol. 2008;295:G598–604.
72. Tessari P. Protein metabolism in liver cirrhosis: from albumin to muscle myofibrils. Curr Opin Clin Nutr Metab Care. 2003;6:79–85.
73. Tessari P, Zanetti M, Barazzoni R, Biolo G, Orlando R, Vettore M, et al. Response of phenylalanine and leucine kinetics to branched chain-enriched amino acids and insulin in patients with cirrhosis. Gastroenterology. 1996;111:127–37.
74. McCullough AJ, Mullen KD, Kalhan SC. Defective nonoxidative leucine degradation and endogenous leucine flux in cirrhosis during an amino acid infusion. Hepatology. 1998;28:1357–64.

75. McCullough AJ, Mullen KD, Tavill AS, Kalhan SC. In vivo differences between the turnover rates of leucine and leucine's ketoacid in stable cirrhosis. Gastroenterology. 1992;103:571–8.
76. Mullen KD, Denne SC, McCullough AJ, Savin SM, Bruno D, Tavill AS, et al. Leucine metabolism in stable cirrhosis. Hepatology. 1986;6:622–30.
77. Morrison WL, Bouchier IA, Gibson JN, Rennie MJ. Skeletal muscle and whole-body protein turnover in cirrhosis. Clin Sci (Lond). 1990;78:613–9.
78. Tsien C, Davuluri G, Singh D, Allawy A, Ten Have GA, Thapaliya S, et al. Metabolic and molecular responses to leucine-enriched branched chain amino acid supplementation in the skeletal muscle of alcoholic cirrhosis. Hepatology. 2015;61:2018–29.
79. Zoli M, Marchesini G, Dondi C, Bianchi GP, Pisi E. Myofibrillar protein catabolic rates in cirrhotic patients with and without muscle wasting. Clin Sci (Lond). 1982;62:683–6.
80. Marchesini G, Zoli M, Angiolini A, Dondi C, Bianchi FB, Pisi E. Muscle protein breakdown in liver cirrhosis and the role of altered carbohydrate metabolism. Hepatology. 1981;1:294–9.
81. Dasarathy S, McCullough AJ, Muc S, Schneyer A, Bennett CD, Dodig M, et al. Sarcopenia associated with portosystemic shunting is reversed by follistatin. J Hepatol. 2011;54:915–21.
82. Davuluri G, Allawy A, Thapaliya S, Rennison JH, Singh D, Kumar A, et al. Hyperammonaemia-induced skeletal muscle mitochondrial dysfunction results in cataplerosis and oxidative stress. J Physiol. 2016;594:7341–60.
83. Davuluri G, Krokowski D, Guan BJ, Kumar A, Thapaliya S, Singh D, et al. Metabolic adaptation of skeletal muscle to hyperammonemia drives the beneficial effects of l-leucine in cirrhosis. J Hepatol. 2016;65:929–37.
84. Nieuwoudt S, Mulya A, Fealy CE, Martelli E, Dasarathy S, Naga Prasad SV, et al. In vitro contraction protects against palmitate-induced insulin resistance in C2C12 myotubes. Am J Physiol Cell Physiol. 2017;313:C575–83.
85. Dasarathy S, Mookerjee RP, Rackayova V, Rangroo Thrane V, Vairappan B, Ott P, et al. Ammonia toxicity: from head to toe? Metab Brain Dis. 2017;32:529–38.
86. Jackson RJ, Hellen CU, Pestova TV. The mechanism of eukaryotic translation initiation and principles of its regulation. Nat Rev Mol Cell Biol. 2010;11:113–27.
87. Tachiyama G, Sakon M, Kambayashi J, Iijima S, Tsujinaka T, Mori T. Endogenous endotoxemia in patients with liver cirrhosis--a quantitative analysis of endotoxin in portal and peripheral blood. Jpn J Surg. 1988;18:403–8.
88. Macallan DC, Cook EB, Preedy VR, Griffin GE. The effect of endotoxin on skeletal muscle protein gene expression in the rat. Int J Biochem Cell Biol. 1996;28:511–20.
89. Chen HW, Dunn MA. Muscle at risk: the multiple impacts of Ammonia on sarcopenia and frailty in cirrhosis. Clin Transl Gastroenterol. 2016;7:e170.
90. Adeva MM, Souto G, Blanco N, Donapetry C. Ammonium metabolism in humans. Metabolism. 2012;61:1495–511.
91. Dimski DS. Ammonia metabolism and the urea cycle: function and clinical implications. J Vet Intern Med. 1994;8:73–8.
92. Schutz Y. Protein turnover, ureagenesis and gluconeogenesis. Int J Vitam Nutr Res. 2011;81:101–7.
93. Rudman D, DiFulco TJ, Galambos JT, Smith RB 3rd, Salam AA, Warren WD. Maximal rates of excretion and synthesis of urea in normal and cirrhotic subjects. J Clin Invest. 1973;52:2241–9.
94. Shangraw RE, Jahoor F. Effect of liver disease and transplantation on urea synthesis in humans: relationship to acid-base status. Am J Phys. 1999;276:G1145–52.
95. Vilstrup H. Synthesis of urea after stimulation with amino acids: relation to liver function. Gut. 1980;21:990–5.
96. Olde Damink SW, Jalan R, Dejong CH. Interorgan ammonia trafficking in liver disease. Metab Brain Dis. 2009;24:169–81.
97. Ganda OP, Ruderman NB. Muscle nitrogen metabolism in chronic hepatic insufficiency. Metabolism. 1976;25:427–35.

98. Lockwood AH, McDonald JM, Reiman RE, Gelbard AS, Laughlin JS, Duffy TE, et al. The dynamics of ammonia metabolism in man. Effects of liver disease and hyperammonemia. J Clin Invest. 1979;63:449–60.

99. Kant S, Davuluri G, Alchirazi KA, Welch N, Heit C, Kumar A, et al. Ethanol sensitizes skeletal muscle to ammonia-induced molecular perturbations. J Biol Chem. 2019;294:7231–44.

100. Ono Y, Sakamoto K. Lipopolysaccharide inhibits myogenic differentiation of C2C12 myoblasts through the toll-like receptor 4-nuclear factor-kappaB signaling pathway and myoblast-derived tumor necrosis factor-alpha. PLoS One. 2017;12:e0182040.

101. de la Garza RG, Morales-Garza LA, Martin-Estal I, Castilla-Cortazar I. Insulin-like growth Factor-1 deficiency and cirrhosis establishment. J Clin Med Res. 2017;9:233–47.

102. Bucuvalas JC, Horn JA, Chernausek SD. Resistance to growth hormone in children with chronic liver disease. Pediatr Transplant. 1997;1:73–9.

103. Sinclair M, Grossmann M, Hoermann R, Angus PW, Gow PJ. Testosterone therapy increases muscle mass in men with cirrhosis and low testosterone: a randomised controlled trial. J Hepatol. 2016;65:906–13.

104. Verboeket-van de Venne WP, Westerterp KR, van Hoek B, Swart GR. Energy expenditure and substrate metabolism in patients with cirrhosis of the liver: effects of the pattern of food intake. Gut. 1995;36:110–6.

105. Berzigotti A, Saran U, Dufour JF. Physical activity and liver diseases. Hepatology. 2016;63:1026–40.

106. Sinclair M, Grossmann M, Gow PJ, Angus PW. Testosterone in men with advanced liver disease: abnormalities and implications. J Gastroenterol Hepatol. 2015;30:244–51.

107. Dasarathy S, Mullen KD, Dodig M, Donofrio B, McCullough AJ. Inhibition of aromatase improves nutritional status following portacaval anastomosis in male rats. J Hepatol. 2006;45:214–20.

108. Kovacheva EL, Hikim AP, Shen R, Sinha I, Sinha-Hikim I. Testosterone supplementation reverses sarcopenia in aging through regulation of myostatin, c-Jun NH2-terminal kinase, notch, and Akt signaling pathways. Endocrinology. 2010;151:628–38.

109. Adamek A, Kasprzak A. Insulin-like growth factor (IGF) system in liver diseases. Int J Mol Sci. 2018;19.

110. Baruch Y, Assy N, Amit T, Krivoy N, Strickovsky D, Orr ZS, et al. Spontaneous pulsatility and pharmacokinetics of growth hormone in liver cirrhotic patients. J Hepatol. 1998;29:559–64.

111. Liu W, Thomas SG, Asa SL, Gonzalez-Cadavid N, Bhasin S, Ezzat S. Myostatin is a skeletal muscle target of growth hormone anabolic action. J Clin Endocrinol Metab. 2003;88:5490–6.

112. Raetz CR, Whitfield C. Lipopolysaccharide endotoxins. Annu Rev Biochem. 2002;71:635–700.

113. Lin RS, Lee FY, Lee SD, Tsai YT, Lin HC, Lu RH, et al. Endotoxemia in patients with chronic liver diseases: relationship to severity of liver diseases, presence of esophageal varices, and hyperdynamic circulation. J Hepatol. 1995;22:165–72.

114. Bode C, Kugler V, Bode JC. Endotoxemia in patients with alcoholic and non-alcoholic cirrhosis and in subjects with no evidence of chronic liver disease following acute alcohol excess. J Hepatol. 1987;4:8–14.

115. Tarabees R, Hill D, Rauch C, Barrow PA, Loughna PT. Endotoxin transiently inhibits protein synthesis through Akt and MAPK mediating pathways in C2C12 myotubes. Am J Physiol Cell Physiol. 2011;301:C895–902.

116. Ghosh S, Lertwattanarak R, Garduno Jde J, Galeana JJ, Li J, Zamarripa F, et al. Elevated muscle TLR4 expression and metabolic endotoxemia in human aging. J Gerontol A Biol Sci Med Sci. 2015;70:232–46.

117. Han HQ, Mitch WE. Targeting the myostatin signaling pathway to treat muscle wasting diseases. Curr Opin Support Palliat Care. 2011;5:334–41.

118. Trendelenburg AU, Meyer A, Rohner D, Boyle J, Hatakeyama S, Glass DJ. Myostatin reduces Akt/TORC1/p70S6K signaling, inhibiting myoblast differentiation and myotube size. Am J Physiol Cell Physiol. 2009;296:C1258–70.

119. Dasarathy S. Myostatin and beyond in cirrhosis: all roads lead to sarcopenia. J Cachexia Sarcopenia Muscle. 2017;8:864–9.
120. Egerman MA, Glass DJ. Signaling pathways controlling skeletal muscle mass. Crit Rev Biochem Mol Biol. 2014;49:59–68.
121. Yoon MS. mTOR as a key regulator in maintaining skeletal muscle mass. Front Physiol. 2017;8:788.
122. Huang J, Manning BD. The TSC1-TSC2 complex: a molecular switchboard controlling cell growth. Biochem J. 2008;412:179–90.
123. Johansen ML, Bak LK, Schousboe A, Iversen P, Sorensen M, Keiding S, et al. The metabolic role of isoleucine in detoxification of ammonia in cultured mouse neurons and astrocytes. Neurochem Int. 2007;50:1042–51.
124. Guan BJ, Krokowski D, Majumder M, Schmotzer CL, Kimball SR, Merrick WC, et al. Translational control during endoplasmic reticulum stress beyond phosphorylation of the translation initiation factor eIF2alpha. J Biol Chem. 2014;289:12593–611.
125. Ron D, Walter P. Signal integration in the endoplasmic reticulum unfolded protein response. Nat Rev Mol Cell Biol. 2007;8:519–29.
126. Dasarathy S, Dodig M, Muc SM, Kalhan SC, McCullough AJ. Skeletal muscle atrophy is associated with an increased expression of myostatin and impaired satellite cell function in the portacaval anastamosis rat. Am J Physiol Gastrointest Liver Physiol. 2004;287:G1124–30.
127. Wek RC, Jiang HY, Anthony TG. Coping with stress: eIF2 kinases and translational control. Biochem Soc Trans. 2006;34:7–11.
128. Dong J, Qiu H, Garcia-Barrio M, Anderson J, Hinnebusch AG. Uncharged tRNA activates GCN2 by displacing the protein kinase moiety from a bipartite tRNA-binding domain. Mol Cell. 2000;6:269–79.
129. Schousboe A, Scafidi S, Bak LK, Waagepetersen HS, McKenna MC. Glutamate metabolism in the brain focusing on astrocytes. Adv Neurobiol. 2014;11:13–30.
130. Kafri M, Metzl-Raz E, Jona G, Barkai N. The cost of protein production. Cell Rep. 2016;14:22–31.
131. Duarte-Rojo A, Ruiz-Margain A, Montano-Loza AJ, Macias-Rodriguez RU, Ferrando A, Kim WR. Exercise and physical activity for patients with end-stage liver disease: improving functional status and sarcopenia while on the transplant waiting list. Liver Transpl. 2018;24:122–39.
132. Lai JC. Editorial: advancing adoption of frailty to improve the Care of Patients with cirrhosis: time for a consensus on a frailty index. Am J Gastroenterol. 2016;111:1776–7.
133. Bay Nielsen H, Secher NH, Clemmesen O, Ott P. Maintained cerebral and skeletal muscle oxygenation during maximal exercise in patients with liver cirrhosis. J Hepatol. 2005;43:266–71.
134. Lunzer M, Newman SP, Sherlock S. Skeletal muscle blood flow and neurovascular reactivity in liver disease. Gut. 1973;14:354–9.
135. Jeppesen JB, Mortensen C, Bendtsen F, Moller S. Lactate metabolism in chronic liver disease. Scand J Clin Lab Invest. 2013;73:293–9.
136. Casaburi R, Oi S. Effect of liver disease on the kinetics of lactate removal after heavy exercise. Eur J Appl Physiol Occup Physiol. 1989;59:89–97.
137. Robin ED. Special report: dysoxia. Abnormal tissue oxygen utilization. Arch Intern Med. 1977;137:905–10.
138. Brownlee EB. The novelty of research--challenging the post-basic student. SA Nurs J. 1977;44:21.

Chapter 5
Prognostic Implications of Physical Frailty and Sarcopenia Pre and Post Transplantation

Stefan Buettner, Jan N. M. IJzermans, and Jeroen L. A. van Vugt

Introduction

In the past 60 years, liver transplantation has become increasingly routine for an increasing number of indications [1]. The main indication in the non-acute setting remains cirrhosis caused by alcoholic liver disease [1]. However, every year a larger proportion of patients develop cirrhosis due to metabolic factors other than alcohol consumption, as a consequence of nonalcoholic steatohepatitis (NASH) [2, 3]. The median age at which this condition develops is usually higher than for classical alcohol or viral hepatitis-induced cirrhosis [4]. Causes for NASH include health disorders such as type II diabetes mellitus, metabolic syndrome, cardiovascular diseases, and renal function impairment [3]. Many of these risk factors are also involved in the causal chain leading to frailty and sarcopenia. Concepts such as "inflammaging" have recently been introduced to describe the conditions in which these diseases of the elderly occur, mostly observing higher levels of pro-inflammatory markers in blood and other tissues [5].

The development of frailty and sarcopenia has many shared risk factors with the occurrence of cirrhosis. Diabetes mellitus and metabolic syndrome are long-known causes for sarcopenia and frailty. Sequelae of diabetes, combined with other factors such as cardiovascular disease, have been shown to explain up to 46% of the variance in muscle quality [6]. Diabetes mellitus and metabolic syndrome are also the main risk factors for developing nonalcoholic liver disease and correlate with the risk and degree of progression of liver disease [7].

Different definitions of frailty and sarcopenia exist and are in use in current literature [8, 9]. Whereas frailty is, by definition, observed in elderly patients, secondary sarcopenia may also be observed in younger patients with chronic diseases such

S. Buettner · J. N. M. IJzermans · J. L. A. van Vugt (✉)
Department of Surgery, Erasmus MC University Medical Center, Rotterdam, The Netherlands
e-mail: s.buttner@erasmusmc.nl; j.ijzermans@erasmusmc.nl; j.l.a.vanvugt@erasmusmc.nl

© Springer Nature Switzerland AG 2020
P. Tandon, A. J. Montano-Loza (eds.), *Frailty and Sarcopenia in Cirrhosis*,
https://doi.org/10.1007/978-3-030-26226-6_5

as cirrhosis [10]. Most criteria defining frailty and sarcopenia are inherent to cirrhosis.

The leading model for defining frailty is the phenotype model, revolving around five factors: weight loss, exhaustion, low activity, slowness, and weakness [11]. The liver has a central position in many metabolism functions [12]. Therefore, loss of liver function directly results in weight loss, only partially compensated by ascites [12, 13]. The loss of nutrient uptake, combined with chronic inflammation processes, has a large toll on patient condition and usually results in exhaustion and dependency in activities of daily living [14, 15].

As previously mentioned, sarcopenia is a condition also observed in younger patients, and its definitions are focused on skeletal muscle mass and function [10]. A causal link between chronic liver disease and sarcopenia has been suggested in murine models [16]. The pathways involved in developing sarcopenia have partially been elucidated and include an upregulation of the ubiquitin-proteasome system and oxidative stress [17, 18]. In clinical studies, NASH and the severity of cirrhosis objectified by the MELD (Model for End-Stage Liver Disease) score were observed to be correlated with sarcopenic obesity, while alcoholic liver disease was associated with sarcopenia [19]. There are indications that sarcopenia, in turn, aggravates insulin resistance and dysglycemia, thus increasing the chance of developing NASH and NASH-induced cirrhosis [20].

While frailty and sarcopenia are linked syndromes, their prevalence and effect on disease course may differ across different etiologies of cirrhosis [21]. In an analysis comparing alcoholic liver disease with NASH, frailty was more prevalent in NASH patients, while sarcopenia was observed more frequently in alcoholic liver disease [21]. The results also suggested that frailty had a larger impact in NASH patients, while sarcopenia was more prognostic in alcoholic liver disease patients [21].

Frailty, Sarcopenia, and Prognosis in Cirrhosis

During the last decade, numerous studies reported the impact of sarcopenia and frailty in liver transplant candidates [8]. However, there is a great variability in the metrics used to define the two syndromes. For frailty, several definitions have been assessed in patients with cirrhosis in recent studies [22]. The self-reported Fried Frailty Criteria, consisting of gait speed, exhaustion, physical activity, unintentional weight loss, and weakness, was prospectively validated for patients with cirrhosis [23]. In the clinical frailty score, patients are categorized by their physician [24]. Finally, the short physical performance battery consists of a series of short physical exercises, while the 6-minute walk test is a measure of maximum walking distance within 6 minutes [25, 26]. While there seems to be consensus that frailty is an important prognostic factor in cirrhosis patients, a definitive method for diagnosing frailty is still unavailable [22].

As described in a recent review, the exact utilized definitions of sarcopenia also greatly differ across studies [9]. Determining muscle wasting solely based on imaging has been popular because it allows researchers to include patients retrospectively.

Metrics such as walking distance and grip strength, though part of most sarcopenia definitions, have in general been neglected. This simpler definition of sarcopenia is often qualified as low skeletal muscle mass [9]. For determining sarcopenia on imaging, several methods enjoy popularity. There is a general distinction between single muscle measurement, as an indicator of general muscle status, and cross-sectional measurement of muscle area on a certain anatomical level [27]. When the choice of which muscles to measure has been made, different cutoffs are commonly used to define low skeletal muscle mass. Methods vary from the lower percentiles of the included cohort to pre-defined criteria. Nevertheless, it remains to be seen which parameter of sarcopenia, skeletal muscle mass or function, has the best predictive value [28].

Many research groups focus on different CT-based measurements. Psoas muscle measurement strategies have consistently proven their correlation with outcomes in cirrhosis patients, mostly advocating the simplicity of measuring a single muscle [9, 16, 27]. Nonetheless, in recent years, a movement toward the use of the cross-sectional muscle area at the level of the 3rd lumbar (L3) vertebra has been observed, because of its demonstrated correlation with whole body muscle mass as calculated by the golden standard dual-energy X-ray absorptiometry (DXA) [29, 30]. Often the cross-sectional muscle area at the level of L3 is normalized for the patient's squared height and called skeletal muscle index (SMI) [9, 29, 31]. The correlation between SMI and single muscle measurements appears to be disappointing in general. Moreover, expert groups consider no single muscle representative of the whole body muscle mass [27, 32, 33]. For example, data from a recent Korean study demonstrates a poor correlation between psoas muscle thickness/height and SMI, with a Pearson's r of 0.5 [16]. The discrepancy between single muscle measurements and SMI is further illustrated by a study specifically focusing on the value of PMI and SMI for predicting mortality in 353 cirrhosis patients [34]. Up to 66% of patients with low skeletal muscle mass might be misclassified using psoas muscle only [34]. A recent study further examined the components of the SMI and concluded that the paraspinal muscles, rather than the abdominal wall muscles, may be correlated with complications and death in cirrhosis patients [35]. Although these results will have to be validated in other cohorts, it proves that a definitive method to estimate muscle wasting, short of automatically measuring whole body muscle mass, is yet to be determined.

Although SMI is the most accepted measurement method among experts, no such consensus exists on the exact definition of low skeletal muscle mass [36]. One of the defining symptoms of cirrhosis is ascites, making weight- or BMI-based cutoffs that are sometimes used in cancer patients less obvious solutions [37, 38]. Sex-specific cutoffs for use specifically in patient on the transplant waitlist for end-stage liver disease have been proposed by Carey and colleagues [36]. These are <50 cm^2/m^2 for men and <39 cm^2/m^2 for women, irrespective of weight or body mass, and have been validated with mixed results [38, 39]. Interestingly, in an analysis of Dutch waitlist patients, we found that the BMI-based sex-specific cutoffs as defined by Martin were more predictive of waitlist mortality, than the Carey cutoffs [38]. Finding an ideal definition of low skeletal muscle mass and sarcopenia remains challenging, due to large differences in population with regard to both body composition and disease characteristics, in particular between Western and Eastern patients [39].

Factors in the causal pathway leading to sarcopenia and frailty have also been associated with poor waitlist outcomes. For example, a recent study described the association between low testosterone levels and sarcopenia in cirrhotic patients [40]. Corrected for a number of confounders, including sex, BMI, MELD score, and reason of cirrhosis, testosterone level proved the most important predictor of sarcopenia [40]. Apart from its predictive value, associations such as these might inform preventive treatment with testosterone to improve outcomes in patients with cirrhosis [40].

The Impact of Frailty and Sarcopenia on Waitlist Outcomes for Liver Transplantation

Drawbacks of the MELD Score

Currently, in the Netherlands and other Eurotransplant countries, the MELD score is employed to prioritize patients for liver transplantation [41]. Although the MELD score strongly predicts waitlist mortality, it inaccurately predicts survival in 15 to 20% of patients due to underestimation of disease severity [42]. One of the frequently mentioned drawbacks of the MELD score is the lack of objective parameters reflecting physical and nutritional status of patients. This led to the development of, for example, the MELDNa and five-variable MELD scores, incorporating sodium and albumin levels, respectively [43–45].

Frailty as Prognostic Factor Independent of the MELD Score

Since robust measurements of frailty and sarcopenia have been developed last decade, interest in these measures as prognostic markers in liver transplant candidates increased concomitantly. Consequently, a wide range of frailty measures has been investigated in liver transplant candidates. The earlier mentioned Fried Frailty Instrument, ranging from 0 to 5 points, was developed to identify vulnerable elders at risk for death, long-term institutionalization, and post surgical complications [46]. Using a cutoff of 3 for the Fried Frailty Instrument, 17% of outpatients listed for liver transplantation (MELD score ≥12) were considered frail. Frail patients had a higher MELD score and significantly higher rates of mild/moderate ascites and moderate hepatic encephalopathy. Waitlist mortality was significantly higher in frail patients (22% versus 10%, $p = 0.03$), and a 1-unit increase in the Fried Frailty scale was associated with 50% waitlist mortality risk, independent of MELD score [23].

Furthermore, hospitalization during waitlist was significantly higher in these patients [47]. Within the same study, other measures of frailty were also assessed. Thirty-one percent of the patients scored low on the short physical performance battery (SPPB), a combination of repeated chair stands, balance testing, and a 13 foot walk [48], 24% had difficulty with at least one activity of daily living (ADL; self-reported daily self-care activities [49]), and 43% scored positive on the instrumental activities of daily living (IADL; self-reported activities that allow an individual to live independently [50]). Patients who died on the waitlist or were delisted had higher rates of frailty, showed higher inactivity rates and higher functional impairment rates, as assessed with the SPPB. The SPPB was independently associated with waitlist mortality with an HR of 1.20, whereas ADL and IADL were not [23].

Although clinical assessment (the "eyeball" test) is subjective and differs per physician, one can accurately predict patients at increased risk for waitlist mortality independent of MELD score [51]. However, a recent study showed that addition of the Liver Frailty Index (LFI) significantly improved the ability to predict waitlist mortality with a reclassification of 34% [52]. Nevertheless, it should be mentioned that a gap exists between clinically assessed physical performance and objective physical activity in liver transplant candidates, a population known for low activity levels [53].

Sarcopenia as Prognostic Factor Independent of the MELD Score

Hitherto, only one meta-analysis pooling the data on the association between sarcopenia and waitlist mortality has been performed. It showed a pooled HR of 1.72 (95% CI 0.99–3.00, $p = 0.050$) with low heterogeneity ($I^2 = 33\%$). However, the evidence is limited as only few studies could be pooled due to the great variety in methodology to measure skeletal muscle mass. Furthermore, data of three out of the four studies that could be pooled originated from one center, and only one of these three studies was included in the meta-analysis [9]. A correlation between sarcopenia and hepatic encephalopathy in particular was also described in a meta-analysis of 1795 patients, observing an odds ratio of 2.38 [54].

In a recent study by Idriss and colleagues, the effect of previous bariatric surgery in cirrhotic patients listed for liver transplantation was investigated [55]. Seventy-eight patients who previously had undergone bariatric surgery were compared with a cohort of 156 patients matched by age, MELD score, and underlying liver disease. Almost 1 in every 2 patients (47.4%) had NASH, which was found to lead to a six-fold increased risk of having sarcopenic obesity in an earlier mentioned cohort of 207 American patients listed for liver transplantation [19]. Notably, BMI was comparable between both the bariatric surgery and non-bariatric surgery groups. The rate of delisting or death was significantly higher among patients who had undergone bariatric surgery compared with patients who did not (33.3% versus 10.1%,

$p = 0.002$), and the transplantation rate was significantly lower (48.9% versus 65.2%, $p = 0.03$). Previous bariatric surgery was independently associated with an increased risk of waitlist death (HR 5.7), which was, however, attenuated by malnutrition. Interestingly, skeletal muscle index (measured on CT) was associated with malnutrition. Furthermore, the skeletal muscle area was significantly lower in the bariatric surgery group, and the prevalence of sarcopenia was significantly higher among delisted patients. Consequently, strict selection in liver transplant patients who previously have undergone bariatric surgery should be opted for.

Incorporating Sarcopenia and Frailty Measures into the MELD Score

Taking into account the results described in the previous paragraph, frail and sarcopenic patients are exposed to an increased risk of waitlist mortality. Indeed, patients with muscle atrophy, which is highly correlated with frailty, malnutrition, and physical impairment, may be underprioritized using the current allocation system [56]. This led to the development of different scores that incorporated skeletal muscle mass into the MELD score. As this subject will be elaborated further in Chap. 13, here we will only mention it briefly.

First, Durand and colleagues developed the MELD-psoas score, using axial and transversal psoas thickness measurements on CT. The discrimination of the MELD-psoas score was superior to that of the MELD score alone, particularly in patients with a low MELD score (i.e., ≤ 25) [56]. In another study, cross-sectional skeletal muscle mass measurements on CT were used to develop the MELD-sarcopenia score with sarcopenia as a dichotomous variable. Prediction of waitlist mortality significantly improved after this modification of the MELD score [57]. This study was externally validated by our group in a cohort of 585 patients listed for transplantation. The results showed that the discriminative performance of the MELD-sarcopenia score (c-index 0.82) for 3-month mortality was lower than for the MELD score alone (c-index 0.84). However, inclusion of sarcopenia in a model together with MELD score, age, and presence of hepatic encephalopathy improved its discriminative performance to a c-index of 0.85. The independent additive predictive effect of sarcopenia was particularly present in patients with low MELD scores (i.e., ≤ 15) again [38]. In conclusion, sarcopenia may be a valuable addition to the MELD score to identify patients with an increased mortality risk that otherwise would be missed.

As mentioned above, factors in the causal pathway of sarcopenia development may also be used to enhance prognostic models. A recent study showed that both sarcopenia and low plasma testosterone levels are associated with waitlist mortality in male cirrhotic patients [58] and testosterone supplementation in these patients showed promising results [59]. The predictive value of low testosterone levels may be stronger than sarcopenia and may be a proper alternative to add to the MELD score [58]. Future studies should determine which factors could be added to improve the predictive value of the MELD score.

Following the study of Lai and colleagues showing the association between frailty and mortality in cirrhotic transplant candidates [23], a frailty index for patients with cirrhosis in particular was developed, since measures such as the Fried Frailty Instrument and SPPB were originally developed in community-dwelling elderly without (liver) disease. In 536 patients with cirrhosis with a median MELDNa score of 18 listed for transplantation, performance-based (gait speed, handgrip strength, chair stands, balance) and self-reported measures (unintentional weight loss, exhaustion, physical activity, activities of daily living, instrumental activities of daily living) were performed. Using a subset Cox regression analysis to select measures with the best predictive value, grip strength, chair stands, and balance were selected to form the Liver Frailty Index (LFI). The c-index to predict 3-month waitlist mortality was 0.80 for the MELDNa score and increased to 0.82 when MELDNa was combined with the newly developed LFI. Using the combination of MELDNa and the LFI, 16% of deaths/delistings were correctly reclassified, resulting in a net reclassification index of 19% [60]. Adjusted for disease severity and baseline physical status, physical function significantly declines during the waitlist period in cirrhotic patients. This functional decline, which has also been correlated with a decrease in skeletal muscle mass [61], is an independent predictor for waitlist mortality [62].

The Economic Burden of Frailty and Sarcopenia in Liver Transplant Candidates

The association of frailty and sarcopenia with waitlist mortality is reflected by a significantly higher number of complications requiring hospitalization. Frailty, as measured by gait speed, was an independent risk factor for hospitalization, and a 0.1 m/s gait speed decrease was associated with 22% more hospital days in an American study of Dunn and colleagues. Similar, but non-significant, results were found for handgrip strength. Moreover, an incremental increase in gait speed was associated with a lower number of hospital days and hospital costs during the listing period: 6.2 days ($24,800/year) in patients with a gait speed of 1 m/s, 21.2 days ($84,800/year) in patients with a gait speed of 0.5 m/s, and 40.2 days ($160,800/year) in patients with a gait speed of 0.25 m/s [25]. In a European study investigating the association between low skeletal muscle mass (CT-assessed skeletal muscle index), similar results were found: median total hospital costs in patients with sarcopenia were €11,294 (IQR 3,570–46,469) compared with €6,878 (IQR 1,305–20,683) in patients without sarcopenia ($p < 0.001$). An incremental increase in skeletal muscle index was independently associated with a decrease in total hospital expenditure (€455 per incremental SMI, 95% CI 11–900, $p = 0.045$) [63]. Interestingly, both studies were performed in tertiary centers and might therefore underestimate the real costs as patients may have been admitted to the referring hospitals without notice.

The Impact of Frailty and Sarcopenia on Outcomes After Liver Transplantation

Efforts have been made to define the impact of sarcopenia and frailty on post-transplantation disease course, which have led to different conclusions. In the post-operative disease course, there are indications that low SMI and psoas muscle area/index are associated with postoperative complications, most commonly bacterial infection, and longer hospital stay [31, 64–67]. One larger American study examining 1-year postoperative complications found that patients with lower psoas muscle area were 1.4 times more likely to experience a complication and 2.8 times more likely to experience failure to rescue, mortality due to a severe complication [66]. A study specifically examining the subject found a fourfold increased chance of severe infection [65]. Frailty as defined by the Karnofsky score was highly associated with postoperative mortality in an American nationwide survey [68]. Interestingly, infection (15.7%), together with cardiovascular factors (25.4%), technical factors (17.9%), and graft failure (16.7%), presented one of the most reported causes of death [68]. Patients with either a frailty or a sarcopenia syndrome might have a higher chance of bacterial infections, sepsis, and multiple organ failure due to links between these syndromes and impaired immunity [69, 70]. The effect of frailty and sarcopenia on graft failure has, to our knowledge, not been reported in current literature.

The MELD-psoas and the MELD-sarcopenia scores that were developed to predict waitlist mortality have not been validated to predict post transplant survival [56, 57]. As the MELD score was developed to predict waitlist mortality rather than post-transplant mortality [42], the development of different predictive tools for post-transplant mortality is required. Primarily the role of sarcopenia has been examined as a postoperative risk factor in a number of retrospective studies. Sarcopenia was not associated with postoperative long-term survival in two studies measuring SMI and one study measuring psoas muscle area [19, 31, 67]. Contrastingly, psoas muscle area as a continuous variable proved most predictive of postoperative survival in a model correcting for other known risk factors (HR per mm^2: 0.27; $p < 0.001$) [71]. This correlation between psoas muscle area and survival was also observed in later studies [64, 72].

Most studies examining postoperative disease course used preoperative measurements as a prognosticator. As a consequence, little is known of the impact of post-transplant developments in both sarcopenia and frailty status. A longitudinal study indicated that frailty worsens initially post-transplant and that pretransplant frailty, as defined by the Liver Frailty Index, predicts postoperative frailty [73]. The same was true for sarcopenia, defined by SMI [19, 31]. There are reports of some patients that developed postoperative sarcopenia, which was correlated with impaired long-term survival in retrospective studies [74–76].

A drawback caused by the retrospective nature of most included studies examining posttransplantation survival is that only patients fit for transplant were included. Because of this selection bias, the role of frailty and sarcopenia on postoperative outcomes may have been underestimated [77]. Although it seems unlikely that many patients have been excluded based on muscle mass only, the features associated with the frailty phenotype may have had an influence on treatment choices [78].

The Economic Burden of Frailty and Sarcopenia in Transplanted Patients

Although costs in patients with sarcopenia and frailty are shown to be higher in patients awaiting transplantation [25, 63], no studies have been performed in patients actually undergoing transplantation. An exploratory analysis was performed, but no significant differences could be demonstrated in our Dutch study, probably due to its inappropriate design for this purpose [63]. Nevertheless, sarcopenia and frailty are strongly associated with post transplant complications, and results may therefore be extrapolated to the post-transplant situation. After all, increased hospital expenditure in patients with sarcopenia has previously been described in various surgical cohorts [79, 80].

Frailty, Sarcopenia, Depression, and Quality of Life

Besides physical complications and mortality, frailty is also associated with mental impairment. The reported prevalence of depression in 500 end-stage liver disease patients screened for transplantation was 39.4%. Frail patients, as assessed with the Fried Frailty Index, were more likely to experience depression (54% versus 29%, $p < 0.001$). A proportional increase in depression symptoms was observed with the severity of frailty; most-frail patients were 3.6 times more likely to experience depression compared with least-frail patients. In this study, frailty and depression were strongly correlated, whereas disease severity was not [81]. Another study among 213 patients listed for liver transplantation showed a significant association between the 6-minute walk distance and health-related qualify of life, assessed by short form 36 (SF-36) questionnaires, whereas this association was not found for sarcopenia [28]. These results warrant awareness for depression and quality of life in the consulting room of the transplant physician. Lastly, in a study including 305 cirrhotic outpatients from Canada, a depression prevalence of 18% was found using the Mini-International Neuropsychiatric Interview (MINI). In these patients, lower baseline health-related quality of life and higher frailty scores were observed [82].

Living-Donor Liver Transplantation

Sarcopenia and Frailty in Living-Donor Liver Transplantation

Living-donor liver transplantation (LDLT) was first described in 1987 by Raia and colleagues [83]. Although the procedure was successful (a mother donated part of her liver to her son), the recipient died shortly after the transplant [83]. The first successful transplantation from mother to son was performed by the Australian surgeon Strong [84]. After refinement of the technique, waitlist-related mortality in children greatly decreased [85, 86]. Nevertheless, when possible deceased donor transplantation remains the option of first choice [85]. After all, potential complications in the healthy donors may be avoided [87, 88]. The first adult-to-adult LDLT was performed in Hong Kong in 1997 [89]. Since, LDLT led to a strong increase in available donor organs. Hence, LDLT is particularly performed in Asia nowadays, where a great shortage in organ donors remains.

During the last few years, multiple studies investigated the impact of sarcopenia in patients undergoing LDLT, which were indeed all performed in Asia [90–98]. Although methodology greatly differs between studies, outcomes were highly comparable showing associations between sarcopenia and post transplant complications and mortality. In the one systematic review and meta-analysis regarding the effect of low skeletal muscle mass in liver transplant patients that has been published [9], a HR of 2.78 (95% CI 1.59–4.85, $p = 0.0003$) with a Z of 3.60, and I^2 of 24%, was shown after pooling data of two studies among LDLT patients using the psoas muscle index to quantify skeletal muscle mass [90, 91].

Modification of the MELD Score for LDLT

Comparable with the MELD-sarcopenia score for patients awaiting orthotopic liver transplantation [38, 57], Hamaguchi and colleagues developed a score to predict overall survival after LDLT called the Muscle-MELD score (i.e., post-transplant) [92]. Using Cox regression analysis, the Muscle-MELD score was created using MELD score, myosteatosis [low intramuscular adipose tissue content (IMAC)] and low skeletal muscle mass [low psoas muscle index (PMI)], which were measured on CT images. Low IMAC and low PMI were calculated using receiver operating characteristics (ROC) curves, and the Muscle-MELD score was calculated as follows: MELD score + 27.0 ∗ low IMAC +25.2 ∗ low PMI. Low Muscle-MELD was also defined using ROC curves. The overall survival was significantly higher in patients with high Muscle-MELD compared with patients with low Muscle-MELD. Muscle-MELD more accurately predicted post transplant survival than MELD score alone at 3, 6, and 12 months after transplantation. The independent odds ratio for mortality at 6 months after transplantation was 6.7 (95% CI 3.3–14.7, $p < 0.001$) for the Muscle-MELD score.

Sarcopenia and Nutrition in LDLT

In a study using bioelectrical impedance analysis (BIA) to measure muscle mass, 21 of 47 patients with sarcopenia and 42 of 77 patients without sarcopenia received perioperative nutritional therapy [98]. Nutritional therapy was started 2 weeks before LDLT and after BIA. It consisted of a nutrient mixture enriched with branched-chain amino acids (BCAAs) or BCAA nutrients as a late evening snack, glutamine-enriched supplementation products, dietary fiber and oligosaccharide three times daily, a lactic fermented beverage containing a *Lactobacillus casei* strain once a day, and zinc supplementation in patients with low serum zinc levels. Postoperatively, enteral nutrition was started within the first 24 hours via tube jejunostomy with a gradually increasing caloric intake until postoperative day 3 aimed at maximization of caloric intake on day 5. Oral nutrition was started after recovery of swallowing ability, usually around day 5. Within the group of patients with low skeletal muscle mass, patients in the perioperative nutritional therapy group showed a significantly better overall survival compared with those who did not. Both groups had comparable preoperative Child-Pugh and MELD scores. Notably, patients with normal/high skeletal muscle mass did not benefit from perioperative nutrition therapy in terms of overall survival. Preoperative low skeletal muscle mass, as well as perioperative nutritional therapy, was found to be an independent risk factor for mortality after transplantation. The main cause of death was sepsis: 9/20 in patients with sarcopenia and 4/11 patients without sarcopenia.

A pilot study investigated the relationship between plasma amino acid levels, post transplant sepsis, and sarcopenia (based on psoas muscle measurements) in patients undergoing LDLT [97]. Indeed, leucine, isoleucine, and glutamine were significantly lower in patients with sarcopenia compared with patients without sarcopenia. Lower plasma glutamine levels were an independent risk factor for post transplant sepsis (OR 5.4, $p = 0.002$). Plasma glutamine levels were significantly lower after LDLT compared with before LDLT in patients with sepsis, whereas levels were comparable in patients without sepsis. In both groups without early nutrition, plasma glutamine levels were significantly decreased after LDLT compared with before LDLT. However, when stratified for sarcopenia, plasma glutamine levels were significantly decreased after LDLT independently of early nutrition in the sarcopenia group, whereas no significant decrease was observed in non-sarcopenic patients with early nutrition. Hence, early postoperative nutrition and supplementation of glutamine may prevent post transplant sepsis and mortality. Further research is therefore warranted.

Sarcopenia and Frailty in Pediatric Liver Transplantation

As such the MELD score lacks objective parameters reflecting patients' physical and nutritional status (i.e., comorbidity and frailty) in adults, so does the Pediatric End-Stage Liver Disease (PELD) score in children. Recently, a study was performed using the five Fried Frailty Criteria (weakness, slowness, shrinkage, exhaustion, and diminished physical activity) [46] in children with compensated chronic liver disease (CCLD) and end-stage liver disease (ESLD) and listed for liver transplantation [99]. The test scores were adjusted for age and sex with a maximum score of 10. It showed that the median frailty score was significantly higher in children with ESLD compared with CCLD (median 5 (IQR 4–7) versus 3 (IQR 2–4), $p < 0.001$). The area under the curve for the frailty score to differentiate between ESLD and CCLD was 0.83 (95% CI 0.73–0.93), which was similar to the PELD and MELDNa scores. In total, 46% of children with ESLD were considered frail using a cutoff of 5. The frailty scores did not correlate with physicians' clinical subjective assessments. Although it was not shown that frailty was predictive for worse outcome, this tool may be used in children to identify the most vulnerable.

Only one study investigating the impact of sarcopenia was performed in pediatric liver transplant recipients [100]. In this Canadian study, DXA was used to measure fat mass, fat-free mass, and skeletal muscle mass on various time points in 58 children aged 0.5–17 years. In total, 41% of the children developed sarcopenia after transplantation with a mean age of sarcopenia detection of 7.6 (SD 3.1) years and a mean time from transplantation of 1.2 (SD 1.9) years. Persistence of sarcopenia after transplantation was associated with poorer growth, recurrent hospitalization (total, intensive care unit, emergency, and readmission), and ventilator dependency, but not with graft rejection or corticosteroid therapy.

Liver Transplantation Beyond the Milan Criteria: Is There a Role for Frailty and Sarcopenia Assessment?

The Milan criteria were introduced to select patients with liver cirrhosis and hepatocellular carcinoma (HCC) eligible for liver transplantation in 1996 [101]. These criteria have universally been accepted since. The Milan criteria state that patients are selected for liver transplantation when there is a single lesion smaller than 5 centimeters or when there are up to three lesions smaller than 3 centimeters, without vascular invasion. Patients meeting the Milan criteria have a 5-year survival rate of at least 70% and recurrence incidence of only 10% [102, 103]. However, in recent years, it has been argued that the Milan criteria are too restrictive. Although most patients with HCC beyond the Milan criteria may experience disease recurrence after liver transplantation leading to decreased 5-year survival rates (53.6% versus 73.3%) [103], a number of patients may still benefit and reach 5-year survival rates that are comparable with recipients fulfilling the Milan criteria. The latest proposal to select eligible patients is known as the up-to-seven rule: the sum of the number of nodule(s) and the maximum diameter of the nodule(s) must not exceed the value of seven which resulted in a 5-year overall survival of 70% inpatients transplanted beyond the Milan criteria [103]. Skeletal muscle mass and frailty may be biomarkers to identify patients with HCC who may or may not benefit from liver transplantation beyond the Milan criteria. Indeed, a recent study among 92 patients undergoing LDLT identified sarcopenia (i.e., height-normalized psoas muscle thickness <15.5 mm/m at the level of L3) as a risk factor for tumor recurrence after transplantation using a competing risk analysis (HR 9.5, 95%CI 1.2–76.3, $p = 0.034$) [104]. Since this was the only study of its kind, its results should be validated.

Interventions

Pretransplant

Prehabilitation in surgical populations increasingly gained interest and priority during recent years [105]. The waitlist period offers a window of opportunity to improve functional status and skeletal muscle mass. The differences in costs between patients with and without frailty and/or sarcopenia justify efforts and the use of resources to seek for therapies and strategies to halt or reverse the processes that make these patients spiraling down a vicious circle [25, 63]. Besides infection control, ascites control, and protection of renal function in liver transplant candidates [106], strategies aimed to reduce sarcopenia and frailty should be multidimensional and, at least, be a combination of nutrition, exercise, and ammonia-lowering therapies with or without novel pharmacological therapy [107]. These will be briefly mentioned here and further elaborated in Chaps. 7 and 8.

Nutrition

Impaired protein synthesis due to hyperammonemia, increased cytokine production and hyperinflammatory state, hormonal abnormalities, direct effects of ethanol, impaired skeletal muscle signaling pathways, and possible splanchnic vasodilatation leading to a hyperdynamic circulation all contribute to the catabolic state of cirrhotic patients [108, 109]. Hence, nutritional supplementation is recommended and ideally guided by indirect calorimetric energy expenditure measurements [110]. However, enteral intake may be hindered by early satiety due to ascites, taste distortions due to zinc deficiency, and encephalopathy. Therefore, nasogastric feeding may be needed to achieve caloric goals [110]. Although evidence is scarce (well-designed clinical trials are lacking) and understanding of the mechanisms involved is poor, some evidence supports the effectiveness of late evening snacks, BCAA supplementation, and high-protein/high-calorie diets [111, 112]. Future studies regarding the effect of nutrition on body composition, physical status, and frailty in cirrhotic patients are highly warranted because current evidence is predominantly of preclinical and experimental [109].

Exercise

Because frailty and sarcopenia are the result of, among others, inactivity and because physical strength, endurance, and balance are significantly associated with frailty [113], exercise interventions obviously may improve physical status, skeletal muscle mass, and frailty. It is recommended to combine exercise with tailored nutritional interventions [114]. Last decade, multiple trials investigating exercise interventions in patients with cirrhosis showed positive results. However, as described by Dunn, "the most formidable challenge to arrest frailty and sarcopenia may be the reluctance of transplant candidates and their caregivers to add another demand, especially exercise, to an already-difficult care regimen" [107].

Pharmacological

Hyperammonemia, leading to impaired skeletal muscle protein synthesis and protein breakdown, plays a key role in skeletal muscle wasting [115]. In experimental animal studies, lowering ammonia by l-ornithine l-aspartate and rifaximin orally for 4 weeks significantly improved lean body mass and grip strength [116]. However, the effect on survival is not known yet and human studies are lacking. Another promising pharmacological intervention to halt cancer cachexia-associated skeletal muscle wasting, which has many overlap with skeletal muscle wasting in cirrhosis, is the inhibition of myostatin by blocking the ActRIIB pathway [117]. However, trials in humans, particularly in those with cirrhosis, are highly warranted. In males with low testosterone levels, testosterone supplementation significantly increases skeletal muscle mass [59]. The effect on survival and complications remains to be investigated.

Cognitive

Since frailty and sarcopenia are associated with depression and decreased quality of life in cirrhotic patients, it seems obvious that these patients may benefit from cognitive and psychological support. Currently, no trials have been performed in liver transplant candidates.

Post transplant

The evidence of post-transplant sarcopenia and its influence on disease outcome remains unknown since studies are heterogeneous with conflicting results [75]. Although some studies showed that skeletal muscle wasting is arrested and frequently improved by liver transplantation, particularly in those with lowest skeletal muscle mass [118], other studies showed that sarcopenia did not restore after transplantation [19]. In a prospective post transplant follow-up of 53 patients (median follow-up time 19.3 months), new-onset post transplant sarcopenia developed in 14 patients (26%). Post transplant skeletal muscle loss was a risk factor for new-onset diabetes mellitus, and a trend towards higher mortality was observed. No correlation with pretransplant characteristics was found [76]. Not only liver transplantation but also transjugular intrahepatic portosystemic shunt (TIPS) creation may lead to skeletal muscle gain with consequent decreased mortality [119].

The previously mentioned study of Lai and colleagues found that the LFI was worse 3 months after transplantation, was comparable at 6 months, and improved 12 months after transplantation compared with pretransplant levels. Pretransplant frailty (i.e., LFI ≤3) was an independent predictor of post transplant robustness (i.e., LFI ≥4.5). Less than 40% of patients, however, reached robustness post transplant [73].

In a study among LDLT patients, skeletal muscle mass worsened after transplantation and did not reach pretransplant levels until 1 year after transplantation. However, grip strength returned to pretransplant levels 6 months after transplantation [95]. Another study showed that trunk muscle mass was successfully restored after LDLT, particularly in patients with lowest skeletal muscle mass [96]. These findings leave room for rehabilitation programs in patients undergoing liver transplantation, and future studies should elucidate its effectiveness.

Ethical Considerations

Due to the general scarcity of liver donors and an increasing number of cirrhosis patients, the ethical aspects of transplantation allocation need to be considered [120]. This is illustrated by the Eurotransplant 2017 report, detailing 2,548 patients on the waitlist in 2017, with 1,674 patients transplanted [121]. Currently, there is no consistent agreement in Western Europe whether the sickest patients or the patients with the most possible health benefit need to be prioritized [120]. Dutch law prescribes a combination of prospect of success and urgency and, only if these factors do not sufficiently differentiate, waiting time period [122]. The principles of urgency and prospect of success are often contradictory, as discussed earlier in this chapter, and this prioritization leaves room for interpretation. The practical approach to these issues is that a combination of waitlist time and MELD score are utilized [41].

The discussion also focuses on the rather high standards patients have to meet in order to be eligible for transplant [120]. In the Netherlands, patients have to be younger than 70 years and cannot have extrahepatic malignancies or multi-organ failure. In addition, the Milan criteria are often applied for transplantation in patients with HCC [101]. The ethical implications of these rather simplistic rules are heavily debated [120]. The case can be made that by focusing on long-term prognosis for inclusion in individual patients, the law, which prescribes the prospect of success and urgency compared to others, is disregarded [120].

The pertinent question in this chapter is whether sarcopenia and frailty metrics need to be entered into the decisions pertaining to organ allocation and eligibility for waitlist placement. In order for the inclusion to be ethical, a number of requirements will have to be met, the most important being discrimination and calibration of the predictions based on sarcopenia and frailty and their applicability to the setting and population in which they are utilized [122]. While there are indications that sarcopenia and frailty impact both waitlist and posttransplantation outcomes, their exact implications are not yet adequately quantified. We therefore believe more, and in particular prospective, research will need to be conducted before these syndromes can be fully considered.

Future Perspectives

Patients with cirrhosis are a vulnerable population, with many risk factors barring successful treatment of their disease. Sarcopenia and physical frailty are two separate yet related syndromes commonly occurring in this patient population and adversely correlated with outcomes. While efforts have been made to quantify the impact of both syndromes, mostly with concordant results, a number of methodological issues and hiatuses in knowledge need to be resolved.

Future trials on prognostication in transplantation patients should be aimed at finding answers to important open questions. One of the objections to the current, primarily retrospectively gathered evidence is that it is unknown whether the impact of frailty and sarcopenia has already been included in the clinical decision-making [77]. Another caveat is that most effects of sarcopenia and frailty described in this chapter are based on association rather than causation. It remains unclear whether sarcopenia and frailty are epiphenomena present in patients in worse clinical condition or whether these syndromes are the cause of the inferior outcomes. This is important for choosing the nature of the intervention: to alleviate the muscle wasting and frailty symptoms or to treat underlying factors.

While mortality in cirrhosis patients appears to be highly correlated with sarcopenia and frailty, a standardized metric of frailty and sarcopenia is required in order to enhance selection of patients and enact interventions [123]. This can be achieved by critically and quantitatively reviewing the current body of evidence, followed by prospective validation efforts. Only then can frailty evaluation (or assessment) be employed to its full potential to improve care in transplantation patients [123, 124].

References

1. Neuberger J. An update on liver transplantation: a critical review. J Autoimmun. 2016;66:51–9.
2. van den Berg EH, Amini M, Schreuder TCMA, Dullaart RPF, Faber KN, Alizadeh BZ, et al. Prevalence and determinants of non-alcoholic fatty liver disease in lifelines: a large Dutch population cohort. PLoS One. 2017;12:e0171502.
3. Younossi ZM, Koenig AB, Abdelatif D, Fazel Y, Henry L, Wymer M. Global epidemiology of nonalcoholic fatty liver disease-meta-analytic assessment of prevalence, incidence, and outcomes. Hepatology. 2016;64:73–84.

4. Sajja KC, Mohan DP, Rockey DC. Age and ethnicity in cirrhosis. J Investigative Med. 2014;62:920–6.
5. Ferrucci L, Fabbri E. Inflammageing: chronic inflammation in ageing, cardiovascular disease, and frailty. Nat Rev Cardiol. 2018;15:505–22.
6. Fukuda T, Bouchi R, Takeuchi T, Nakano Y, Murakami M, Minami I, et al. Association of diabetic retinopathy with both sarcopenia and muscle quality in patients with type 2 diabetes: a cross-sectional study. BMJ Open Diabetes Research & Amp Care. 2017:5.
7. Marchesini G, Marzocchi R. Metabolic syndrome and NASH. Clin Liver Dis. 2007;11:105–17.
8. Cederholm T. Overlaps between frailty and sarcopenia definitions. Nestle Nutr Inst Workshop Ser. 2015;83:65–9.
9. van Vugt JL, Levolger S, de Bruin RW, van Rosmalen J, Metselaar HJ, JN IJ. Systematic review and meta-analysis of the impact of computed tomography-assessed skeletal muscle mass on outcome in patients awaiting or undergoing liver transplantation. Am J Transplant. 2016;16:2277–92.
10. Cruz-Jentoft AJ, Baeyens JP, Bauer JM, Boirie Y, Cederholm T, Landi F, et al. Sarcopenia: European consensus on definition and diagnosis: report of the European working group on sarcopenia in older people. Age Ageing. 2010;39:412–23.
11. Fried LP, Tangen CM, Walston J, Newman AB, Hirsch C, Gottdiener J, et al. Frailty in older adults: evidence for a phenotype. J Gerontol A Biol Sci Med Sci. 2001;56:M146–56.
12. Kalaitzakis E, Simrén M, Olsson R, Henfridsson P, Hugosson I, Bengtsson M, et al. Gastrointestinal symptoms in patients with liver cirrhosis: associations with nutritional status and health-related quality of life. Scand J Gastroenterol. 2006;41:1464–72.
13. Pedersen JS, Bendtsen F, Møller S. Management of cirrhotic ascites. Ther Adv Chronic Dis. 2015;6:124–37.
14. Swain MG. Fatigue in liver disease: pathophysiology and clinical management. Can J Gastroenterol. 2006;20:181–8.
15. Kalaitzakis E, Josefsson A, Castedal M, Henfridsson P, Bengtsson M, Hugosson I, et al. Factors related to fatigue in patients with cirrhosis before and after liver transplantation. Clin Gastroenterol Hepatol. 2012;10:174–81.e1.
16. Campos F, Abrigo J, Aguirre F, Garces B, Arrese M, Karpen S, et al. Sarcopenia in a mice model of chronic liver disease: role of the ubiquitin-proteasome system and oxidative stress. Pflugers Arch. 2018;470:1503.
17. Philippe AB, Erin SC, Simon SW. The ubiquitin proteasome system in atrophying skeletal muscle: roles and regulation. Am J Phys Cell Phys. 2016;311:C392–403.
18. Scicchitano BM, Pelosi L, Sica G, Musarò A. The physiopathologic role of oxidative stress in skeletal muscle. Mech Ageing Dev. 2018;170:37–44.
19. Carias S, Castellanos AL, Vilchez V, Nair R, Dela Cruz AC, Watkins J, et al. Nonalcoholic steatohepatitis is strongly associated with sarcopenic obesity in patients with cirrhosis undergoing liver transplant evaluation. J Gastroenterol Hepatol. 2016;31:628–33.
20. Srikanthan P, Hevener AL, Karlamangla AS. Sarcopenia exacerbates obesity-associated insulin resistance and Dysglycemia: findings from the National Health and nutrition examination survey III. PLoS One. 2010;5:e10805.
21. Bhanji RA, Narayanan P, Moynagh MR, Takahashi N, Angirekula M, Kennedy CC, et al. Differing impact of sarcopenia and frailty in non-alcoholic steatohepatitis (NASH) and alcoholic liver disease (ALD). Liver Transpl. 2018.
22. Kok B, Tandon P. Frailty in patients with cirrhosis. Curr Treat Options Gastroenterol. 2018;16:215–25.
23. Lai JC, Feng S, Terrault NA, Lizaola B, Hayssen H, Covinsky K. Frailty predicts waitlist mortality in liver transplant candidates. Am J Transplant. 2014;14:1870–9.
24. Tandon P, Tangri N, Thomas L, Zenith L, Shaikh T, Carbonneau M, et al. A rapid bedside screen to predict unplanned hospitalization and death in outpatients with cirrhosis: a prospective evaluation of the clinical frailty scale. Am J Gastroenterol. 2016;111:1759–67.

25. Dunn MA, Josbeno DA, Tevar AD, Rachakonda V, Ganesh SR, Schmotzer AR, et al. Frailty as tested by gait speed is an independent risk factor for cirrhosis complications that require hospitalization. Am J Gastroenterol. 2016;111:1768–75.
26. Carey EJ, Steidley DE, Aqel BA, Byrne TJ, Mekeel KL, Rakela J, et al. Six-minute walk distance predicts mortality in liver transplant candidates. Liver Transpl. 2010;16:1373–8.
27. Baracos VE. Psoas as a sentinel muscle for sarcopenia: a flawed premise. J Cachexia Sarcopenia Muscle. 2017;8:527–8.
28. Yadav A, Chang YH, Carpenter S, Silva AC, Rakela J, Aqel BA, et al. Relationship between sarcopenia, six-minute walk distance and health-related quality of life in liver transplant candidates. Clin Transpl. 2015;29:134–41.
29. Mourtzakis M, Prado CM, Lieffers JR, Reiman T, McCargar LJ, Baracos VE. A practical and precise approach to quantification of body composition in cancer patients using computed tomography images acquired during routine care. Appl Physiol Nutr Metab. 2008;33:997–1006.
30. Holt DQ, Strauss BJ, Lau KK, Moore GT. Body composition analysis using abdominal scans from routine clinical care in patients with Crohn's disease. Scand J Gastroenterol. 2016;51:842–7.
31. Montano-Loza AJ, Meza-Junco J, Baracos VE, Prado CM, Ma M, Meeberg G, et al. Severe muscle depletion predicts postoperative length of stay but is not associated with survival after liver transplantation. Liver Transpl. 2014;20:640–8.
32. Cesari M, Fielding RA, Pahor M, Goodpaster B, Hellerstein M, van Kan GA, et al. Biomarkers of sarcopenia in clinical trials-recommendations from the international working group on sarcopenia. J Cachexia Sarcopenia Muscle. 2012;3:181–90.
33. Bahat G, Tufan A, Tufan F, Kilic C, Akpinar TS, Kose M, et al. Cut-off points to identify sarcopenia according to European working group on sarcopenia in older people (EWGSOP) definition. Clin Nutr. 2016;35:1557–63.
34. Ebadi M, Wang CW, Lai JC, Dasarathy S, Kappus MR, Dunn MA, et al. Poor performance of psoas muscle index for identification of patients with higher waitlist mortality risk in cirrhosis. J Cachexia Sarcopenia Muscle. 2018.
35. Engelmann C, Schob S, Nonnenmacher I, Werlich L, Aehling N, Ullrich S, et al. Loss of paraspinal muscle mass is a gender-specific consequence of cirrhosis that predicts complications and death. Aliment Pharmacol Ther:0.
36. Carey EJ, Lai JC, Wang CW, Dasarathy S, Lobach I, Montano-Loza AJ, et al. A multicenter study to define sarcopenia in patients with end-stage liver disease. Liver Transpl. 2017;23:625–33.
37. Martin L, Birdsell L, Macdonald N, Reiman T, Clandinin MT, McCargar LJ, et al. Cancer cachexia in the age of obesity: skeletal muscle depletion is a powerful prognostic factor, independent of body mass index. J Clin Oncol. 2013;31:1539–47.
38. van Vugt JLA, Alferink LJM, Buettner S, Gaspersz MP, Bot D, Darwish Murad S, et al. A model including sarcopenia surpasses the MELD score in predicting waiting list mortality in cirrhotic liver transplant candidates: a competing risk analysis in a national cohort. J Hepatol. 2017.
39. Kang SH, Jeong WK, Baik SK, Cha SH, Kim MY. Impact of sarcopenia on prognostic value of cirrhosis: going beyond the hepatic venous pressure gradient and MELD score. J Cachexia Sarcopenia Muscle. 2018;9:860–70.
40. Moctezuma-Velazquez C, Low G, Mourtzakis M, Ma M, Burak KW, Tandon P, et al. Association between Low testosterone levels and sarcopenia in cirrhosis: a Cross-sectional study. Ann Hepatol. 2018;17:615–23.
41. Cholongitas E, Burroughs AK. The evolution in the prioritization for liver transplantation. Ann Gastroenterol. 2012;25:6.
42. Kamath PS, Kim WR, Advanced Liver Disease Study G. The model for end-stage liver disease (MELD). Hepatology. 2007;45:797–805.

43. Kim WR, Biggins SW, Kremers WK, Wiesner RH, Kamath PS, Benson JT, et al. Hyponatremia and mortality among patients on the liver-transplant waiting list. N Engl J Med. 2008;359:1018–26.

44. Myers RP, Shaheen AA, Faris P, Aspinall AI, Burak KW. Revision of MELD to include serum albumin improves prediction of mortality on the liver transplant waiting list. PLoS One. 2013;8:e51926.

45. Myers RP, Tandon P, Ney M, Meeberg G, Faris P, Shaheen AA, et al. Validation of the five-variable model for end-stage liver disease (5vMELD) for prediction of mortality on the liver transplant waiting list. Liver Int. 2014;34:1176–83.

46. Fried LP, Tangen CM, Walston J, Newman AB, Hirsch C, Gottdiener J, et al. Frailty in older adults: evidence for a phenotype. J Gerontol A Biol Sci Med Sci. 2001;56:M146–56.

47. Sinclair M, Poltavskiy E, Dodge JL, Lai JC. Frailty is independently associated with increased hospitalisation days in patients on the liver transplant waitlist. World J Gastroenterol. 2017;23:899–905.

48. Guralnik JM, Simonsick EM, Ferrucci L, Glynn RJ, Berkman LF, Blazer DG, et al. A short physical performance battery assessing lower extremity function: association with self-reported disability and prediction of mortality and nursing home admission. J Gerontol. 1994;49:M85–94.

49. Katz S, Ford AB, Moskowitz RW, Jackson BA, Jaffe MW. Studies of illness in the aged. The index of Adl: a standardized measure of biological and psychosocial function. JAMA. 1963;185:914–9.

50. Lawton MP, Brody EM. Assessment of older people: self-maintaining and instrumental activities of daily living. Gerontologist. 1969;9:179–86.

51. Lai JC, Covinsky KE, Hayssen H, Lizaola B, Dodge JL, Roberts JP, et al. Clinician assessments of health status predict mortality in patients with end-stage liver disease awaiting liver transplantation. Liver Int. 2015;35:2167–73.

52. Lai JC, Covinsky KE, McCulloch CE, Feng S. The liver frailty index improves mortality prediction of the subjective clinician assessment in patients with cirrhosis. Am J Gastroenterol. 2018;113:235–42.

53. Dunn MA, Josbeno DA, Schmotzer AR, Tevar AD, DiMartini AF, Landsittel DP, et al. The gap between clinically assessed physical performance and objective physical activity in liver transplant candidates. Liver Transpl. 2016;22:1324–32.

54. Chang KV, Chen JD, Wu WT, Huang KC, Lin HY, Han DS. Is sarcopenia associated with hepatic encephalopathy in liver cirrhosis? A systematic review and meta-analysis. J Formos Med Assoc. 2018.

55. Idriss R, Hasse J, Wu T, Khan F, Saracino G. McKenna G, et al. Liver Transpl: Impact of prior bariatric surgery on perioperative liver transplant outcomes; 2018.

56. Durand F, Buyse S, Francoz C, Laouenan C, Bruno O, Belghiti J, et al. Prognostic value of muscle atrophy in cirrhosis using psoas muscle thickness on computed tomography. J Hepatol. 2014;60:1151–7.

57. Montano-Loza AJ, Duarte-Rojo A, Meza-Junco J, Baracos VE, Sawyer MB, Pang JX, et al. Inclusion of sarcopenia within MELD (MELD-sarcopenia) and the prediction of mortality in patients with cirrhosis. Clin Transl Gastroenterol. 2015;6:e102.

58. Sinclair M, Grossmann M, Angus PW, Hoermann R, Hey P, Scodellaro T, et al. Low testosterone as a better predictor of mortality than sarcopenia in men with advanced liver disease. J Gastroenterol Hepatol. 2016;31:661–7.

59. Sinclair M, Grossmann M, Hoermann R, Angus PW, Gow PJ. Testosterone therapy increases muscle mass in men with cirrhosis and low testosterone: a randomised controlled trial. J Hepatol. 2016;65:906–13.

60. Lai JC, Covinsky KE, Dodge JL, Boscardin WJ, Segev DL, Roberts JP, et al. Development of a novel frailty index to predict mortality in patients with end-stage liver disease. Hepatology. 2017;66:564–74.

61. Dolgin NH, Smith AJ, Harrington SG, Movahedi B, PNA M, Bozorgzadeh A. Association between sarcopenia and functional status in liver transplant patients. Exp Clin Transplant. 2018.
62. Lai JC, Dodge JL, Sen S, Covinsky K, Feng S. Functional decline in patients with cirrhosis awaiting liver transplantation: results from the functional assessment in liver transplantation (FrAILT) study. Hepatology. 2016;63:574–80.
63. van Vugt JLA, Buettner S, Alferink LJM, Bossche N, de Bruin RWF, Darwish Murad S, et al. Low skeletal muscle mass is associated with increased hospital costs in patients with cirrhosis listed for liver transplantation-a retrospective study. Transpl Int. 2018;31:165–74.
64. Golse N, Bucur PO, Ciacio O, Pittau G, Sa Cunha A, Adam R, et al. A new definition of sarcopenia in patients with cirrhosis undergoing liver transplantation. Liver Transpl. 2017;23:143–54.
65. Krell RW, Kaul DR, Martin AR, Englesbe MJ, Sonnenday CJ, Cai S, et al. Association between sarcopenia and the risk of serious infection among adults undergoing liver transplantation. Liver Transpl. 2013;19:1396–402.
66. Underwood PW, Cron DC, Terjimanian MN, Wang SC, Englesbe MJ, Waits SA. Sarcopenia and failure to rescue following liver transplantation. Clin Transpl. 2015;29:1076–80.
67. Valero V 3rd, Amini N, Spolverato G, Weiss MJ, Hirose K, Dagher NN, et al. Sarcopenia adversely impacts postoperative complications following resection or transplantation in patients with primary liver tumors. J Gastrointest Surg. 2015;19:272–81.
68. Dolgin NH, Martins PN, Movahedi B, Lapane KL, Anderson FA, Bozorgzadeh A. Functional status predicts postoperative mortality after liver transplantation. Clin Transpl. 2016;30:1403–10.
69. Merli M, Lucidi C, Giannelli V, Giusto M, Riggio O, Falcone M, et al. Cirrhotic patients are at risk for health care-associated bacterial infections. Clin Gastroenterol Hepatol. 2010;8:979–85.
70. Cosqueric G, Sebag A, Ducolombier C, Thomas C, Piette F, Weill-Engerer S. Sarcopenia is predictive of nosocomial infection in care of the elderly. Br J Nutr. 2006;96:895–901.
71. Englesbe MJ, Patel SP, He K, Lynch RJ, Schaubel DE, Harbaugh C, et al. Sarcopenia and mortality after liver transplantation. J Am Coll Surg. 2010;211:271–8.
72. Kalafateli M, Mantzoukis K, Choi Yau Y, Mohammad AO, Arora S, Rodrigues S, et al. Malnutrition and sarcopenia predict post-liver transplantation outcomes independently of the model for end-stage liver disease score. J Cachexia Sarcopenia Muscle. 2017;8:113–21.
73. Lai JC, Segev DL, McCulloch CE, Covinsky KE, Dodge JL, Feng S. Physical frailty after liver transplantation. Am J Transplant. 2018;18:1986–94.
74. Jeon JY, Wang HJ, Ock SY, Xu W, Lee JD, Lee JH, et al. Newly developed sarcopenia as a prognostic factor for survival in patients who underwent liver transplantation. PLoS One. 2015;10:e0143966.
75. Dasarathy S. Posttransplant sarcopenia: an underrecognized early consequence of liver transplantation. Dig Dis Sci. 2013;58:3103–11.
76. Tsien C, Garber A, Narayanan A, Shah SN, Barnes D, Eghtesad B, et al. Post-liver transplantation sarcopenia in cirrhosis: a prospective evaluation. J Gastroenterol Hepatol. 2014;29:1250–7.
77. Clark K, Cross T. Sarcopenia and survival after liver transplantation. Liver Transpl. 2014;20:1423.
78. Montano-Loza AJ. Severe muscle depletion predicts postoperative length of stay but is not associated with survival after liver transplantation. Liver Transpl. 2014;20:1424.
79. Norman K, Otten L. Financial impact of sarcopenia or low muscle mass - A short review. Clin Nutr. 2018.
80. Koter S, Cohnert TU, Hindermayr KB, Lindenmann J, Bruckner M, Oswald WK, et al. Increased hospital costs are associated with low skeletal muscle mass in patients undergoing elective open aortic surgery. J Vasc Surg. 2018.

81. Cron DC, Friedman JF, Winder GS, Thelen AE, Derck JE, Fakhoury JW, et al. Depression and frailty in patients with end-stage liver disease referred for transplant evaluation. Am J Transplant. 2016;16:1805–11.
82. Buganza-Torio E, Mitchell N, Abraldes JG, Thomas L, Ma M, Bailey RJ, et al. Depression in cirrhosis - a prospective evaluation of the prevalence, predictors and development of a screening nomogram. Aliment Pharmacol Ther. 2019;49:194–201.
83. Raia S, Nery JR, Mies S. Liver transplantation from live donors. Lancet. 1989;2:497.
84. Strong RW, Lynch SV, Ong TH, Matsunami H, Koido Y, Balderson GA. Successful liver transplantation from a living donor to her son. N Engl J Med. 1990;322:1505–7.
85. Broering DC, Mueller L, Ganschow R, Kim JS, Achilles EG, Schafer H, et al. Is there still a need for living-related liver transplantation in children? Ann Surg. 2001;234:713–21. discussion 21-2
86. Sugawara Y, Makuuchi M. Living donor liver transplantation: present status and recent advances. Br Med Bull. 2005;75-76:15–28.
87. Abbasoglu O. Liver transplantation: yesterday, today and tomorrow. World J Gastroenterol. 2008;14:3117–22.
88. Malago M, Burdelski M, Broelsch CE. Present and future challenges in living related liver transplantation. Transplant Proc. 1999;31:1777–81.
89. Lo CM, Fan ST, Liu CL, Wei WI, Lo RJ, Lai CL, et al. Adult-to-adult living donor liver transplantation using extended right lobe grafts. Ann Surg. 1997;226:261–9. discussion 9-70
90. Hamaguchi Y, Kaido T, Okumura S, Fujimoto Y, Ogawa K, Mori A, et al. Impact of quality as well as quantity of skeletal muscle on outcomes after liver transplantation. Liver Transpl. 2014;20:1413–9.
91. Masuda T, Shirabe K, Ikegami T, Harimoto N, Yoshizumi T, Soejima Y, et al. Sarcopenia is a prognostic factor in living donor liver transplantation. Liver Transpl. 2014;20:401–7.
92. Hamaguchi Y, Kaido T, Okumura S, Kobayashi A, Shirai H, Yagi S, et al. Proposal of muscle-MELD score, including muscularity, for prediction of mortality after living donor liver transplantation. Transplantation 2016; 100: 2416–2423.
93. Izumi T, Watanabe J, Tohyama T, Takada Y. Impact of psoas muscle index on short-term outcome after living donor liver transplantation. Turk J Gastroenterol. 2016;27:382–8.
94. Hammad A, Kaido T, Hamaguchi Y, Okumura S, Kobayashi A, Shirai H, et al. Impact of sarcopenic overweight on the outcomes after living donor liver transplantation. Hepatobiliary Surg Nutr. 2017;6:367–78.
95. Kaido T, Tamai Y, Hamaguchi Y, Okumura S, Kobayashi A, Shirai H, et al. Effects of pre-transplant sarcopenia and sequential changes in sarcopenic parameters after living donor liver transplantation. Nutrition. 2017;33:195–8.
96. Onuma T, Kamishima T, Shimamura T, Kawamura N, Yamashita K, Sutherland K, et al. Longitudinal CT study of sarcopenia due to hepatic failure after living donor liver transplantation. Quant Imaging Med Surg. 2018;8:25–31.
97. Toshima T, Shirabe K, Kurihara T, Itoh S, Harimoto N, Ikegami T, et al. Profile of plasma amino acids values as a predictor of sepsis in patients following living donor liver transplantation: special reference to sarcopenia and postoperative early nutrition. Hepatol Res. 2015;45:1170–7.
98. Kaido T, Ogawa K, Fujimoto Y, Ogura Y, Hata K, Ito T, et al. Impact of sarcopenia on survival in patients undergoing living donor liver transplantation. Am J Transplant. 2013;13:1549–56.
99. Lurz E, Quammie C, Englesbe M, Alonso EM, Lin HC, Hsu EK, et al. Frailty in children with liver disease: a prospective multicenter study. J Pediatr. 2018;194:109–15. e4
100. Mager DR, Hager A, Ooi PH, Siminoski K, Gilmour SM, Yap JYK. Persistence of sarcopenia after pediatric liver transplantation is associated with poorer growth and recurrent hospital admissions. JPEN J Parenter Enteral Nutr. 2018.
101. Mazzaferro V, Regalia E, Doci R, Andreola S, Pulvirenti A, Bozzetti F, et al. Liver transplantation for the treatment of small hepatocellular carcinomas in patients with cirrhosis. N Engl J Med. 1996;334:693–9.

102. Mazzaferro V, Bhoori S, Sposito C, Bongini M, Langer M, Miceli R, et al. Milan criteria in liver transplantation for hepatocellular carcinoma: an evidence-based analysis of 15 years of experience. Liver Transpl. 2011;17(Suppl 2):S44–57.
103. Mazzaferro V, Llovet JM, Miceli R, Bhoori S, Schiavo M, Mariani L, et al. Predicting survival after liver transplantation in patients with hepatocellular carcinoma beyond the Milan criteria: a retrospective, exploratory analysis. Lancet Oncol. 2009;10:35–43.
104. Kim YR, Park S, Han S, Ahn JH, Kim S, Sinn DH, et al. Sarcopenia as a predictor of post-transplant tumor recurrence after living donor liver transplantation for hepatocellular carcinoma beyond the Milan criteria. Sci Rep. 2018;8:7157.
105. Wynter-Blyth V, Moorthy K. Prehabilitation: preparing patients for surgery. BMJ. 2017;358:j3702.
106. Kogiso T, Tokushige K. Key roles of hepatologists in successful liver transplantation. Hepatol Res. 2018;48:608–21.
107. Dunn MA. The cost of sarcopenia. Transpl Int. 2018;31:155–6.
108. Laube R, Wang H, Park L, Heyman JK, Vidot H, Majumdar A, et al. Frailty in advanced liver disease. Liver Int. 2018.
109. Anand AC. Nutrition and muscle in cirrhosis. J Clin Exp Hepatol. 2017;7:340–57.
110. Plauth M, Merli M, Kondrup J, Weimann A, Ferenci P, Muller MJ, et al. ESPEN guidelines for nutrition in liver disease and transplantation. Clin Nutr. 1997;16:43–55.
111. Sinclair M, Gow PJ, Grossmann M, Angus PW. Review article: sarcopenia in cirrhosis-aetiology, implications and potential therapeutic interventions. Aliment Pharmacol Ther. 2016;43:765–77.
112. Plank LD, Gane EJ, Peng S, Muthu C, Mathur S, Gillanders L, et al. Nocturnal nutritional supplementation improves total body protein status of patients with liver cirrhosis: a randomized 12-month trial. Hepatology. 2008;48:557–66.
113. Lai JC, Volk ML, Strasburg D, Alexander N. Performance-based measures associate with frailty in patients with end-stage liver disease. Transplantation. 2016;100:2656–60.
114. Duarte-Rojo A, Ruiz-Margain A, Montano-Loza AJ, Macias-Rodriguez RU, Ferrando A, Kim WR. Exercise and physical activity for patients with end-stage liver disease: improving functional status and sarcopenia while on the transplant waiting list. Liver Transpl. 2018;24:122–39.
115. Dasarathy S, Merli M. Sarcopenia from mechanism to diagnosis and treatment in liver disease. J Hepatol. 2016;65:1232–44.
116. Kumar A, Davuluri G, Silva RNE, Engelen M, Ten Have GAM, Prayson R, et al. Ammonia lowering reverses sarcopenia of cirrhosis by restoring skeletal muscle proteostasis. Hepatology. 2017;65:2045–58.
117. Zhou X, Wang JL, Lu J, Song Y, Kwak KS, Jiao Q, et al. Reversal of cancer cachexia and muscle wasting by ActRIIB antagonism leads to prolonged survival. Cell. 2010;142:531–43.
118. Bergerson JT, Lee JG, Furlan A, Sourianarayanane A, Fetzer DT, Tevar AD, et al. Liver transplantation arrests and reverses muscle wasting. Clin Transpl. 2015;29:216–21.
119. Jahangiri Y, Pathak P, Tomozawa Y, Li L, Schlansky BL, Farsad K. Muscle gain after Transjugular intrahepatic portosystemic shunt creation: time course and prognostic implications for survival in cirrhosis. J Vasc Interv Radiol. 2019;30:866.
120. Lauerer M, Kaiser K, Nagel E. Organ transplantation in the face of donor shortage - ethical implications with a focus on liver allocation. Visc Med. 2016;32:278–85.
121. Wet op de orgaandonatie (Law on organ donation) 1996, 24 May. Accessed 13-11-2018.
122. Cohen IG, Amarasingham R, Shah A, Xie B, Lo B. The legal and ethical concerns that Arise from using complex predictive analytics in health care. Health Aff. 2014;33:1139–47.
123. Kahn J, Wagner D, Homfeld N, Muller H, Kniepeiss D, Schemmer P. Both sarcopenia and frailty determine suitability of patients for liver transplantation-a systematic review and meta-analysis of the literature. Clin Transpl. 2018;32:e13226.
124. Lai JC. Editorial: advancing adoption of frailty to improve the Care of Patients with cirrhosis: time for a consensus on a frailty index. Am J Gastroenterol. 2016;111:1776.

Chapter 6
Nutritional Therapy in the Management of Physical Frailty and Sarcopenia

Manuela Merli, Barbara Lattanzi, Daria D'Ambrosio, Nicoletta Fabrini, and Alice Liguori

Introduction

In patients with liver cirrhosis, progressive liver insufficiency is associated with multiple extra-hepatic alterations. Among these alterations, a gradual decline of muscle mass and function and the deterioration of physical performance are frequently recognized [1–3]. Sarcopenia and/or frailty are negative prognostic factors for morbidity and mortality in liver cirrhosis. For these reasons, the diagnosis, prevention, and treatment of these conditions are of great importance.

Despite the high prevalence and the clinical impact of sarcopenia and frailty in patients with liver disease, to date, these two entities are not included in the prognostic and severity scores of liver cirrhosis [4]. As a consequence, sarcopenia and frailty are not systematically investigated and may go even under-recognized in liver patients.

Being potentially reversible conditions [5–7], early identification of physical frailty and sarcopenia could help to plan early management of these conditions [8, 9]. However, there are few clinical studies specifically focused on the management of sarcopenia and physical frailty in patients with a diagnosis of liver cirrhosis.

What Can We Derive from the Results of Nutritional Intervention in Elderly Patients: Some Certainties

In elderly patients, the main therapeutic approaches that have been proposed to improve sarcopenia and frailty are adequate nutrition and cognitive and physical training [7, 10].

M. Merli (✉) · B. Lattanzi · D. D'Ambrosio · N. Fabrini · A. Liguori
Gastroenterology and Hepatology Unit, Department of Translation and Precision Medicine, Sapienza University of Rome, Rome, Italy
e-mail: Manuela.merli@uniroma1.it

© Springer Nature Switzerland AG 2020   77
P. Tandon, A. J. Montano-Loza (eds.), *Frailty and Sarcopenia in Cirrhosis*,
https://doi.org/10.1007/978-3-030-26226-6_6

Some evidence suggests amelioration of frailty in older people with cognitive training and physical exercise [11–15]; other studies were mainly focused on nutritional interventions [16–21]. In a recent study conducted in 256 older adults, patients were randomized to five different 6-month interventions. These included nutritional supplementation (supplying 300 kcal in the form of carbohydrate, fat, protein, + vitamins), cognitive training, physical training, combination treatment, and usual care (controls). Results indicate that all the active treatments' approaches were effective in reducing frailty vs controls. However, the best results were obtained in patients receiving the combination treatment [7].

Concerning the amelioration of sarcopenia, data are more encouraging, and specific nutritional interventions showed a significant amelioration in muscle mass and function in older adults, mainly when combined with physical exercise [5, 22]. In particular, a daily protein intake of 1.0 g/kg has been identified as the minimum amount required to maintain muscle mass in old age [22]. According to the available evidence, older people should, therefore, be encouraged to eat between 1.0 and 1.5 g/kg of proteins daily [23].

A large ongoing phase III, multi-center randomized controlled trial ("Sarcopenia and Physical Frailty in older people: multi-component Treatment strategies"(SPRINTT)) is testing long-term structured physical activity and nutritional counseling/dietary intervention to prevent mobility disability in community-dwelling older people with physical frailty and sarcopenia [24]. The results of this study will possibly increase our knowledge in this field in the near future.

Nutritional Intervention in the Management of Physical Frailty and Sarcopenia in Cirrhotic Patients: More Uncertainties

While in mixed patients' populations, the benefits of nutritional therapy are evidenced by a reduction in mortality, infections, systemic inflammation, and hospital length of stay [5]; in cirrhotic patients, similar results have been limited by small cohort size and lack of randomized trials; therefore evidence-based efficacy of nutritional interventions is often lacking. The end points of these studies are frequently heterogeneous (muscle strength and/or muscle mass, mortality, complications of portal hypertension, etc.) which make the results difficult to analyze [25]. With regard to frailty, the Liver Frailty Index [15] has been only recently proposed and is not commonly utilized; consequently, studies evaluating the effect of nutritional supplementation on physical frailty in cirrhotic patients are still lacking. Nutritional treatment approaches in cirrhotic patients, have focused on different strategies: calories or protein supplementation, stimulation of protein synthesis, reinforcement to increase exercise and physical activity, and use of anabolic hormones and ammonia-lowering strategies. The use of anabolic hormones and the ammonia-lowering strategies will not be dealt with in this chapter.

Calories and Protein Supplementation

A crucial aspect of nutritional management is to ensure that the patient's rehabilitative diet contains the correct amount of each essential nutrient or macromolecule [26]. The approach of most nutritional intervention studies in liver cirrhosis is to supply at least 35 kcal/kg/d [26]. It is also recommended to shorten the duration of fasting periods during the day, and there is evidence that a late evening and an early morning snack containing proteins are likely to have the greatest benefit in preventing muscle loss in cirrhosis [27].

Since caloric and protein intakes are frequently decreased in patients with liver cirrhosis, regimens providing extra calories via high caloric oral nutritional supplements (ONS) feeding and/or enteral feeding have been proposed to increase the suboptimal oral intake. Results have, however, been controversial. Nutritional support with enteral nutrition in hospitalized malnourished cirrhotic patients [28] and perioperative nutrition in cirrhotic patients undergoing surgery for hepatocellular carcinoma were found to improve patients' survival [29]. On the other hand, long-term nutritional supplementation before liver transplantation [30] and an immuno-nutrition supplement provided before and perioperatively to liver transplant patients [31] failed to obtain any significant improvement in survival and outcomes in treated patients vs controls, in randomized controlled trials. Therefore, despite promising results in some studies, systematic meta-analyses could not clearly demonstrate a significant benefit of nutritional therapy on survival [32–34]. Results have been conflicting also regarding the benefits of parenteral nutritional supplementation in patients with cirrhosis [35]. However, during prolonged periods of poor oral intake or fasting as in severe hepatic encephalopathy, gastrointestinal bleeding, and impaired gut motility or ileus, to provide nutritional support is considered to be beneficial by most authors [36].

An important strategy to approach malnutrition and sarcopenia in cirrhotic patients is protein supplementation. Adequate protein intake, to meet the increased protein requirements in patients with a diagnosis of liver cirrhosis with malnutrition, has been defined as 1.2–1.5 g/kg body weight daily by the EASL guidelines [26].

In the past, there has been controversy about whether protein intake could favor the development of hepatic encephalopathy (HE) in cirrhotic patients. Indeed, in the majority of patients suffering from HE, a transient protein restriction was recommended, in order to limit the synthesis of ammonia induced by protein deamination and impaired urea synthesis. Later on, a number of studies have shown that normal to high protein intake does not precipitate HE [37] and may even improve mental status [38, 39]. Furthermore, recovery from an acute episode of HE with standard pharmacologic treatment was found to be similar in patients with normal protein intake vs those following severe protein restriction [40]. At the same time, protein-restriction induced protein catabolism which is detrimental [40]. In cirrhotic patients hospitalized for HE, a hyper-caloric and hyper-proteic oral diet has been found to be beneficial [50], and protein refeeding is an important target for malnourished cirrhotic patients [41].

Branched-Chain Amino Acid (BCAA), Leucine, and HMB Supplementation

Hepatic damage causes an increase in aromatic amino acids (produced by decreased liver clearance) and a decrease in branched-chain amino acids (due to increased utilization as the energy source). BCAA supplementation is a strategy that has been initially utilized for the treatment of acute HE based on the false neurotransmitter hypothesis [42]. However, old studies supplementing BCAA in patients with HE did not investigate the effects of BCAA on nutritional status or muscle mass [43, 44]. Later on, long-term oral BCAA consumption was proposed to increase protein intake in those cirrhotic patients who are intolerant to normal dietary proteins [45]. Two randomized, double-blind, multicenter studies in advanced cirrhotic patients reported an improvement in muscle mass following a 12-month BCAA oral supplement [45, 46]. Further studies reported similar encouraging results, although important biases were present such as small cohorts of patients, lack of patients' randomization, short-term observation time, and different kinds of nutritional supplements. Furthermore, BCAA are not freely available in many countries, and results are mainly reported where these supplements are most used [47–50] (Table 6.1).

Leucine directly activates mTORC1 that stimulates protein synthesis and decreases autophagy in muscle [51]. In a recent study, six alcoholic cirrhotics and eight healthy controls received a single oral BCAA mixture enriched with leucine, and muscle biopsies were obtained before and 7 h after the nutritional supplement [52]. The oral BCAA/LEU mixture improved mTOR1 signaling and increased autophagy in the skeletal muscle of cirrhotic patients showing a possible physio-pathological mechanism for a beneficial effect of BCAA.

Some studies suggested a beneficial effect of exercise training associated with BCAA supplements in improving nutritional status in cirrhotic patients [49]. A small randomized pilot trial, while giving leucine supplements 10 g/day orally for 12 weeks in all participants, proposed exercise training in eight and no physical intervention in nine cirrhotic patients (controls). Lower thigh circumference and the 6-min walking test both improved significantly ($P = 0.01$) only in those cirrhotic patients combining exercise training with leucine supplements [53].

Beta-hydroxy-beta-methyl butyrate (HMB) is a metabolite of leucine with the potential to increase muscle's performance and tropism. Studies on experimental models of cachexia have reported an increase in phosphorylation and activation of mTOR secondary to the use of HMB [54]. Experimental studies performed on cell cultures of myoblasts also showed an increase in IGF-1 and inhibition of the ubiquitin-proteasome secondary to treatment with HMB [55, 56]. This evidence confirms the anabolic properties of HMB. The association of anabolic properties targeting mTOR and anti-proteolytic effect makes HMB a potentially effective supplement for the treatment of sarcopenia in the patient with liver cirrhosis. There are currently no data in the literature on the use of HMB in cirrhotic patients, but two studies are ongoing, and two studies are registered on clinicaltrial.gov.

Table 6.1 Effect of an adequate oral dietary intake with or without nutritional supplements enriched with BCAA on muscle mass or function in patients with liver cirrhosis (recent studies)

	Study type	Patients	Treatment	Aims	Results
Ruiz-Margain (2018) [47]	Randomized, open-label study	72 cirrhotic patients	Intervention group: high-protein, high-fiber diet (HPHF) with 1.2 g/kg protein and 30 g of fiber + nutritional supplement (500 kcal, protein 18.6 g (BCAA 9.5 g) daily. Control group: HPHF. Time: 6 months	To evaluate the effect of a combination of a high-protein, high-fiber diet plus nutritional supplementation enriched with BCAA on the nutritional status	Nutritional supplementation enriched with BCAA increased muscle mass evaluated by MAMC ($p < 0.001$). No significant changes in Psychometric Hepatic Encephalopathy Score or Critical Flicker Frequency Score in either group
Haraoka (2017) [49]	Interventional study	33 cirrhotic patients	Nutritional supplement package (protein 13.5 g (BCAA 5.55 g), 210 kcal) once daily as a late evening snack + walking exercise (additional 2000 steps/day). Time: 12 weeks	To evaluate the improvement of muscle volume (BIA) and function (leg strength and hand-grip strength)	Muscle volume and leg strength and hand-grip strength both increased ($p < 0.01$)
K tajima (2017) [48]	Interventional study	21 cirrhotic patients	Patient received a standard diet of 25–35 kcal/kg/day and protein intake of 1.0–1.4 g/kg/day plus BCAA granules three times daily (12 g/day). Time: 24 weeks	To evaluate the effects of dietary BCAAs on systemic glucose metabolism, skeletal muscle, and prognosis	BCAAs supplementation increased albumin levels in patients with hypoalbuminemia (3.1 ± 0.3 to 3.4 ± 0.3 $p < 0.01$) and was associated to decreased fat accumulation in skeletal muscle detected by CT scan ($p < 0.05$)
Uojima H (2017) [50]	Interventional study	82 cirrhotic patients	Control: 28-day pretreatment observation period. Treatment: nutritional supplement package (protein 13.5 g/day (BCAA 5.56 g), 210 kcal) twice daily. Time: 24 weeks	To evaluate the effect of nutritional supplements enriched with BCAA on muscle strength and muscle mass	Nutritional supplementation enriched with BCAA induced a significant increase in hand-grip strength (22.2 ± 6.3 kg vs. 23.9 ± 6.4 kg; $p < 0.001$).
Maharshi S (2016) [38]	Randomized clinical trial	73 cirrhotic patients with MHE	Intervention group: nutritional therapy (30–35 kcal/kg/day, 1.0–1.5 g vegetable protein/kg/day). Control group: patients continued on their same diet. Time: 6 months	To assess the effects of nutritional therapy on cognitive functions and HRQOL	MAMC, hand-grip strength, serum albumin, skeletal muscle mass, and creatinine height index improved in the intervention group ($p < 0.05$)

Abbreviation: *BCAA* branched-chain amino acids, *BIA* bioelectrical impedance analysis, *DEXA* dual-energy X-ray absorptiometry, *MAMC* mid-arm muscle circumference

MHE minimal hepatic encephalopathy, *HRQOL* health-related quality of life

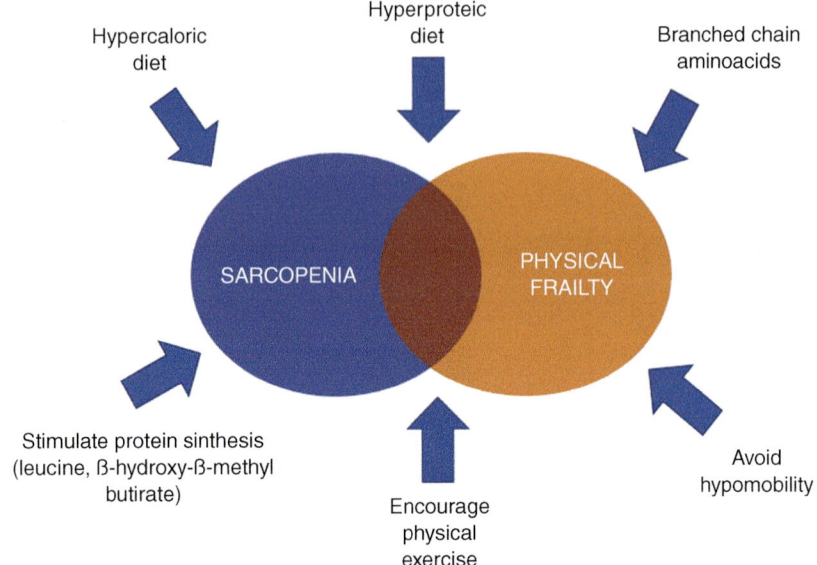

Fig. 6.1 Interactions and possible strategies to manage sarcopenia and physical frailty

Conclusions

In conclusion, cirrhotic patients are at high risk of developing sarcopenia and frailty that represents negative prognostic features in cirrhosis. Being potentially modifiable conditions, the prevention of further worsening or even an improvement of skeletal muscle mass and frailty in patients with cirrhosis could lead to decreased morbidity and mortality. To date, there are no established protocols to reverse or prevent deterioration of nutritional status and frailty in patients with liver cirrhosis. Nutritional intervention and individual counseling to achieve adequate amounts of calories and proteins are recommended (Fig. 6.1). Oral nutritional supplementations with BCAA or leucine, combined with exercise training, are promising measures, but more studies are needed to define the best way and time to adopt this approach. Moreover, taking into account the improving knowledge about the molecular mechanisms of sarcopenia, target therapies may be promising for the future.

References

1. Lai JC, Covinsky KE, Dodge JL, Boscardin WJ, Segev DL, Roberts JP, Feng S. Development of a novel frailty index to predict mortality in patients with end-stage liver disease. Hepatology. 2017;66(2):564–74.
2. Montano-Loza AJ, Meza-Junco J, Prado CM, Lieffers JR, Baracos VE, Bain VG, et al. Muscle wasting is associated with mortality in patients with cirrhosis. Clin Gastroenterol Hepatol. 2012;10:166–173 e161.

3. Merli M, Riggio O, Dally L. Does malnutrition affect survival in cirrhosis? PINC (Policentrica Italiana Nutrizione Cirrosi). Hepatology. 1996;23:1041–6.
4. van Vugt JLA, Alferink LJM, Buettner S, Gaspersz MP, Bot D, Murad SD, et al. A model including sarcopenia surpasses the MELD score in predicting waiting list mortality in cirrhotic liver transplant candidates. J Hepatol. 2017;68:707–14.
5. McClave SA, Di Baise JK, Mullin GE, Martindale RG. ACG Clinical Guideline: Nutrition therapy in the adult hospitalized patient. Am J Gastroenterol. 2016.
6. Tarazona-Santabalbina FJ, Gómez-Cabrera MC, Pérez-Ros P, Martínez-Arnau FM, Cabo H, Tsaparas K, Salvador-Pascual A, Rodriguez-Mañas L, Viña J. A multicomponent exercise intervention that reverses frailty and improves cognition, emotion, and social networking in the community-dwelling frail elderly: a randomized clinical trial. J Am Med Dir Assoc. 2016;17:426–33.
7. Ng TP, Feng L, Nyunt MS, Feng L, Niti M, Tan BY, Chan G, Khoo SA, Chan SM, Yap P, Yap KB. Nutritional, physical, cognitive, and combination interventions and frailty reversal among older adults: a randomized controlled trial. Am J Med. 2015;128:1225–1236.e1.
8. Kok B, Tandon P. Frailty in patients with cirrhosis. Curr Treat Options Gastroenterol. 2018;16:215–25.
9. Lattanzi B, D'Ambrosio D, Fedele F, Merli M. Nutritional assessment and management for hospitalized patients with cirrhosis. Current Hepatology Reports. 2018; https://doi.org/10.1007/s11901-018-0398-6.
10. Laube R, Wang H, Park L, Heyman JK, Vidot H, Majumdar A, Strasser SI, McCaughan GW, Liu K. Frailty in advanced liver disease. Liver Int. 2018;38:2117–28.
11. Smith-Ray RL, Hughes SL, Prohaska TR, Little DM, Jurivich DA, Hedeker D. Impact of cognitive training on balance and gait in older adults. J Gerontol B Psychol Sci Soc Sci. 2015;70(3):357–66.
12. Li KZ, Roudaia E, Lussier M, Bherer L, Leroux A, McKinley PA. Benefits of cognitive dual task training on balance performance in healthy older adults. J Gerontol A Biol Sci Med Sci. 2010;65(12):1344–52.
13. Theou O, Stathokostas L, Roland K, et al. The effectiveness of exercise interventions for the management of frailty: a systematic review. J Aging Res. 2011;2011:569194.
14. Willis SL, Tennstedt SL, Marsiske M, et al. Long-term effects of cognitive training on everyday functional outcomes in older adults. JAMA. 2006;296(23):2805–14.
15. Doumas M, Rapp MA, Krampe RT. Working memory and postural control: adult age differences in potential for improvement, task priority, and dual tasking. J Gerontol B Psychol Sci Soc Sci. 2009;64(2):193–201.
16. Kim CO, Lee KR. Preventive effect of protein-energy supplementation on the functional decline of frail older adults with low socioeconomic status: a community-based randomized controlled study. J Gerontol A Biol Sci Med Sci. 2013;68(3):309–16.
17. Rosendahl E, Lindelöf N, Littbrand H, et al. High-intensity functional exercise program and protein-enriched energy supplement for older persons dependent in activities of daily living: a randomised controlled trial. Aust J Physiother. 2006;52(2):105–13.
18. Milne AC, Avenell A, Potter J. Meta-analysis: protein and energy supplementation in older people. Ann Intern Med. 2006;144(1):37–48.
19. Payette H, Boutier V, Coulombe C, Gray-Donald K. Benefits of nutritional supplementation in free-living, frail, undernourished elderly people: a prospective randomized community trial. J Am Diet Assoc. 2002;102(8):1088–95.
20. Fiatarone MA, O'Neill EF, Ryan ND, et al. Exercise training and nutritional supplementation for physical frailty in very elderly people. N Engl J Med. 1994;330(25):1769–75.
21. Park Y, Choi JE, Hwang HS. Protein supplementation improves muscle mass and physical performance in undernourished prefrail and frail elderly subjects: a randomized, double-blind, placebo-controlled trial. Am J Clin Nutr. 2018;108:1026–33.
22. Calvani R, Miccheli A, Landi F, Bossola M, Cesari M, Leeuwenburgh C, Sieber CC, Bernabei R, Marzetti E. Current nutritional recommendations and novel dietary strategies to manage sarcopenia. J Frailty Aging. 2013;2:38–53.

23. Malafarina V, Uriz-Otano F, Iniesta R, Gil-Guerrero L. Effectiveness of nutritional supplementation on muscle mass in the treatment of sarcopenia in old age: a systematic review. J Am Med Dir Assoc. 2013;14(1):10–7.

24. Marzetti E, Cesari M, Calvani R, Msihid J, Tosato M, Rodriguez-Mañas L, Lattanzio F, Cherubini A, Bejuit R, Di Bari M, Maggio M, Vellas B, Dantoine T, Cruz-Jentoft AJ, Sieber CC, Freiberger E, Skalska A, Grodzicki T, Sinclair AJ, Topinkova E, Rýznarová I, Strandberg T, AMWJ S, JMGA S, Roller-Wirnsberger R, Jónsson PV, Ramel A, Del Signore S, Pahor M, Roubenoff R, Bernabei R, Landi F. SPRINTT Consortium. The "Sarcopenia and Physical fRailty IN older people: multi-componenT Treatment strategies" (SPRINTT) randomized controlled trial: Case finding, screening, and characteristics of eligible participants. Exp Gerontol. 2018;113:48–57.

25. Ooi PH, Gilmour SM, Yap J, Mager DR. Effects of branched chain amino acid supplementation on patient care outcomes in adults and children with liver cirrhosis: a systematic review. Clin Nutr ESPEN. 2018;28:41–51.

26. European Association for the Study of the Liver. EASL Clinical Practice Guidelines on nutrition in chronic liver disease. J Hepatol. 2019;70(1):172–93.

27. Tsien CD, McCullough AJ, Dasarathy S. Late evening snack: exploiting a period of anabolic opportunity in cirrhosis. J Gastroenterol Hepatol. 2012;27:430–41.

28. Cabre E, Gonzalez-Huix F, Abad-Lacruz A, Esteve M, Acero D, Fernandez-Bañares F, et al. Effect of total enteral nutrition on the short-term outcome of severely malnourished cirrhotics. A randomized controlled trial. Gastroenterology. 1990;98(3):715–20. PMID: 2105256.

29. Fan ST, Lo CM, Lai EC, Chu KM, Liu CL, Wong J. Perioperative nutritional support in patients undergoing hepatectomy for hepatocellular carcinoma. N Engl J Med. 1994;331(23):1547–52.

30. Le Cornu KA, McKiernan FJ, Kapadia SA, Neuberger JM. A prospective randomized study of preoperative nutritional supplementation in patients awaiting elective orthotopic liver transplantation. Transplantation. 2000;69(7):1364–9.

31. Plank LD, Mathur S, Gane EJ, Peng SL, Gillanders LK, McIlroy K, Chavez CP, Calder PC, McCall JL. Perioperative immunonutrition in patients undergoing liver transplantation: a randomized double-blind trial. Hepatology. 2015;61(2):639–47.

32. Fialla AD, Israelsen M, Hamberg O, Krag A, Gluud LL. Nutritional therapy in cirrhosis or alcoholic hepatitis: a systematic review and meta-analysis. Liver Int. 2015;35(9):2072–8.

33. Koretz RL, Avenell A, Lipman TO. Nutritional support for liver disease. Cochrane Database Syst Rev. 2012;5:CD008344.

34. Antar R, Wong P, Ghali P. A meta-analysis of nutritional supplementation for management of hospitalized alcoholic hepatitis. Can J Gastroenterol. 2012;26(7):463–7.

35. Koretz RL, Avenell A, Lipman TO. Nutritional support for liver disease. Cochrane Database Syst Rev. 2012;5:CD008344.

36. Plauth M, Cabré E, Campillo B, Kondrup J, Marchesini G, Schütz T, Shenkin A, Wendon J, ESPEN. ESPEN guidelines on parenteral nutrition: hepatology. Clin Nutr. 2009;28:436–44. https://doi.org/10.1016/j.clnu.2009.04.019. Epub 2009 Jun 11.

37. Bianchi GP, Marchesini G, Fabbri A, Rondelli A, Bugianesi E, Zoli M, Pisi E. Vegetable versus animal protein diet in cirrhotic patients with chronic encephalopathy. A randomized cross-over comparison. J Intern Med. 1993;233(5):385–92.

38. Maharshi S, Sharma BC, Sachdeva S, Srivastava S, Sharma P. Efficacy of nutritional therapy for patients with cirrhosis and minimal hepatic encephalopathy in a randomized trial. Clin Gastroenterol Hepatol. 2016;14(3):454–460.e3.

39. Gheorghe L, Iacob R, Vădan R, Iacob S, Gheorghe C. Improvement of hepatic encephalopathy using a modified high-calorie high-protein diet. Rom J Gastroenterol. 2005;14(3):231–8.

40. Córdoba J, López-Hellín J, Planas M, Sabín P, Sanpedro F, Castro F, Esteban R, Guardia J. Normal protein diet for episodic hepatic encephalopathy: results of a randomized study. Jm Hepatol. 2004;41(1):38–43.

41. Kondrup J, Müller MJ. Energy and protein requirements of patients with chronic liver disease. J Hepatol. 1997;27(1):239–47. Review. PMID: 9252101.

42. Gluud LL, Dam G, Les I, Marchesini G, Borre M, Aagaard NK, Vilstrup H. Branched-chain amino acids for people with hepatic encephalopathy. Cochrane Database Syst Rev. 2017;5:CD001939.
43. Horst D, Grace ND, Conn HO, Schiff E, Schenker S, Viteri A, Law D, Atterbury CE. Comparison of dietary protein with an oral, branched chain-enriched amino acid supplement in chronic portal-systemic encephalopathy: a randomized controlled trial. Hepatology. 1984;4(2):279–87.
44. Christie ML, Sack DM, Pomposelli J, Horst D. Enriched branched-chain amino acid formula versus a casein-based supplement in the treatment of cirrhosis. JPEN J Parenter Enteral Nutr. 1985;9(6):671–8.
45. Marchesini G, Bianchi G, Merli M, Amodio P, Panella C, Loguercio C, Rossi Fanelli F, Abbiati R, Italian BCAA Study Group. Nutritional supplementation with branched-chain amino acids in advanced cirrhosis: a double-blind, randomized trial. Gastroenterology. 2003;124(7):1792–801.
46. Les I, Doval E, García-Martínez R, Planas M, Cárdenas G, Gómez P, Flavià M, Jacas C, Mínguez B, Vergara M, Soriano G, Vila C, Esteban R, Córdoba J. Effects of branched-chain amino acids supplementation in patients with cirrhosis and a previous episode of hepatic encephalopathy: a randomized study. Am J Gastroenterol. 2011;106(6):1081–8.
47. Ruiz-Margáin A, Macías-Rodríguez RU, Ríos-Torres SL, Román-Calleja BM, Méndez-Guerrero O, Rodríguez-Córdova P, Torre A. Effect of a high-protein, high-fiber diet plus supplementation with branched-chain amino acids on the nutritional status of patients with cirrhosis. Rev Gastroenterol Mex. 2018;83(1):9–15.
48. Kitajima Y, Takahashi H, Akiyama T, Murayama K, Iwane S, Kuwashiro T, Tanaka K, et al. Supplementation with branched-chain amino acids ameliorates hypoalbuminemia, prevents sarcopenia, and reduces fat accumulation in the skeletal muscles of patients with liver cirrhosis. J Gastroenterol. 2017;24.
49. Hiraoka A, Michitaka K, Kiguchi D, Izumoto H, Ueki H, Kaneto M, et al. Efficacy of branched-chain amino acid supplementation and walking exercise for preventing sarcopenia in patients with liver cirrhosis. Eur J Gastroenterol Hepatol. 2017;29(12):1416–23.
50. Uojima H, Sakurai S, Hidaka H, Kinbara T, Sung JH, Ichita C, Tokoro S, Masuda S, Sasaki A, Koizumi K, Egashira H, Kako M, Kobayashi S. Effect of branched-chain amino acid supplements on muscle strength and muscle mass in patients with liver cirrhosis. Eur J Gastroenterol Hepatol. 2017;29(12):1402–7.
51. Carroll B, Korolchuk VI, Sarkar S. Amino acids and autophagy: cross-talk and co-operation to control cellular homeostasis. Amino Acids. 2015;47:2065–88. https://doi.org/10.1007/s00726-014-1775-2.
52. Tsien C, Davuluri G, Singh D, Allawy A, Ten Have GA, Thapaliya S, et al. Metabolic and molecular responses to leucine enriched branched chain amino acid supplementation in the skeletal muscle of alcoholic cirrhosis. Hepatology. 2015;61(6):2018–29.
53. Román E, Torrades MT, Nadal MJ, Cárdenas G, Nieto JC, Vidal S, Bascuñana H, Juárez C, Guarner C, Córdoba J, Soriano G. Randomized pilot study: effects of an exercise programme and leucine supplementation in patients with cirrhosis. Dig Dis Sci. 2014;59(8):1966–75.
54. Aversa Z, Bonetto A, Costelli P, Minero VG, Penna F, Baccino FM, Lucia S, Rossi Fanelli F, Muscaritoli M. β-Hydroxy-β-methylbutyrate (HMB) attenuates muscle and body weight loss in experimental cancer cachexia. Int J Oncol. 2011;38(3):713–20.
55. Kornasio R, Riederer I, Butler-Browne G, Mouly V, Uni Z, Halevy O. Beta-hydroxy-betamethylbutyrate (HMB) stimulates myogenic cell proliferation, differentiation, and survival via the MAPK/ERK and PI3K/Akt pathways. Biochim Biophys Acta. 2009;1793(5):755–63.
56. Smith HJ, Mukerji P, Tisdale MJ. Attenuation of proteasome-induced proteolysis in skeletal muscle by {beta}-hydroxy-{beta}-methylbutyrate in cancer-induced muscle loss. Cancer Res. 2005;65(1):277–83.

Chapter 7
Exercise Training in Patients with Cirrhosis

Graeme M. Purdy, Kenneth J. Riess, Kathleen P. Ismond, and Puneeta Tandon

Introduction

Cirrhosis is a chronic progressive disease that affects not only the liver but also multiple other organ systems, including both the neuromuscular and cardiorespiratory systems [1]. As reviewed in other chapters, a multitude of factors inherent to the disease lead to significant deconditioning, sarcopenia, and frailty, which impacts the patients' activities of daily living. Patients living with cirrhosis have an aerobic capacity (as measured by peak VO_2) 60–82% lower than healthy, aged-matched adults [2]. Patients also experience significant peripheral muscle dysfunction [3], bone density loss [4], fatigue [5], and increased fall risk [6]. Exercise programming can target these impairments and contribute to the improved function of patients with cirrhosis [7].

G. M. Purdy
Department of Physical Therapy, Faculty of Rehabilitation Medicine, University of Alberta, Edmonton, AB, Canada

K. J. Riess
Department of Physical Therapy, Faculty of Rehabilitation Medicine, University of Alberta, Edmonton, AB, Canada

School of Health and Life Sciences, Northern Alberta Institute of Technology, Edmonton, AB, Canada

K. P. Ismond
Division of Gastroenterology, Department of Medicine, Faculty of Medicine and Dentistry, University of Alberta, Edmonton, AB, Canada

P. Tandon (✉)
Division of Gastroenterology, Department of Medicine, Faculty of Medicine and Dentistry, University of Alberta, Edmonton, AB, Canada

Department of Medicine, Cirrhosis Care Clinic, University of Alberta, Edmonton, AB, Canada
e-mail: ptandon@ualberta.ca

© Springer Nature Switzerland AG 2020
P. Tandon, A. J. Montano-Loza (eds.), *Frailty and Sarcopenia in Cirrhosis*,
https://doi.org/10.1007/978-3-030-26226-6_7

With liver disease, patients experience what has been described as "a downward spiral of deconditioning" [8] attributed to low levels of physical activity and high levels of sedentary behaviour [9, 10]. Contributing factors include [11–13]:

– A lack of cirrhosis- or chronic disease-specific programming
– High levels of fatigue and impaired exercise tolerance
– A paucity of evidence-based tools for clinicians to inform prescribing and monitoring of safe, effective programming
– Concurrent cognitive impairment related to hepatic encephalopathy
– Lack of self-efficacy

In other chronic disease populations (e.g., cancer, diabetes, cardiac disease, pulmonary hypertension), specific exercise guidelines have been published [14–19]. The American Association for the Study of Liver Diseases has recommended personalized exercise interventions for patients with cirrhosis [3]. Moreover, it is recommended that patients awaiting solid organ transplantation complete exercise training [5, 20–23]. However, the clinical application of exercise programming in cirrhosis has been slow to be integrated into routine care [24–28].

This chapter will briefly review sarcopenia and frailty as they relate to exercise, provide an overview of the literature about the role of exercise in attenuating cirrhosis-related complications, outline a recommendation on how to screen and assess patients before initiating an exercise programme, and offer practical, evidence-based exercise programming considerations and examples pertinent for a range of patient levels. The measurement tools used to assess the impact of an exercise programme on sarcopenia and frailty have been covered in other chapters and will not be reviewed in great detail here.

The operationalization of this chapter's recommendations into a clinical context will vary from centre to centre largely dependent upon the resources available to the clinician. Ideally, all patients will have access to an exercise specialist to guide them through a safety screen, physical assessment, and testing for sarcopenia and frailty culminating in a personalized exercise prescription. Recognizing that this is not a reality for most clinical settings, and recognizing that many primary care physicians also may have a level of discomfort prescribing exercise to patients with cirrhosis, we include resources so that clinicians can provide patients with the basic information required to safely incorporate exercise and increased activity into their lives.

Sarcopenia and Frailty in Relation to Exercise

Sarcopenia

Sarcopenia is defined as the loss of muscle mass, strength, and function leading to adverse health outcomes [29]. Cirrhosis-induced sarcopenia affects 30–50% of end-stage liver disease patients [30–33] and is most prevalent in those with advanced disease [34, 35]. As detailed in previous chapters, the pathology inherent with liver disease directly leads to impaired protein synthesis and muscle contractility as well as increased muscle breakdown. Changes in muscle mass are predictive of mortality, independent of the Model for End-Stage Liver Disease (MELD) score [34]. Evidence suggests that sarcopenia may be reversible in patients with cirrhosis after exercise rehabilitation [36–40].

Frailty

In cirrhosis, physical frailty is characterized by sarcopenia, malnutrition, and physical deconditioning [7]. Frailty is defined in many ways, but for cirrhosis patients, it is likely best defined as a low physiologic reserve and decreased functional status [4], which leaves patients vulnerable to health stressors, leading to physical dependency and death [41]. Roughly 20% of patients with cirrhosis are classified as frail, while 40% are functionally limited [42]. Patients are at an increased risk for falls, fractures, hospitalization, and limited recovery from health complications [42, 43]. Tests of frailty have been correlated with poor clinical outcomes in the cirrhosis population. Newly developed indices of frailty can improve the prognostic ability of conventional status scores including the Model for End-Stage Liver Disease (MELD) and Child-Pugh [42, 44]. Given that frailty in cirrhosis is characterized by declines in multiple systems, the benefits of exercise are of clinical interest to guard against health declines and to improve overall health.

Exercise Training in Cirrhosis

Rationale for Exercise Training

Physical inactivity and sedentary behaviour are strong predictors of poor health outcomes, such as cardiovascular disease, malignancy, musculoskeletal disease, and metabolic disorders [45]. In cirrhosis, physical inactivity exacerbates other existing poor health conditions, such as decreased protein synthesis, hypermetabolism, increased inflammatory cytokines, hyperammonemia, and low testosterone levels [7, 46]. Together, these factors lead to cardiovascular and skeletal muscle deconditioning, characterized by sarcopenia and frailty. Exercise improves skeletal muscle mass, strength, endurance, and cardiopulmonary function. Given that cirrhosis-related impairment is founded on muscle dysfunction and cardiopulmonary deconditioning, exercise is a promising therapy for patients living with liver disease. In other chronic disease populations, exercise-related benefits have been noted independent of the degree of physical deconditioning [47]. As the majority of studies in cirrhosis have been performed in patients with compensated disease, the degree of response expected across the strata of disease severity and physical deconditioning in cirrhosis remains to be evaluated [7, 12].

Safety Concerns

A major concern regarding exercise in cirrhosis is a rise in the hepatic venous pressure gradient (HVPG), an accurate surrogate measure of portal hypertension. Rises in the HVPG put patients at risk for variceal bleeding [48, 49]. An early study found that the HVPG increased in patients with cirrhosis and portal hypertension during exercise [49]. However, a follow-up study showed that, with the use of non-selective beta-blocker medication, a decrease in the HVPG occurs during exercise [48]. Further, evidence from more recent years has failed to prove that patients with cirrhosis and portal hypertension are at increased risk for adverse events when performing exercise [50–52]. Indeed, a randomized controlled trial combining moderate aerobic and resistance exercise training resulted in decreases in the HVPG over the long term [53]. A subsequent randomized controlled trial confirmed this finding using a lifestyle intervention which involved both light-moderate exercise training and diet modification in cirrhosis patients with portal hypertension [36].

A recent meta-analysis of four randomized controlled trials performed with patients awaiting liver transplantation found that exercise programmes do not worsen Child-Pugh or Model for End-stage Liver Disease (MELD) scores [54]. Further, no adverse events occurred during these interventions. Other studies involving non-transplant wait-listed cirrhosis patients have found similar results [7]. The evidence has notable limitations, focusing largely on compensated cirrhosis patients and has included a small sample size per study [Table 7.1]. Future large-scale studies are needed to confirm that exercise is safe, particularly in decompensated patients.

Effects on Sarcopenia and Frailty

Sarcopenia can be assessed by measuring muscle mass using computed tomography (CT) scan, DEXA, or ultrasound each with their inherent advantages and disadvantages. It can also be indirectly measured using bioelectrical impedance or measures of muscle strength, like handgrip strength. Although no studies have evaluated the effects of exercise on muscle mass using cross-sectional imaging (CT or MRI scans), several studies have shown improvements in both muscle mass and strength through supervised and home-based exercise training [50, 51, 55–57]. Improvements in muscle mass can also be complemented by decreases in fat mass [36, 52, 56, 58].

Cardiopulmonary endurance/function is often assessed by either cardiopulmonary exercise testing or the 6-minute walk test. Frailty can be assessed by composite tests, including the Short Physical Performance Battery (comprised of gait speed, balance, and repeated sit to stand) or the Liver Frailty Index (including

Table 7.1 Exercise type and principles from the available literature on the effects of exercise on cirrhosis-related complications

Author (year) Study design Aetiology and Child-Pugh (n)	Intervention and cohorts (n) Duration	Training principles Time, frequency (Adherence %)	Sarcopenia or frailty outcomes
Pattullo (2013) Prospective cohort study Hepatitis C; non-cirrhotic ($n = 10$), Child-Pugh A ($n = 5$) or B ($n = 1$)	Aerobic step count goals ($n = 16$) 12 weeks	Achieve 3000 steps/day above baseline step count, each day, light-moderate (Adherence 100%)	↓ body weight ↓ fat mass (measured by skinfold caliper)
Debette-Gratien (2014) Prospective cohort study Child-Pugh A ($n = 5$), B ($n = 1$), or C ($n = 2$). Mean MELD = 13	Supervised aerobic and resistance exercise ($n = 8$) 12 weeks	Aerobic: 20+ min, 2×/week, moderate intensity Resistance: 20 min, 2×/week, 70–80% max, 3 sets of 8–10 (Adherence "good")	↑ VO$_2$ peak ↑ 6MWT ↑ quadriceps muscle strength
Roman (2014) RCT Child-Pugh A ($n = 7$) or B ($n = 1$). Mean MELD = 9.5	Supervised aerobic and resistance exercise ($n = 8$) standard care ($n = 9$) 12 weeks	Aerobic: 10–15 min increasing to 25–30 min, 3×/week, 60–70% of max Resistance: 5–10 min weights and 10–15 min balance/stretching, intensity based on patient tolerance, last 6 weeks of programme (Adherence: 83.3%)	Between group: n.s. 6MWT n.s. thigh circumference Within group: ↑ 6MWT ↑ thigh circumference
Macias-Rodriguez (2016) RCT Child-Pugh A and B (median = 6). Median MELD = 9	Supervised aerobic and resistance exercise + nutritional therapy ($n = 11$) nutritional therapy ($n = 11$) 14 weeks	Aerobic: 40 min, 3×/week, 60–80% maximum, 14 weeks Resistance: 30 minutes, 3×/week, RPE 12–14 (Adherence: 97%)	Between group: n.s. VO$_2$ peak n.s. body weight
Roman (2016) RCT Previously decompensated cirrhosis (mean Child-Pugh = 5.4, MELD = 8.2)	Supervised aerobic and resistance exercise ($n = 14$) relaxation programme ($n = 9$) 12 weeks	Aerobic: 10–15 min increasing to 25–30 min, 3×/week, 60–70% of max exertion Resistance: 5–10 min weights and 10–15 min balance/stretching, intensity based on patient tolerance, last 6 weeks of programme (Adherence: 93.6%)	Between group: n.s. body composition (measured by dual X-ray absorptiometry) n.s. VO$_2$ peak Within group: n.s. VO$_2$ peak ↑ muscle mass ↓ fat mass (measured by dual X-ray absorptiometry) ↓ timed up and go
Zenith (2016) RCT Child-Pugh A or B (mean = 6.2); mean MELD = 9.7	Supervised aerobic exercise ($n = 9$) standard care ($n = 10$) 8 weeks	30 min increasing to 50 min, 3×/week, 60–80% of max (Adherence: not reported)	Between group: ↑ VO$_2$peak ↑ 6MWT ↑ thigh circumference

(continued)

Table 7.1 (continued)

Author (year) Study design Aetiology and Child-Pugh (n)	Intervention and cohorts (n) Duration	Training principles Time, frequency (Adherence %)	Sarcopenia or frailty outcomes
Berzigotti (2017) Prospective study Child-Pugh A ($n = 46$) or B (≤ 8 pts.; $n = 4$)	Supervised aerobic and resistance exercise ($n = 50$) 16 weeks	60 minute sessions, 1×/ week, RPE 10–12 (Adherence: 88%)	↓ body weight ↓ fat mass (measured by bioelectrical impedance analysis) n.s. muscle mass (measured by dual X-ray absorptiometry) ↑ VO$_2$ peak
Kruger et al. (2018) RCT Child-Pugh A ($n = 14$) or B ($n = 6$), mean MELD = 9.05	Unsupervised aerobic exercise ($n = 19$) standard care ($n = 18$) 8 weeks	30 min increasing to 60 min, 3×/week, 60–80% max, (Adherence: 61.1%)	Between group: n.s. VO$_2$peak Within group: ↑ VO$_2$peak ↑ thigh circumference n.s. thigh muscle thickness

Abbreviations: ↓ significant decrease ($P < 0.05$), ↑ significant increase ($P < 0.05$), *n.s.* non significant, *6MWT* 6-minute walk test, *RCT* randomized controlled trial, *RPE* rating of perceived exertion

balance, repeated sit to stand, and handgrip strength tests). Trials in cirrhosis have shown that exercise training can reduce the risk of falls [56], decrease fatigue [50], and improve exercise capacity as well as physiologic reserve [36, 50–53, 55, 56]. Further research is required to explore the effects of exercise training on additional frailty metrics.

Although the evidence supports the use of exercise training to attenuate sarcopenia and frailty in patients with liver disease, there is much variability in the frequency, intensity, time, and type of exercise showing effects in the literature. Trials have ranged from progressive step goals for aerobic exercise to supervised randomized controlled trials using both aerobic and resistance exercise [Table 7.1]. The exercise parameters vary considerably, yet it is clear that both resistance and aerobic exercise show promise in targeting sarcopenia and frailty in this population.

Pre-exercise Screening and Assessment

There are several recommended pre-exercise health safety screens that should be performed before initiating an exercise programme. As described by Tandon et al., pre-exercise screening can be divided into three categories: cirrhosis-related safety considerations, cardiopulmonary safety screening, and other considerations [12].

Cirrhosis-Related Safety Considerations

The 2015 Baveno VI Consensus recommends that patients with a FibroScan score ≥ 20 kPa or platelet count $\leq 150,000/\mu l$ be screened for varices [59]. Thrombocytopenia (low platelet count) is not a contraindication to exercise per se, but exercises with high risk of injury or falling should be avoided, particularly when platelets are $<20,000/\mu l$. In this situation, it is recommended that the patient is prescribed exercises that incorporate a stable support surface. Patients with high-risk varices or those who have had a previous variceal bleed should be on primary or secondary variceal prophylaxis prior to exercise initiation [60].

Beyond varices, no other cirrhosis-related considerations are absolute contraindications to activity that is low-moderate intensity. However, a number of other complications can impact exercise tolerability, adherence, and efficacy [2]. These include large volume ascites, pedal oedema, and hepatic encephalopathy. Patients with ascites typically experience impaired exercise capacity, and it may be challenging to perform certain exercises. Exercises should be progressed on days where ascites accumulation is minimal. Exercises where pressure is put on the abdomen (i.e. prone exercise or straining abdominal exercises) should be avoided. For patients with overt hepatic encephalopathy, their readiness to engage, understand, and perform exercise directions should be considered. At the very least, a caregiver should be present during exercise sessions. Finally, patients on diuretic therapy may be at risk of volume depletion or hypotension following exercise. These patients should consume water during their exercise sessions, monitor symptoms of dizziness [61], and end the exercise session immediately if they feel faint.

Cardiopulmonary Safety Screening

Prevalence of cardiovascular risk factors in the liver disease population is high, but the link between these factors and events is low. The current American College of Sports Medicine (ACSM) guidelines recommends "medical clearance" for those starting a moderate intensity programme with signs, symptoms, or a history of cardiovascular, metabolic, or renal disease. Medical clearance should be obtained if the patient presents with any of the following signs or symptoms: chest discomfort with exertion, unreasonable breathlessness, dizziness, fainting, blackouts, heart palpitations, lower limb claudication, or heart murmur [62]. Likewise, medical clearance should be obtained if the patient has a history of the following: heart attack, heart surgery, cardiac catheterization or coronary angioplasty, pacemaker, heart valve disease, heart failure, heart transplantation, congenital heart disease, diabetes, or renal disease. The procedure for medical clearance is left up to the clinician.

ACSM defines moderate intensity as 40–59% heart rate reserve, a VO_2 reserve of 3.0–5.9 metabolic equivalent (METs), or a rating of perceived exertion (RPE) of 12–13 on the 6–20 Borg scale or 5–6 on the 0–10 scale.

In our opinions, asymptomatic patients wanting to pursue low-moderate activity should adhere to a "start low and progress slow" approach to training [7] and do not require a pre-participation cardiac clearance [63]. In symptomatic patients, it may be beneficial to conduct additional testing, including cardiopulmonary exercise testing. At the very least, approval for participation should be obtained from the patient's clinician prior to exercise training initiation.

Other Safety Considerations

Patients should be asked if they experience exertional symptoms that limit their activities of daily living. This can help identify factors (e.g. muscle cramping, claudication, joint pain, restricted range of motion) that may require exercise programme modification or additional therapeutic intervention before exercise initiation [19]. During physical performance assessments, fall risk can be assessed using balance testing included in the Short Performance Physical Battery or Liver Frailty Index. Those at high risk of falling should perform supported activity (e.g. seated or standing with a support). Caregiver supervision is also recommended. If the patient has additional comorbidities, the recent ACSM guidelines should be consulted for safety implications [19]. Lastly, for patients who are identified as having an increased risk of falling, careful consideration is needed before progressing the patient to unsupported exercises.

Exercise Prescription

Encourage Non-exercise Activity Thermogenesis (NEAT)

Describing the simple principles of NEAT to patients is a way to encourage them to increase the amount of physical activity that they do outside of scheduled exercise programming. NEAT activities involve making the "less convenient" choice, with a goal to increase activity, for example, stepping in place while watching TV instead of sitting on the couch, climbing stairs instead of taking the elevator, or parking in a spot further away from their destination instead of the closest spot [64].

Scheduled Exercise Programming

On the basis of the available literature, 30- to 60-minute sessions of both aerobic and resistance training are recommended with the goal being to achieve 150+ minutes/week of moderate intensity exercise. For an exercise training programme to be effective, it should last at least 3 months to facilitate physiological gains [65].

Table 7.2 Aerobic and resistance exercise training recommendations

	Exercise targets	
Characteristics	Aerobic exercise	Resistance exercise
Goal	Increase endurance, stamina, and energy	Increase muscle mass, strength, and function
Frequency	3–7 days/week	2–4 days/week
Intensity	2–3 on the 10-point Borg scale Increase to 3–5 on the 10-point Borg scale	1 to 3 sets of 10–15 Increase sets to 2 and then to 3
Time	2–10 or more minutes/session Increase to 30–60 minutes/session Goal: 150 minutes/week	3–4 exercises/session Increase to 8 exercises/session Goal: 120 minutes/week
Type	Walking, cycling, elliptical, water aerobics, dancing	Progressive free weight or band resistance

Resistance exercise should always be prescribed as it has an important role in preventing or attenuating muscle loss. Aerobic exercise compounds the effects of resistance exercise by improving physiological reserve and functioning of patients. Flexibility and balance exercise can complement these two primary training modes by maintaining joint function and balance. Table 7.2 outlines the ideal frequency, intensity, time (duration), and type of exercise that are effective in targeting sarcopenia and frailty and explain how exercise can be progressed for patients with liver disease. These recommendations are adapted from Tandon et al. [12].

Aerobic Exercise

Aerobic exercise plays an important role in targeting sarcopenia and frailty in the cirrhosis population. When progressing in aerobic exercise training, it is easiest to start by increasing the frequency at which the exercise sessions are being done. If short sessions are well tolerated, the duration of sessions can be slowly progressed in small increments (e.g., ~2 minutes at a time). If further progression is required, intensity of exercise can then be increased.

Resistance Exercise

Resistance exercise poses as a unique strategy that will specifically target and build musculature, thus targeting both sarcopenia and frailty in this population.

There are a countless number of resistance/weights exercises that patients could choose from to enact physiological gains. Table 7.3 outlines resistance exercises that are appropriate for this patient population. Together, these series of exercises target all major muscle groups in the body that have been adapted from Tandon

Table 7.3 Proposed muscle strengthening and resistance exercises

Target	Level	Exercise
Shoulders	Level 1	Seated lateral arm raise
	Level 2	Standing lateral arm raise
	Level 3	Lateral arm raise in ¼ squat
Chest	Level 1	Seated pec fly
	Level 2	Standing pec fly
	Level 3	Supine pec fly
Back	Level 1	Seated row
	Level 2	Reverse fly
	Level 3	Dumbbell row
Arms	Level 1	Seated biceps curl
	Level 2	Standing biceps curl
	Level 3	Biceps curl in ¼ squat
Arms	Level 1	Seated triceps extension
	Level 2	Triceps kickback
	Level 3	Triceps pressdown in ¼ squat
Thigh	Level 1	Seated march
	Level 2	Sit to stand
	Level 3	Split squat
Thigh	Level 1	Seated hamstring curl
	Level 2	Wall squat
	Level 3	Wall sit
Glutes/low back	Level 1	Bridging
	Level 2	Bridging with band
	Level 3	Bridging with leg raise
Lower leg/thigh	Level 1	Calf raise
	Level 2	Calf raise on step
	Level 3	Plie squat
Balance	Level 1	Tree pose
	Level 2	Standing single leg raise
	Level 3	Single leg alphabet
Flexibility	Hamstrings	
	Quadriceps	
	Lower leg	
	Glutes	
	Triceps	
	Shoulders	
	Chest	

et al. [12]. Patients can progress slowly through these exercises with guidance from the recommendations in Table 7.2. When choosing which exercise level a patient should start their programme at, the Short Physical Performance Battery [66] or Liver Frailty Index [44] provides useful information, as does a 6-minute walk test. The subjective, clinician-assigned Clinical Frailty Scale (CFS) can also be used but would not be sufficiently sensitive to monitor changes over time [67, 68]. The starting level of exercise remains at the specialist's judgement based upon the information gathered by a detailed assessment. If in doubt, patients should be started at

Level 1. If scores on the Short Physical Performance Battery are above 4 or if either the Liver Frailty Index or Clinical Frailty Scale demonstrates that the patient is not frail, then the patient may be able to progress quickly from Levels 1 to 2 or even start at Level 2.

Flexibility and Balance

Flexibility and balance are important components of exercise training for frail patients. Completing light stretching following each exercise session will improve joint mobility while helping patients remain mobile and functional. Cirrhosis patients are at an increased risk of falling due to a variety of complications associated with liver disease including muscle weakness, hepatic encephalopathy, and autonomic dysfunction [6, 42, 43]. Balance training can specifically target the increased fall risk observed in frail patients. Flexibility and balance training should be performed at least 2 days per week and can be included as a cool-down following an exercise session [Table 7.3]. Stretching should be to the point of feeling tightness or tension and involve slow, controlled movement, holding the end points. Patients should aim to stretch each major muscle group for 60 seconds by completing 2–3 sets of 20–30-second holds. Exercises should challenge the patient's balance, but not put them at undue risk of falling. Dynamic balance exercises can be more favourable than static ones as they are more functional, but patients should begin with a static, two foot balance exercise, with a sturdy support nearby.

Additional Considerations

–   All exercise sessions should involve an active warm-up (~5 minutes) and end with a cool-down phase (5–10 minutes), a good opportunity to perform flexibility and balance exercises.
–   Patients should be taught to evaluate how they are feeling before, during, and after each exercise session. If they feel tired or unwell beforehand, they may choose to perform the exercises at either a lower intensity or do less repetitions. If muscle soreness is excessive or persists beyond 48 hours after a session, intensity should be decreased, and rest for 1–2 days should be allowed.
–   Patients should stop exercising if they notice a racing or abnormal pulse, fever, sudden shortness of breath, sudden severe fatigue, chest pain, dizziness, headache or blurred vision, nausea, or confusion, or disorientation.
–   In other chronic disease populations, exercise programming paired with nutritional intervention achieved better health outcomes than exercise alone [69]. The majority of exercise studies in cirrhosis have been performed in concert with a nutritional intervention. As such, it is suggested to combine exercise and nutritional interventions to achieve the greatest benefits [12].

SAMPLE LEVEL 1 EXERCISE PROGRAM – each activity can be done starting from 1 set of 10-15 x increasing to 2 and then 3 sets as tolerated

Target	Exercise Name	Images	Description
Shoulders	Seated Lateral Arm Raise		Equipment: Dumbbells & Chair Description: Sitting tall in a chair, grasp a dumbbell in each hand. With your arms straight, raise the dumbbells up to shoulder height, then lower them back down. Repeat this motion as prescribed.
Chest	Seated Pec Fly		Equipment: Band & Chair Description: Sitting in chair with band secured behind, grab hold of each end of the band. Begin with arms at shoulder height to your sides. Bring arms directly in front of you. Repeat motion as prescribed.

Table 7.4 Sample exercise routines – Level 1 (seated, easiest), Level 2, and Level 3. Sample Level 1 exercise programme – each activity can be done starting from 1 set of 10–15× increasing to 2 and then 3 sets as tolerated

			Equipment: Band & Chair Description: Sitting in chair with band secured in front of you just below shoulder height, grab hold of each end of the band. Begin with arms straight in front of you. Pull band backward, squeezing shoulder blades together. Repeat motion as prescribed.
Back	Seated Row		
Arms	Seated Biceps Curl		Equipment: Dumbbells & Chair Description: Sit in a chair with a dumbbell in each hand. With elbows close to your sides, curl the weights up to shoulder height. Then slowly return them back to the starting position. Repeat motion as prescribed.

Table 7.4 (continued)

Table 7.4 (continued)

| Arms | Seated Triceps Extension | | Equipment: Dumbbell & Chair

Description: sitting in chair and begin by bending elbow and raise towards ceiling. Keep elbow in position with the guidance of the other hand. Extend elbow, raising the dumbbell to the ceiling, then return to the starting position. Repeat motion with each arm as prescribed. |
| Thigh | Seated March | | Equipment: Chair

Description: Start with your feet flat sitting in a chair. Raise one knee and opposing arm at the same time. Lower them back to the starting position as you raise the other leg and arm. Repeat this pattern at a comfortable pace for a full minute. Complete twice. |

				Equipment: Band
Thigh	Seated Hamstring Curl			Description: Secure a band in front of you and sit tall in a chair. Wrap the band and one foot with your knee straight. With your knees side-by-side, curl your lower leg back under the chair then slowly return to the starting position. Repeat as prescribed for each leg.
Glutes/Low Back	Bridging			Equipment: Mat Description: Begin by lying on your back, knees bent and feet flat on the floor. Squeezing your core and buttock, lift your hips off the mat and slowly return them down. Repeat motion as prescribed.

Table 7.4 (continued)

Table 7.4 (continued)

Lower Leg	Calf Raise		Equipment: none Description: Either standing on flat ground or near a supportive surface, begin by pressing through the balls of your feet to lift your heels as high as you can. Slowly return your heel back to the ground. Repeat motion as prescribed.
Balance	Tree Pose		Equipment: Chair Description: Find a sturdy object like a chair or counter. With light pressure on the surface, raise one leg up so it touches the other leg. Hold your balance on one leg using the sturdy surface as needed. Hold for set amount of time and repeat with each leg as prescribed.

LEVEL 2 EXERCISE PROGRAM -- each activity can be done starting from 1 set of 10-15 x increasing to 2 and then 3 sets as tolerated

Target	Exercise Name	Images	Description
Shoulders	Standing Lateral Arm Raise		Equipment: Dumbbells Description: Grasp a dumbbell in each hand. With your arms straight, raise the dumbbells up to shoulder height, then lower them back down. Repeat this motion as prescribed.
Chest	Standing Pec Fly		Equipment: Band Description: Loop a band behind your back and grab hold of each end of the band. Begin with arms at shoulder height to your sides. Bring arms directly in front of you. Repeat motion as prescribed.

Table 7.4 (continued)

Table 7.4 (continued)

| Back | Reverse Fly | | Equipment: Band

Description: Grab hold of a band just less than shoulder width apart. Raise the band in front of you to shoulder height. Starting with your arms straight, pull the band apart, arcing your arms backwards, squeezing your shoulder blades together. Return to the starting position and repeat the motion as prescribed. |
| Arms | Standing Biceps Curl | | Equipment: Dumbbells

Description: Grab a dumbbell in each hand. With elbows close to your sides, curl the weights up to shoulder height. Then slowly return them back to the starting position. Repeat motion as prescribed. |

| Arms | Tricep Kickback | | Equipment: Dumbbell

Description: On all four, grab a dumbbell in one hand. With your elbow tucked to your side, extend your forearm straight back, keeping your elbow and shoulder in the same position. Lower back to the starting position, and repeat as prescribed for each arm. |
| Thigh | Sit to Stand | | Equipment: Chair

Description: Sit in a chair. To make this exercise harder, you can choose to add dumbbells in each hand. With a slight forward lean, stand up, then sit back down again. Repeat the motion as prescribed. |

Table 7.4 (continued)

Table 7.4 (continued)

Thigh	Wall Squat		Equipment: Wall Description: Stand about a foot away from the wall with your back flat against the wall. Slowly squat down, keeping your back against the wall. Once your knees reach 90 degrees, slowly rise back up. Repeat the motion as prescribed.
Glutes/Low Back	Bridging with Band		Equipment: Band & Mat Description: Tie a band around your thighs just above the knee and lie on your back, knees bent and feet flat on the floor. Squeezing your core and buttock, lift your hips off the mat and slowly return them down. While doing this, keep the band from bringing your knees inward. Repeat motion as prescribed.

| Lower Leg | Calf Raise on Step | | Equipment: Step

Description: Stand on the edge of a step, with just the forefront of your feet on the step. Rise up onto your toes, then lower down till your heels are below the step. Repeat this motion as prescribed. |
|---|---|---|---|
| Balance | Standing Single Leg Raise | | Equipment: none

Description: Stand with your hands on your hips with one foot flat, the other toe pointed. Slowly raise the non-planted leg up, and return back to the ground. Slightly tap the ground, and repeat the motion from the beginning. Repeat motion as prescribed for each leg. |

Table 7.4 (continued)

Table 7.4 (continued)

LEVEL 3 EXERCISE PROGRAM — each activity can be done starting from 1 set of 10-15 x increasing to 2 and then 3 sets as tolerated

Target	Exercise Name	Images	Description
Shoulders	Lateral Arm Raise in ¼ Squat		Equipment: Dumbbells Description: Grasp a dumbbell in each hand. Squat down slightly so your knees are moderately bent. With your arms straight, raise the dumbbells up to shoulder height, then lower them back down. Repeat this motion as prescribed.
Chest	Supine Chest Fly		Equipment: Dumbbell & Mat Description: Lay on your back, knees bent, feet flat on the floor. Begin with the dumbbell directly upward. Slowly lower the dumbbells to your side, then bring them in an arc-like motion back to the top. Repeat this motion as prescribed.

Back	Dumbbell Row		Equipment: Dumbbell Description: On all four, grab a dumbbell in one hand. Lift the weight straight up off the ground, leading with your elbow. Lower the weight back down. Repeat motion as prescribed.
Arms	Biceps Curl in ¼ Squat		Equipment: Dumbbells Description: Grab a dumbbell in each hand. Bend your knees until you have a moderate bend, then maintain that position for the full exercise. With elbows close to your sides, curl the weights up to shoulder height. Then slowly return them back to the starting position. Repeat motion as prescribed.

Table 7.4 (continued)

Table 7.4 (continued)

Arms	Tricep Preessdown in ¼ Squat		Equipment: Band Description: Secure a band up high. Grab hold of each end of the band and bend your knees into a quarter squat. With your elbows tucked to your sides, extend your elbows down then slowly return back up to the starting position. Repeat motion as prescribed.
Thigh	Split Squat		Equipment: none Description: Stagger your stance so your feet are 2-3 feet apart. With slightly more weight on your front foot, lower your body down, leading with your back knee. Just before touching the floor, come back up. Repeat this motion as prescribed with each foot forward. Be sure to keep your chest up throughout the exercise.

| Thigh | Wall Sit | | Equipment: Wall

Description: Stand about a foot away from a sturdy wall. Lean backward into the wall so your back is flat, then slowly lower yourself until your knees are between 120 and 90 degrees. Hold your body here for 30-45 seconds. Repeat as prescribed. |
| Glutes/Low Back | Bridging with Leg Raise | | Equipment: Mat

Description: This exercise is similar to the traditional glute bridge (see level 1 exercise) with one additional component. Starting on your back, lift your hips up off the mat. Once raised, raise one leg up into the chair. Return your foot to the floor then lower your hips back down. Repeat motion as prescribed. |

Table 7.4 (continued)

Table 7.4 (continued)

Thigh & Lower Leg	Plie Squat			Equipment: Dumbbell Description: Stand with feet shoulder width apart, toes pointed outward. With a dumbbell in your hands directly in front of you, squat down and back up. Repeat motion as prescribed.
Balance	Single Leg Alphabet			Equipment: none Description: Standing on one leg, try to draw each letter of the alphabet with your other leg. Try to get through the whole alphabet without losing your balance. Repeat with each leg the prescribed number of repetitions.

Conclusion

Overall, with appropriate pre-exercise screening and safety considerations, exercise shows promise as a safe and effective way to attenuate declines in function in cirrhosis patients. Future larger-scale randomized controlled trials in the area will allow us to establish clinical safety and determine the degree of benefit across the strata of liver disease severity and physical deconditioning. As with other chronic diseases, exercise therapy in cirrhosis will have an effect in rebuilding muscle mass and restoring functional capacity. Making exercise and nutritional intervention a routine part of cirrhosis care will require additional large-scale clinical trials supporting safety and efficacy, formal guidelines in the area, and the enthusiastic backing of clinicians to champion these interventions. We have concluded the chapter with sample exercise routines for Level 1, 2, and 3 participants [Table 7.4], increasing in difficulty with each level. More exercises and routines will be updated and available at the authors' website resource – www.wellnesstoolbox.ca.

References

1. Dasarathy S. Consilience in sarcopenia of cirrhosis. J Cachexia Sarcopenia Muscle. 2012;3:225–37.
2. Jones JC, Coombes JS, Macdonald GA. Exercise capacity and muscle strength in patients with cirrhosis. Liver Transpl. 2012;18:146–51.
3. Chen H-W, Dunn MA. Arresting frailty and sarcopenia in cirrhosis: future prospects. Clinical Liver Disease. 2018;11:52–7.
4. Trivedi HD, Tapper EB. Interventions to improve physical function and prevent adverse events in cirrhosis. Gastroenterol Rep (Oxf). 2018;6:13–20.
5. van den Berg-Emons R, Kazemier G, van Ginneken B, Nieuwenhuijsen C, Tilanus H, Stam H. Fatigue, level of everyday physical activity and quality of life after liver transplantation. J Rehabil Med. 2006;38:124–9.
6. Ezaz G, Murphy SL, Mellinger J, Tapper EB. Increased morbidity and mortality associated with falls among patients with cirrhosis. Am J Med. 2018;131:645–650.e642.
7. Duarte-Rojo A, Ruiz-Margáin A, Montaño-Loza AJ, Macías-Rodríguez RU, Ferrando A, Kim WR. Exercise and physical activity for patients with end-stage liver disease: improving functional status and sarcopenia while on the transplant waiting list. Liver Transpl. 2018;24:122–39.
8. Painter P. Exercise for patients with chronic disease: physician responsibility. Curr Sports Med Rep. 2003;2:173–80.
9. Wallen MP, Skinner TL, Pavey TG, Hall A, Macdonald GA, Coombes JS. Safety, adherence and efficacy of exercise training in solid-organ transplant candidates: a systematic review. Transplant Rev (Orlando). 2016;30:218–26.
10. Dunn MA, Josbeno DA, Schmotzer AR, Tevar AD, DiMartini AF, Landsittel DP, et al. The gap between clinically assessed physical performance and objective physical activity in liver transplant candidates. Liver Transpl. 2016;22:1324–32.
11. Ney M, Gramlich L, Mathiesen V, Bailey RJ, Haykowsky M, Ma M, et al. Patient-perceived barriers to lifestyle interventions in cirrhosis. Saudi J Gastroenterol. 2017;23:97–104.
12. Tandon P, Ismond KP, Riess K, Duarte-Rojo A, Al-Judaibi B, Dunn MA, et al. Exercise in cirrhosis: translating evidence and experience to practice. J Hepatol. 2018;69:1164–77.

13. Malini FM, Lourenço RA, Lopes CS. Prevalence of fear of falling in older adults, and its associations with clinical, functional and psychosocial factors: the frailty in Brazilian older people-Rio de Janeiro study. Geriatr Gerontol Int. 2016;16:336–44.
14. Schmitz KH, Courneya KS, Matthews C, Demark-Wahnefried W, Galvão DA, Pinto BM, et al. American College of Sports Medicine roundtable on exercise guidelines for cancer survivors. Med Sci Sports Exerc. 2010;42:1409–26.
15. Sigal RJ, Armstrong MJ, Bacon SL, Boulé NG, Dasgupta K, Kenny GP, et al. Physical activity and diabetes. Can J Diabetes. 2018;42(Suppl 1):S54–63.
16. Thomas RJ, King M, Lui K, Oldridge N, Piña IL, Spertus J, et al. AACVPR/ACCF/AHA 2010 Update: Performance Measures on Cardiac Rehabilitation for Referral to Cardiac Rehabilitation/Secondary Prevention Services Endorsed by the American College of Chest Physicians, the American College of Sports Medicine, the American Physical Therapy Association, the Canadian Association of Cardiac Rehabilitation, the Clinical Exercise Physiology Association, the European Association for Cardiovascular Prevention and Rehabilitation, the Inter-American Heart Foundation, the National Association of Clinical Nurse Specialists, the Preventive Cardiovascular Nurses Association, and the Society of Thoracic Surgeons. J Am Coll Cardiol. 2010;56:1159–67.
17. Galie N, Manes A, Palazzini M. Exercise training in pulmonary hypertension: improving performance but waiting for outcome. Eur Heart J. 2016;37:45–8.
18. Wickerson L, Rozenberg D, Janaudis-Ferreira T, Deliva R, Lo V, Beauchamp G, et al. Physical rehabilitation for lung transplant candidates and recipients: an evidence-informed clinical approach. World J Transplant. 2016;6:517–31.
19. Medicine ACoS, Moore GE, Durstine JL, Painter PL. ACSM's exercise management for persons with chronic diseases and disabilities. 4th ed. Champaign: Human Kinetics; 2016.
20. Didsbury M, McGee RG, Tong A, Craig JC, Chapman JR, Chadban S, et al. Exercise training in solid organ transplant recipients: a systematic review and meta-analysis. Transplantation. 2013;95:679–87.
21. Griffith K, Wenzel J, Shang J, Thompson C, Stewart K, Mock V. Impact of a walking intervention on cardiorespiratory fitness, self-reported physical function, and pain in patients undergoing treatment for solid tumors. Cancer. 2009;115:4874–84.
22. Kjaer M, Beyer N, Secher NH. Exercise and organ transplantation. Scand J Med Sci Sports. 1999;9:1–14.
23. Mathur S, Janaudis-Ferreira T, Wickerson L, Singer LG, Patcai J, Rozenberg D, et al. Meeting report: consensus recommendations for a research agenda in exercise in solid organ transplantation. Am J Transplant. 2014;14:2235–45.
24. Anastácio LR, Ferreira LG, Ribeiro HS, Liboredo JC, Lima AS, Correia MI. Metabolic syndrome after liver transplantation: prevalence and predictive factors. Nutrition. 2011;27:931–7.
25. Krasnoff JB, Vintro AQ, Ascher NL, Bass NM, Paul SM, Dodd MJ, et al. A randomized trial of exercise and dietary counseling after liver transplantation. Am J Transplant. 2006;6:1896–905.
26. Bergasa NV, Mehlman J, Bir K. Aerobic exercise: a potential therapeutic intervention for patients with liver disease. Med Hypotheses. 2004;62:935–41.
27. Galant LH, Forgiarini LA, Dias AS. The aerobic capacity and muscle strength are correlated in candidates for liver transplantation. Arq Gastroenterol. 2011;48:86–8.
28. Foroncewicz B, Mucha K, Szparaga B, Raczyńska J, Ciszek M, Pilecki T, et al. Rehabilitation and 6-minute walk test after liver transplantation. Transplant Proc. 2011;43:3021–4.
29. Cederholm T, Barazzoni R, Austin P, Ballmer P, Biolo G, Bischoff SC, et al. ESPEN guidelines on definitions and terminology of clinical nutrition. Clin Nutr. 2017;36:49–64.
30. Vintro AQ, Krasnoff JB, Painter P. Roles of nutrition and physical activity in musculoskeletal complications before and after liver transplantation. AACN Clin Issues. 2002;13:333–47.
31. Painter P. The importance of exercise training in rehabilitation of patients with end-stage renal disease. Am J Kidney Dis. 1994;24:S2–9; discussion S31–32.
32. Montano-Loza AJ, Meza-Junco J, Prado CM, Lieffers JR, Baracos VE, Bain VG, et al. Muscle wasting is associated with mortality in patients with cirrhosis. Clin Gastroenterol Hepatol. 2012;10:166–173.e161.

33. Golse N, Bucur PO, Ciacio O, Pittau G, Sa Cunha A, Adam R, et al. A new definition of sarcopenia in patients with cirrhosis undergoing liver transplantation. Liver Transpl. 2017;23:143–54.
34. van Vugt JL, Levolger S, de Bruin RW, van Rosmalen J, Metselaar HJ, IJzermans JN. Systematic review and meta-analysis of the impact of computed tomography-assessed skeletal muscle mass on outcome in patients awaiting or undergoing liver transplantation. Am J Transplant. 2016;16:2277–92.
35. Carey EJ, Lai JC, Wang CW, Dasarathy S, Lobach I, Montano-Loza AJ, et al. A multi-center study to define sarcopenia in patients with end-stage liver disease. Liver Transpl. 2017;23:625–33.
36. Berzigotti A, Albillos A, Villanueva C, Genescá J, Ardevol A, Augustín S, et al. Effects of an intensive lifestyle intervention program on portal hypertension in patients with cirrhosis and obesity: the SportDiet study. Hepatology. 2017;65:1293–305.
37. Vandenborne K, Elliott MA, Walter GA, Abdus S, Okereke E, Shaffer M, et al. Longitudinal study of skeletal muscle adaptations during immobilization and rehabilitation. Muscle Nerve. 1998;21:1006–12.
38. Herbison GJ, Talbot JM. Muscle atrophy during space flight: research needs and opportunities. Physiologist. 1985;28:520–7.
39. Osawa Y, Azuma K, Tabata S, Katsukawa F, Ishida H, Oguma Y, et al. Effects of 16-week high-intensity interval training using upper and lower body ergometers on aerobic fitness and morphological changes in healthy men: a preliminary study. Open Access J Sports Med. 2014;5:257–65.
40. Hayashi F, Matsumoto Y, Momoki C, Yuikawa M, Okada G, Hamakawa E, et al. Physical inactivity and insufficient dietary intake are associated with the frequency of sarcopenia in patients with compensated viral liver cirrhosis. Hepatol Res. 2013;43:1264–75.
41. Morley JE, Vellas B, van Kan GA, Anker SD, Bauer JM, Bernabei R, et al. Frailty consensus: a call to action. J Am Med Dir Assoc. 2013;14:392–7.
42. Lai JC, Feng S, Terrault NA, Lizaola B, Hayssen H, Covinsky K. Frailty predicts waitlist mortality in liver transplant candidates. Am J Transplant. 2014;14:1870–9.
43. Tandon P, Tangri N, Thomas L, Zenith L, Shaikh T, Carbonneau M, et al. A rapid bedside screen to predict unplanned hospitalization and death in outpatients with cirrhosis: a prospective evaluation of the clinical frailty scale. Am J Gastroenterol. 2016;111:1759–67.
44. Lai JC, Covinsky KE, Dodge JL, Boscardin WJ, Segev DL, Roberts JP, et al. Development of a novel frailty index to predict mortality in patients with end-stage liver disease. Hepatology. 2017;66:564–74.
45. Biswas A, Oh PI, Faulkner GE, Bajaj RR, Silver MA, Mitchell MS, et al. Sedentary time and its association with risk for disease incidence, mortality, and hospitalization in adults: a systematic review and meta-analysis. Ann Intern Med. 2015;162:123–32.
46. Tandon P, Raman M, Mourtzakis M, Merli M. A practical approach to nutritional screening and assessment in cirrhosis. Hepatology. 2017;65:1044–57.
47. Stout NL, Baima J, Swisher AK, Winters-Stone KM, Welsh J. A systematic review of exercise systematic reviews in the Cancer literature (2005-2017). PM R. 2017;9:S347–84.
48. Bandi JC, García-Pagán JC, Escorsell A, François E, Moitinho E, Rodés J, et al. Effects of propranolol on the hepatic hemodynamic response to physical exercise in patients with cirrhosis. Hepatology. 1998;28:677–82.
49. García-Pagàn JC, Santos C, Barberá JA, Luca A, Roca J, Rodriguez-Roisin R, et al. Physical exercise increases portal pressure in patients with cirrhosis and portal hypertension. Gastroenterology. 1996;111:1300–6.
50. Zenith L, Meena N, Ramadi A, Yavari M, Harvey A, Carbonneau M, et al. Eight weeks of exercise training increases aerobic capacity and muscle mass and reduces fatigue in patients with cirrhosis. Clin Gastroenterol Hepatol. 2014;12:1920–1926.e1922.
51. Román E, Torrades MT, Nadal MJ, Cárdenas G, Nieto JC, Vidal S, et al. Randomized pilot study: effects of an exercise programme and leucine supplementation in patients with cirrhosis. Dig Dis Sci. 2014;59:1966–75.

52. Pattullo V, Duarte-Rojo A, Soliman W, Vargas-Vorackova F, Sockalingam S, Fantus IG, et al. A 24-week dietary and physical activity lifestyle intervention reduces hepatic insulin resistance in the obese with chronic hepatitis C. Liver Int. 2013;33:410–9.
53. Macías-Rodríguez RU, Ilarraza-Lomelí H, Ruiz-Margáin A, Ponce-de-León-Rosales S, Vargas-Voráčková F, García-Flores O, et al. Changes in hepatic venous pressure gradient induced by physical exercise in cirrhosis: results of a pilot randomized open clinical trial. Clin Transl Gastroenterol. 2016;7:e180.
54. Brustia R, Savier E, Scatton O. Physical exercise in cirrhotic patients: towards prehabilitation on waiting list for liver transplantation. A systematic review and meta-analysis. Clin Res Hepatol Gastroenterol. 2018;42:205–15.
55. Debette-Gratien M, Tabouret T, Antonini MT, Dalmay F, Carrier P, Legros R, et al. Personalized adapted physical activity before liver transplantation: acceptability and results. Transplantation. 2015;99:145–50.
56. Román E, García-Galcerán C, Torrades T, Herrera S, Marín A, Doñate M, et al. Effects of an exercise programme on functional capacity, body composition and risk of falls in patients with cirrhosis: a randomized clinical trial. PLoS One. 2016;11:e0151652.
57. Hiraoka A, Michitaka K, Kiguchi D, Izumoto H, Ueki H, Kaneto M, et al. Efficacy of branched-chain amino acid supplementation and walking exercise for preventing sarcopenia in patients with liver cirrhosis. Eur J Gastroenterol Hepatol. 2017;29:1416–23.
58. Konishi I, Hiasa Y, Tokumoto Y, Abe M, Furukawa S, Toshimitsu K, et al. Aerobic exercise improves insulin resistance and decreases body fat and serum levels of leptin in patients with hepatitis C virus. Hepatol Res. 2011;41:928–35.
59. de Franchis R, Faculty BV. Expanding consensus in portal hypertension: report of the Baveno VI consensus workshop: stratifying risk and individualizing care for portal hypertension. J Hepatol. 2015;63:743–52.
60. Garcia-Tsao G, Abraldes JG, Berzigotti A, Bosch J. Portal hypertensive bleeding in cirrhosis: risk stratification, diagnosis, and management: 2016 practice guidance by the American association for the study of liver diseases. Hepatology. 2017;65:310–35.
61. Sawka MN, Burke LM, Eichner ER, Maughan RJ, Montain SJ, Stachenfeld NS, et al. American College of Sports Medicine position stand. Exercise and fluid replacement. Med Sci Sports Exerc. 2007;39:377–90.
62. Riebe D, Franklin BA, Thompson PD, Garber CE, Whitfield GP, Magal M, et al. Updating ACSM's recommendations for exercise Preparticipation health screening. Med Sci Sports Exerc. 2015;47:2473–9.
63. Colberg SR, Sigal RJ, Yardley JE, Riddell MC, Dunstan DW, Dempsey PC, et al. Physical activity/exercise and diabetes: a position statement of the American Diabetes Association. Diabetes Care. 2016;39:2065–79.
64. Villablanca PA, Alegria JR, Mookadam F, Holmes DR, Wright RS, Levine JA. Nonexercise activity thermogenesis in obesity management. Mayo Clin Proc. 2015;90:509–19.
65. Chodzko-Zajko WJ, Proctor DN, Fiatarone Singh MA, Minson CT, Nigg CR, Salem GJ, et al. American College of Sports Medicine position stand. Exercise and physical activity for older adults. Med Sci Sports Exerc. 2009;41:1510–30.
66. Treacy D, Hassett L. The short physical performance battery. J Physiother. 2018;64:61.
67. Rockwood K, Song X, MacKnight C, Bergman H, Hogan DB, McDowell I, et al. A global clinical measure of fitness and frailty in elderly people. CMAJ. 2005;173:489–95.
68. Searle SD, Mitnitski A, Gahbauer EA, Gill TM, Rockwood K. A standard procedure for creating a frailty index. BMC Geriatr. 2008;8:24.
69. Fiatarone MA, O'Neill EF, Ryan ND, Clements KM, Solares GR, Nelson ME, et al. Exercise training and nutritional supplementation for physical frailty in very elderly people. N Engl J Med. 1994;330:1769–75.

Part II
The Challenges

Chapter 8
Sex-, Age-, and Ethnicity-Dependent Variation in Body Composition: Can There Be a Single Cutoff?

Maria Cristina Gonzalez, Jingjie Xiao, and Ilana Roitman Disi

Introduction

Body composition measurements are an essential component for the evaluation of nutritional and health status in clinical assessment [1]. The association between body fat and health risks is well known, and body mass index (BMI) is commonly used as a marker of increased body fat. The progress of the techniques to analyze body composition has enabled the accurate quantification of its compartments and increased the importance of body composition as a key determinant not only of health but also as a prognostic factor in several clinical conditions. It is also highlighted that muscle mass is the major determinant of negative outcomes in clinical settings [2]. Although BMI has a good correlation with increased body fat at the population level, there are several conditions, like aging or chronic diseases, where low muscle can occur in obese individuals (sarcopenic obesity), and BMI alone cannot identify it [3]. For this reason, weight and BMI are not enough to identify body composition abnormalities at the individual level, particularly in clinical situations.

M. C. Gonzalez (✉)
Catholic University of Pelotas, Pelotas, RS, Brazil

J. Xiao
Department of Agricultural, Food and Nutritional Science, University of Alberta, Edmonton, AB, Canada

Division of Palliative Care Medicine, Department of Oncology, University of Alberta, Edmonton, AB, Canada

Covenant Health Palliative Institute, Edmonton, AB, Canada
e-mail: jingjie1@ualberta.ca

I. R. Disi
Division of Anesthesia, Faculty of Medicine Foundation of the University of Sao Paulo, Cancer Institute of Sao Paulo, Sao Paulo, SP, Brazil
e-mail: ilana.roitman@usp.br

© Springer Nature Switzerland AG 2020
P. Tandon, A. J. Montano-Loza (eds.), *Frailty and Sarcopenia in Cirrhosis*,
https://doi.org/10.1007/978-3-030-26226-6_8

119

Several body composition methods can be used to assess muscle mass compartments. Depending on the employed technology, different terminologies can be used to identify muscularity. The most commonly used terms are skeletal muscle mass [from computerized tomography (CT) and magnetic resonance imaging (MRI)], appendicular lean mass or appendicular lean soft tissue, a marker of appendicular skeletal muscle mass [from dual X-ray absorptiometry (DXA)], and fat-free mass [from DXA, air displacement plethysmography (ADP), and bioelectrical impedance analysis (BIA)] [2]. In all these assessments, muscle mass is usually adjusted for body size, using height squared to create an index (cm^2/m^2 or kg/m^2).

Determinants of Body Composition Variability

There are several determinants of body composition variability (Fig. 8.1), and the most studied are: sex, age, and ethnicity. The objective of the current review was to

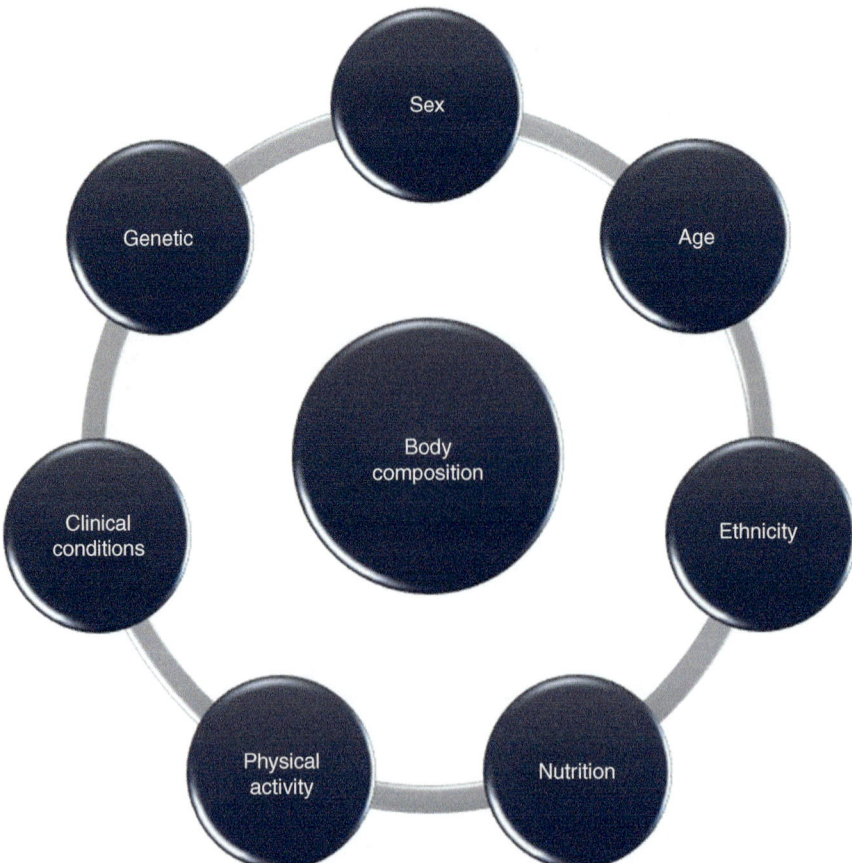

Fig. 8.1 Determinants of body composition variability

describe the role of age, sex, and ethnicity on body composition variability. For the purposes of brevity and clarity in the following sections, we will focus this discussion on muscle mass instead of all body composition components, noting the growing body of literature suggesting that the definition of low muscle mass (i.e., myopenia) should be justified by age, sex, and ethnicity.

Sex as a Determinant of Body Composition Variability

The differences in body composition by sex can be noted since birth. Boys in general have an increased lean mass (mainly due to muscle mass) compared to girls resulting in a heavier weight from birth to the first decade of life [4]. The dimorphism in body composition becomes more notable under the hormonal influence during adolescence, when girls increase their weights due to increments in fat mass, while boys increase their lean mass, leading to a higher lean to fat ratio in boys than in girls. This distinctive pattern of body mass accretion is also found in adulthood, with women having a lower percentage of lean mass, regardless of ethnicity [4]. Another sex-related body composition difference is the muscle mass distribution. In all ages during adulthood, men have a greater muscularity of the upper body compared to women. Although men also have a greater muscularity in the lower body until the fifth decade, the difference between the sexes decreases because of the steeper decline in this regional muscle mass in men. From the fourth to ninth decade, quadriceps thickness assessed by ultrasound reduces by 50% in men and 30% in women, resulting in similar amounts of this muscle in men and women after the eighth decade [5].

The sex-related differences in body composition are usually recognized, and most of the cutoffs to identify low muscularity are specific for sex. The only exception is the recommendation from the new European Working Group on Sarcopenia in Older People (EWGSOP) consensus for calf circumference measurement, a marker of muscle mass used in epidemiological studies [6]. Despite all the very well-known sex-related differences in muscle mass, they still recommend a single cutoff, derived from a study performed only in women, notwithstanding other studies have showed that this measurement is also different in older men and women [7, 8].

Age as a Determinant of Body Composition Variability

The age-related changes in muscle mass have a negative impact on health and quality of life of the elderly. These alterations start very early, in the third decade, but muscle mass loss and its consequences are usually evident only after the fifth decade [9]. The main factors accounting for age-related variations in body composition seem to be hormonal changes and decline in physical activity.

The loss of muscle mass is positively associated with the loss of muscle strength in a nonlinearly relation, with muscle strength declining at a faster rate than muscle mass [10]. While the depletion of muscle mass after the fifth decade is at an annual rate of 1%, the annual decline rate for muscle strength is 1.5% between the fifth and sixth decade and 3% from the seventh decade onwards [11]. The greater impact of age on muscle strength than mass can be explained by remodeling in muscle composition with aging, such as an increased conversion of type II muscle fibers (fast) into type I (slow) and the increase in fat deposition within the muscle fibers (i.e., myosteatosis). These age-related alterations promote a decrease in muscle quality, which may precede the loss of muscle mass.

There is also a difference in the rates of age-associated muscle mass depletion between sexes. Although men had more muscle mass, mainly in the upper limbs, they also have a steeper decrease after the fourth decade. This decrease is even more pronounced in lower limb muscles [5, 12, 13]. The modifying effect of sex on age-related muscle loss has been demonstrated by muscle mass assessment from different body composition analysis methods, including ultrasound, DXA, and calf circumference measurement. Ethnicity may also modify the effect of sex in muscle mass depletion with aging. The age-related decline in muscle mass in African American, Whites, and Asians men is two times faster than in women, but in Hispanic men this rate could be three to four times higher than in Hispanic women [14, 15]. An exception to this age-related decline in muscle mass was found in Asian women from China, who didn't show any relationship between muscle mass and age [16]. All these sex, age, and ethnicity interactions should be considered during the identification of low muscularity.

The term *sarcopenia*, defined by a progressive loss of muscle mass and muscle strength, was initially implemented to name this age-related muscle loss, but sarcopenia is now considered a muscle disease, where both muscle quantity and quality are diminished, and loss of muscle strength is recognized as its key component for negative outcomes [6].

Ethnicity as a Determinant of Body Composition Variability

Another important determinant of body composition variability is ethnicity. Ethnic differences are associated with environmental conditions and genetic polymorphism [17]. African Americans have the highest amount of muscle mass, followed by Whites, Hispanic, and Asians, as demonstrated by several studies using different techniques [10, 14, 15]. One hypothesis explaining these differences would be the longer extremities of African Americans compared to that of other ethnicities, as muscularity is usually assessed by appendicular lean mass from DXA. However, this hypothesis was rejected when the analysis was controlled by appendicular bone lengths [18]. Besides the modification effect of age on muscle loss between sexes as discussed above, ethnicity also impact the rates of decline in muscle mass among women and men. African American women and Hispanic men have the highest age-associated decline rate of muscle mass across ethnicities and sex, respectively [15].

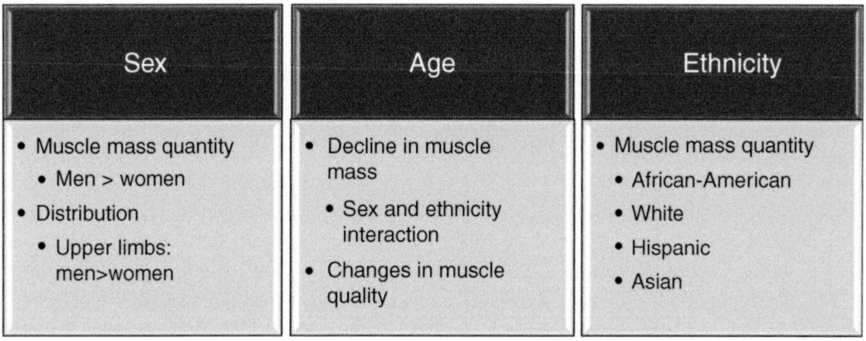

Sex	Age	Ethnicity

• Muscle mass quantity
  • Men > women
• Distribution
  • Upper limbs:
    men>women
	• Decline in muscle mass
	  • Sex and ethnicity interaction
	• Changes in muscle quality
		• Muscle mass quantity
		  • African-American
		  • White
		  • Hispanic
		  • Asian

Fig. 8.2 Main effects of sex, age, and ethnicity in body composition variability

Variations in muscle mass among different countries from East to South and West Asia have also been reported. Therefore, reference values to define low muscularity (myopenia) can differ among these regions [19]. The use of a cutoff value not specific for ethnicity may result in an over- or underestimation of myopenia prevalence.

A summary of the effects of sex, age, and ethnicity in body composition variability is showed at (Fig. 8.2).

Determination of Cutoffs to Identify Low Muscularity

Different approaches are used to define the normality thresholds and therefore identify low muscularity or myopenia. The consensus from EWGSOP recommended that cutoff should be determined as two standard deviations below the mean reference value (i.e., normative values for healthy young adults) [6]. Another commonly used approach is the identification of the lowest muscle percentiles (usually quintiles). Optimal stratification or receive operator curve are also used to generate sex-specific cutoffs in a sample of subjects with a disease. These cutoff values separate individuals with a lower amount of muscle mass who are at a higher risk for a specific adverse outcome (e.g., mortality or disability) [20]. Although these cutoffs seem to be more disease-specific, they cannot assure a good external validity. This means that these cutoffs will only have the same prognostic performance if the studied populations have the same ethnicity and age distribution from which the cutoffs have been derived from, in addition to the same disease and body composition assessment technique.

Low muscularity has been associated with several adverse outcomes in patients with cirrhosis, such as survival and hepatic encephalopathy, and this association seems to be independent of the severity of the liver disease [21]. Nevertheless, there is not a standardization for low muscularity definition in this group of patients, and several body composition analysis techniques and cutoffs have been used. Tables 8.1 and 8.2 show the recommended cutoffs from three Working Group on Sarcopenia [6, 22, 23] and the most often used cutoffs in studies in patients with cirrhosis.

Table 8.1 Suggested cut-off values for muscle mass (appendicular muscle mass/height^2) according to different consensus

	DXA (ASMI)[a]	BIA (ASMI)
AWGS	Men: 7.0 kg/m^2 Women: 5.4 kg/m^2	Men: 7.0 kg/m^2 Women: 5.7 kg/m^2
EWGSOP	Men: 7.0 kg/m^2	
	Women: 5.5 kg/m^2	
IWGS	Men: 7.23 kg/m^2 Women: 5.67 kg/m^2	

DXA dual X-ray absorptiometry, *ASMI* appendicular skeletal muscle index, *BIA* bioelectrical impedance analysis, *AWGS* Asian Working Group for Sarcopenia, *EWGSOP* European Working Group on Sarcopenia in Older People, *IWGS* International Working Group in Sarcopenia; [a]Appendicular lean mass from DXA is used as a marker of appendicular skeletal muscle

Table 8.2 Suggested cut-off values for muscle mass used to define low muscle mass in patients with cirrhosis

Author, year Country	Tool	Cut-off values	Age[a] (y)	Clinical condition
Prado, 2008 Canada	CT	W: SMI[b] < 38.5 cm^2/m^2 M: SMI[b] < 52.4 cm^2/m^2	W: 64.6 ± 10.2 M: 63.2 ± 10.5	Obesity + GI or lung cancer
Martin, 2013 Canada	CT	W: SMI[b] < 41 cm^2/m^2 M: SMI[b] < 43 cm^2/m^2 (BMI < 25) SMI[b] < 53 cm^2/m^2 (BMI ≥ 25)	W: 64.8 ± 11.5 M: 64.7 ± 11.2	GI or lung cancer
Benjamin, 2017 India	CT	W: SMI[c] < 30.21 cm^2/m^2 M: SMI[c] < 36.54 cm^2/m^2	32 ± 9.8	Healthy controls
Carey, 2017 USA	CT	W: SMI[d] < 39 cm^2/m^2 M: SMI[d] < 50 cm^2/m^2	W: 57 (50-62) M: 58 (52-61)	End-stage liver stage disease
Lucidi, 2018 Italy	Anthropometry	MAMC[e] <5th percentile	49.7 ± 16	Cirrhosis with sepsis
van Vugt, 2018 The Netherlands	CT	W: SMI[f] < 37.9 cm^2/m^2 M: SMI[f] < 44.1 cm^2/m^2	56 (48-62)	Cirrhosis (liver transplantation)
Derstine et al. 2018	CT	W: SMI[c] < 34.4 cm^2/m^2	W: 31.2 ± 6.1	Healthy controls
USA		M: SMI[c] < 45.4 cm^2/m^2	M: 30.9 ± 6.1	
Van de Werf et al. 2018	CT	W: SMI[g] < 32.0 cm^2/m^2	W: 54 ± 11	Healthy controls
The Netherlands		M: SMI[g] < 41.6 cm^2/m^2	M: 52 ± 12	

W women, *M* men, *SMI* Lumbar skeletal muscle index from muscle area; [a]Mean ± sd or median (IQR); [b]Cut-off obtained from optimal stratification; [c]Cut-off obtained as less than two standard deviations below the mean of healthy controls; [d]Cut-off obtained from log-rank test statistics for survival; [e]MAMC: Mid-arm muscle circumference from general population matched for age and sex; [f]Cut-off obtained from the sex-specific lowest quartile; [g]Cut-off defined as value below p5 of healthy controls

Most of the studies in patients with cirrhosis used the term *sarcopenia* to define low muscularity. The variability found among the cutoff values may reflect the differences in sex, age, and ethnicity characteristics of the studies they derived from or the approach used for their definition. Most of the studies in patients with cirrhosis used CT images for skeletal mass assessment and specific disease cutoffs (cancer or end-stage liver disease) [24–26]. As discussed in the section above, this approach lacks external validity unless it is applied in a population similar in age, sex, and ethnicity distribution to which the cutoffs were developed. The acquisition of normative values from the healthy population using CT assessment is difficult because the CT scan is not a routine exam and might not be appropriate to perform for body composition measurement purpose due to CT radiation exposure. For this reason, most of the studies where CT is employed for body composition assessment were performed retrospectively in patients who already have a CT scan, like cancer or chronic liver disease patients. Only three studies from India, USA, and The Netherlands used normative values from healthy controls (adult organ donors) [27–29]. Another approach would be the use of appendicular lean mass (ALM) assessment obtained from DXA. This technique is radiation-free, and it is easier to generate normative values from a healthy population. Furthermore, it was already shown that DXA assesses ALM in cirrhotic patients even in the presence of ascites [30].

Studies using cutoffs without a justification of age, sex, and ethnicity to identify myopenia should be interpreted with caution because there is a risk of misclassification of the studied population.

In conclusion, a single cutoff for body composition assessment cannot be generalized across sex, age, and ethnicity. The normative reference values, specific for sex and population, obtained from healthy young subjects are the optimal approach to determine low muscularity thresholds. It is essential to standardize sarcopenia definition and assessment in cirrhosis, to enable prevalence comparisons and its association with adverse outcomes in these patients.

References

1. Thibault R, Genton L, Pichard C. Body composition: why, when and for who? Clin Nutr. 2012;31(4):435–47.
2. Prado CM, Purcell SA, Alish C, et al. Implications of low muscle mass across the continuum of care: a narrative review. Ann Med. 2018:1–19.
3. Gonzalez MC, Correia M, Heymsfield SB. A requiem for BMI in the clinical setting. Curr Opin Clin Nutr Metab Care. 2017;20(5):314–21.
4. Wells JC. Sexual dimorphism of body composition. Best Pract Res Clin Endocrinol Metab. 2007;21(3):415–30.
5. Arts IM, Pillen S, Overeem S, et al. Rise and fall of skeletal muscle size over the entire life span. J Am Geriatr Soc. 2007;55(7):1150–2.
6. Cruz-Jentoft AJ, Bahat G, Bauer J, et al. Sarcopenia: revised European consensus on definition and diagnosis. Age Ageing. 2018.
7. Barbosa-Silva TG, Menezes AM, Bielemann RM, et al. Enhancing SARC-F: improving sarcopenia screening in the clinical practice. J Am Med Dir Assoc. 2016;17(12):1136–41.
8. Kawakami R, Murakami H, Sanada K, et al. Calf circumference as a surrogate marker of muscle mass for diagnosing sarcopenia in Japanese men and women. Geriatr Gerontol Int. 2015;15(8):969–76.

9. Shaw SC, Dennison EM, Cooper C. Epidemiology of sarcopenia: determinants throughout the Life course. Calcif Tissue Int. 2017;101(3):229–47.

10. Goodpaster BH, Park SW, Harris TB, et al. The loss of skeletal muscle strength, mass, and quality in older adults: the health, aging and body composition study. J Gerontol A Biol Sci Med Sci. 2006;61(10):1059–64.

11. von Haehling S, Morley JE, Anker SD. An overview of sarcopenia: facts and numbers on prevalence and clinical impact. J Cachexia Sarcopenia Muscle. 2010;1(2):129–33.

12. Clark P, Denova-Gutierrez E, Ambrosi R, et al. Reference values of Total lean mass, appendicular lean mass, and fat mass measured with dual-energy X-ray absorptiometry in a healthy Mexican population. Calcif Tissue Int. 2016;99(5):462–71.

13. Landi F, Calvani R, Tosato M, et al. Age-related variations of muscle mass, strength, and physical performance in community-dwellers: results from the Milan EXPO survey. J Am Med Dir Assoc. 2017;18(1):88 e17–24.

14. He Q, Heo M, Heshka S, et al. Total body potassium differs by sex and race across the adult age span. Am J Clin Nutr. 2003;78(1):72–7.

15. Silva AM, Shen W, Heo M, et al. Ethnicity-related skeletal muscle differences across the lifespan. Am J Hum Biol. 2010;22(1):76–82.

16. Xiao Z, Guo B, Gong J, et al. Sex- and age-specific percentiles of body composition indices for Chinese adults using dual-energy X-ray absorptiometry. Eur J Nutr. 2017;56(7):2393–406.

17. Wulan SN, Westerterp KR, Plasqui G. Ethnic differences in body composition and the associated metabolic profile: a comparative study between Asians and Caucasians. Maturitas. 2010;65(4):315–9.

18. Gallagher D, Visser M, De Meersman RE, et al. Appendicular skeletal muscle mass: effects of age, gender, and ethnicity. J Appl Physiol (1985). 1997;83(1):229–39.

19. Alkahtani SA. A cross-sectional study on sarcopenia using different methods: reference values for healthy Saudi young men. BMC Musculoskelet Disord. 2017;18(1):119.

20. Bosy-Westphal A, Muller MJ. Identification of skeletal muscle mass depletion across age and BMI groups in health and disease--there is need for a unified definition. Int J Obes. 2015;39(3):379–86.

21. Ebadi M, Montano-Loza AJ. Insights on clinical relevance of sarcopenia in patients with cirrhosis and sepsis. Liver Int. 2018;38(5):786–8.

22. Chen LK, Liu LK, Woo J, et al. Sarcopenia in Asia: consensus report of the Asian working Group for Sarcopenia. J Am Med Dir Assoc. 2014;15(2):95–101.

23. Fielding RA, Vellas B, Evans WJ, et al. Sarcopenia: an undiagnosed condition in older adults. Current consensus definition: prevalence, etiology, and consequences. International working group on sarcopenia. J Am Med Dir Assoc. 2011;12(4):249–56.

24. Carey EJ, Lai JC, Wang CW, et al. A multicenter study to define sarcopenia in patients with end-stage liver disease. Liver Transpl. 2017;23(5):625–33.

25. Martin L, Birdsell L, Macdonald N, et al. Cancer cachexia in the age of obesity: skeletal muscle depletion is a powerful prognostic factor, independent of body mass index. J Clin Oncol. 2013;31(12):1539–47.

26. Prado CM, Lieffers JR, McCargar LJ, et al. Prevalence and clinical implications of sarcopenic obesity in patients with solid tumours of the respiratory and gastrointestinal tracts: a population-based study. Lancet Oncol. 2008;9(7):629–35.

27. Benjamin J, Shasthry V, Kaal CR, et al. Characterization of body composition and definition of sarcopenia in patients with alcoholic cirrhosis: a computed tomography based study. Liver Int. 2017;37(11):1668–74.

28. Derstine BA, Holcombe SA, Ross BE, et al. Skeletal muscle cutoff values for sarcopenia diagnosis using T10 to L5 measurements in a healthy US population. Sci Rep. 2018;8(1):11369.

29. van der Werf A, Langius JAE, de van de Schueren MAE, et al. Percentiles for skeletal muscle index, area and radiation attenuation based on computed tomography imaging in a healthy Caucasian population. Eur J Clin Nutr. 2018;72(2):288–96.

30. Belarmino G, Gonzalez MC, Sala P, et al. Diagnosing sarcopenia in male patients with cirrhosis by dual-energy X-ray absorptiometry estimates of appendicular skeletal muscle mass. JPEN J Parenter Enteral Nutr. 2018;42(1):24–36.

Chapter 9
Muscle Mass Versus Muscle Strength and Performance: Is Muscle Mass Measurement Alone Enough?

Matthew R. Kappus and Pranab Barman

Introduction

Patients with cirrhosis are susceptible to significant symptoms of decompensation which have a significant impact on both quality of life and survival. These symptoms often lead to frequent hospitalizations which can lead to decreased quality of life and increased morbidity and mortality in this patient population. Liver-specific conditions known to be associated with these increased hospitalizations include encephalopathy, ascites, and variceal bleeding [1]. Additional systemic complications such as reduced muscle mass, physical frailty, malnutrition, metabolic syndrome, and immune dysregulation and functional immunosuppression increase the susceptibility of poor outcomes in cirrhosis [2]. Sarcopenia, defined as low muscle mass, is a lethal complication of cirrhosis. This condition in liver transplantation independently associates with waitlist mortality, as well as posttransplant outcomes such as prolonged hospital and intensive care unit stay, increased infection, and post-LT mortality [3–6]. Frailty is often considered the "functional" component of reduced muscle mass. The concept of frailty has been newly applied to patients with cirrhosis and is generally defined as a decline in physiologic reserve resulting in an increased susceptibility to stressors. It has been notoriously difficult to objectively define, although this has changed with the advent of objective measures such as the Liver Frailty Index (LFI) [7].

As a major component to frailty, sarcopenia is tightly linked to this construct and generally one cannot be addressed without the other. With advancing stages of liver disease, there is an increased rate of frailty and sarcopenia, both of which are independently associated with decompensated cirrhosis and mortality [2]. Frailty currently does not have a gold standard assessment tool given its global nature. The currently accepted measurement tools collectively assess for indices in weight loss,

M. R. Kappus (✉) · P. Barman
Division of Gastroenterology and Hepatology, Duke University Hospital, Durham, NC, USA
e-mail: matthew.kappus@duke.edu

© Springer Nature Switzerland AG 2020
P. Tandon, A. J. Montano-Loza (eds.), *Frailty and Sarcopenia in Cirrhosis*,
https://doi.org/10.1007/978-3-030-26226-6_9

127

physical stamina, and function. Sarcopenia, on the other hand, involves the quantification of muscle mass, and is characterized by the loss of muscle mass and resultant loss of muscle strength. This has also been challenging to objectively measure over the years. However, more recently, the European Working Group on Sarcopenia in Older People (EWGSOP) proposed a definition of sarcopenia that includes the loss of muscle mass plus the presence of low muscle strength or low physical performance [8]. In this chapter, we aim to outline the objective measures of muscle mass and muscle function and review the strengths and weaknesses of each.

Assessment of Sarcopenia

As defined by the EWGSOP, a working definition of sarcopenia includes the presence of both low muscle mass and low muscle function. The latter is defined as strength or performance [8]. Most studies focus on objective measures of muscle mass alone; for example, in the aging population, sarcopenia is defined as loss of muscle mass two standard deviations below the mean. The gold standard of measuring muscle mass relies on skeletal muscle imaging with computed tomography (CT) or magnetic resonance (MR) imaging techniques, which can precisely separate fat from other soft tissues. The location of measurement has varied by study, with L3 (third lumbar vertebrae) or psoas muscle level being commonly used. Limitations to CT and MR include the high cost of imaging, somewhat limited access to image analysis software and concerns regarding radiation exposure over time with CT. However, this modality is becoming more accepted as patients with cirrhosis are generally receiving cross-sectional imaging at frequent intervals for hepatocellular cancer screening and presurgical planning. Dual energy x-ray absorptiometry (DXA) is an alternative method to distinguish fat from other lean tissues while exposing the patient to minimal radiation. DXA equipment is largely not portable, rendering it useful in specific locations that already have the equipment.

Alternative methods to muscle mass measurement include bioimpedance analysis and total or partial body potassium per fat-free soft tissue. Bioimpedance analysis (BIA) has been in use for a longer period of time and can estimate volumes of fat and lean body mass. It is considered to be easy to use and inexpensive, and one of its hallmarks is its appropriateness for both ambulatory and hospitalized patients [8]. It correlates well with MR-based predictions and is validated in multiethnic adult populations [8]. BIA takes fat mass and subtracts it from total body weight in order to estimate lean mass. It is limited in patients with ascites whose total body weight is affected not by fat or muscle but rather by water volume. Body potassium measurements are considered the classic measurement of skeletal muscle as >50% of the body's potassium pool is located in skeletal muscle. It is not used routinely. Finally, measurements of arm or calf circumference have been used, but changes in fat content and skin elasticity have made this an unreliable measure in older and obese people and thus vulnerable to error [9]. With the wide availability of imaging techniques in cirrhotic patients, these alternative methods have not been widely studied in patients with cirrhosis.

Assessment of Muscle Strength

Measuring muscle strength has proven to be more difficult as there are less well-validated measurements, and factors unrelated to muscle strength, such as pain or posture, can interfere with the correct measurement of strength. Handgrip strength via dynamometer is an easy-to-use, widely available tool that correlates with lower extremity muscle power, knee extension torque, and calf cross-sectional muscle area, all of which are more relevant for gait and overall physical function [10]. In older adults, low handgrip strength was noted to be a better predictor of clinical outcomes than low muscle mass itself [10]. This measurement of muscle strength is predicated upon the belief that muscle strength across different body compartments is generally well correlated.

An important caveat in the measurement of muscle strength is also that of muscle power, a measurement of work per unit time. There is data that suggests power is a better predictor of certain functional activities [8]. This is centered around leg extensor power that can be measured isometrically or isokinetically, the latter of which is more closely associated with every day muscle function. This measurement tool is limited to research settings due to the need for specialized equipment and expert training. Finally, in patients without lung disease, peak expiratory flow measures the strength of respiratory muscles. However, data on its relationship to sarcopenia is limited, and it is not necessarily a valid measurement tool in patients with cirrhosis, who may have occult pulmonary disease.

Assessment of Muscle Function

With only limited, specialized tools to measure strength, more focus has turned toward measuring muscle function, providing a more global picture of a patient's physical performance incorporating strength, balance, and coordinated muscle movement. Implicitly, these tests also indirectly assess difficult to measure components of muscle use including neurologic connectivity, coordination, balance, and stamina. A number of tests are available and have been used in patients with end-stage liver disease.

The Short Physical Performance Battery (SPPB) examines a patient's ability to stand with feet together in three different positions (side-by-side, semi-tandem, and tandem), time to walk 8 feet, and rise from a seated position five times. There has been an established relationship between gait speed and leg strength, which suggests that small changes in physiologic reserve may have tremendous effects on performance in frail patients. As a component of the SPPB, gait speed can also be used on its own and carries predictive value for the onset of disability, mobility limitations, and mortality [8]. Finally, the timed get up and go test (TUG) requires a patient to rise from a seated chair; walk a short, defined distance; turn around; and return to a seated position. This tests for the additional component of balance, with a mid-test 180-degree turn. Importantly, these tests represent a composite measure of physical performance as opposed to static measurements of muscle mass, are easy to perform in clinic, and do not require any specialized equipment or training to administer.

Because a significant number of patients with end-stage liver disease fulfill criteria for frailty, additional tests for this specific population include the Fried Frailty Index (FFI), LFI, activities of daily living (ADL) scale, Braden Scale, and 6-minute walk test (6MWT) [2]. The FFI measures unintentional weight loss, hand grip exhaustion (via dynamometer), and low-activity gait speed to derive a composite score, with a higher score being more frail. The LFI, created specifically for patients with cirrhosis, combines grip strength, chair stands, and balance and places a patient on a scale from robust to frail [7]. These two frailty scales can be performed in the ambulatory setting (as long as a dynamometer is available) in less than 5 minutes. They are slightly more difficult to perform in the inpatient setting due to less availability of a dynamometer, potential physical limitations such as hepatic encephalopathy, and competing care priorities. These tests are limited in the encephalopathic patient, those with limited mobility, although, admittedly, we would not expect this type of patient to score "robust" utilizing any measure. The ADL scale measures the need for assistance with ADLs and assigns a score commensurate to the level of independence for each ADL. Finally, the 6-minute walk test can also be completed in the outpatient setting and increase the accessibility of a diagnosis of frailty in routine clinical care. The challenge in using these measures for both sarcopenia and frailty lies in the implementation and integration into clinical practice.

Muscle Mass and End-Stage Liver Disease

Prioritization for liver transplantation currently relies on the Model for End-Stage Liver Disease (MELD), which is based on a "sickest-first" policy; however, it is thought that the MELD score may not accurately capture the true prognosis of patients with cirrhosis. MELD does not capture certain measures which may affect quality of life and function such as ascites, malnutrition, and severe muscle wasting. However, in order to further optimize this score, modifications to this score have been studied over the years, with one such successful example being the addition of sodium level to generate the MELD-Na score. Muscle mass is one of these areas that can carry promising prognostic value.

In patients with cirrhosis, subjective measures such as BMI and anthropometric measures are limited by salt/water retention and subjectivity in measurement. With routine cross-sectional imaging being performed for HCC surveillance, sarcopenia can objectively be determined and defined using sex-specific cutoffs. Many early studies simply applied definitions used in oncology literature and were limited in scope and influence. It was not clear that these definitions were accurate in the population with cirrhosis and thus were felt to misclassify patients. Recently, Carey et al. performed a multicenter image analysis study that yielded skeletal muscle index

(SMI) cutoffs of 50 cm^2/m^2 for men and 39 cm^2/m^2 for women, which best correlated with waitlist mortality [13]. Through a variety of mechanisms, not discussed here, sarcopenia has a clear relationship with the development of hepatic encephalopathy (HE) and large volume ascites. Using anthropometric measurements, two separate studies independently found that sarcopenia predicted the presence of HE, adjusting for age, Child-Turcotte-Pugh (CTP) score and diabetes [14, 15].

While promising, the influence of sarcopenia has been shown to be greater on true waitlist and posttransplant outcomes. In an early study [11], patients with cirrhosis had SMI measured at the level of L3 vertebrae. Sarcopenia was identified as an independent predictor of mortality, with a median decrease in survival time of 15 months when compared to nonsarcopenic patients. Interestingly, there was a low level of correlation between sarcopenia and liver dysfunction scoring systems (CTP & MELD). Furthermore, it was seen that sarcopenia was associated with a higher frequency of sepsis-related death, which is consistent with earlier literature demonstrating that sarcopenia might have increased associations with infections in patients with cirrhosis [16]. This also further suggests that conventional scoring systems may not accurately capture true mortality risk. One can argue that an all-comer population of cirrhosis will have a proportion of patients with exceedingly low muscle mass which could skew results, favoring the impact of sarcopenia. A follow-up study from the same group, using the same methodology, determined that sarcopenia is independently associated with a 2.4-fold increased risk of waitlist mortality after adjusting for age and MELD score [17]. Notably, patients with a MELD <15 with sarcopenia had similar survival curves as patients with MELD >15 with and without sarcopenia. This suggests patients with less severe liver disease suffer the greatest impact from sarcopenia and would be an appropriate patient population to target sarcopenic-reversing interventions – nutrition- and exercise-based therapy [17]. Montano-Loza et al. further determined that a "MELD-sarcopenia" score improved upon the predictive power of the MELD alone score especially in those patients with a low MELD score. The authors estimated that sarcopenia adds 10 points to the MELD score [18]. Additionally, this impact was also felt to be greatest in patients with refractory ascites, which contributes to the development of sarcopenia through abdominal distension and thinning of the parietal muscles.

Some of the biggest theoretical limitations to utilizing imaging-based SMI are the time, software, and expertise required. Even though patients with cirrhosis undergo cross-sectional imaging routinely, a center must have the proper software and time needed in order to fully calculate a patient's muscle mass. The standard algorithm uses computer software to differentiate skeletal muscle from adipose tissue using Hounsfield units and automatically compute cross-sectional areas by summing tissue pixels and multiplying by pixel surface area and standardizing to patient height [11]. It has been shown that calculating the SMI in this manner at the L3 level with a single cross-sectional image correlates well to total body skeletal muscle [19]. However, this method requires specific software and technical skills in order to accurately make the calculations. In order to evaluate a simpler single-image method, Durand and colleagues measured psoas muscle thickness on a single image at the level of the umbilicus, approximately at the same vertical level of L3 [20]. The benefit of this anatomic level is that the psoas muscle is easily identified and not prone to alterations by the presence of ascites, and psoas muscle thickness can be measured on any picture archiving and communication system (PACS), ubiquitous in today's era of electronic medical record systems. This study demonstrated that psoas thickness was predictive of wait list mortality, independent of the MELD score and a MELD-psoas score performed better than the MELD-Na in patients with a MELD <25 [20]. This again suggested the impact of sarcopenia is strongest in patients with less advanced liver disease. Regarding waitlist mortality, there have been some studies that have not shown an impact on outcome; in 2016, a systematic review was performed to investigate the influence of skeletal muscle mass who were being evaluated for liver transplant [5], which concluded that sarcopenia was associated with waitlist mortality with a hazard ratio of 2, an effect that was independent of MELD [5].

Sarcopenia has also been shown to be linked with worse outcomes after liver transplantation. An early study demonstrated that pretransplant sarcopenia, as defined by psoas muscle area, correlated poorly with MELD score and was associated with increased posttransplant mortality [3]. This impact has also been shown in the living donor liver transplant recipients, who generally have a lower MELD score at the time of transplant and a lower risk of mortality. In two separate cohorts, skeletal muscle mass [21] and psoas muscle index [22] were predictive of survival after living donor liver transplantation. In a more recent study evaluating the quality of muscle tissue, low SMI and high intramuscular adipose tissue content were independently identified as risk factors for death after living donor liver transplant [23]. Finally, a recent meta-analysis by Vugt et al. demonstrated that sarcopenia carried a hazard ratio of 1.84 for posttransplant survival. This effect increased when removing transplants done primarily for malignancy to a hazard ratio of 2.03 [5]. There are a limited number of studies examining this relationship, but the work by Vugt et al. shows that studies in which cross-sectional muscle area was calculated yielded a higher impact on overall survival. In those studies where SMI was the primary variable calculated, the forest plots favored higher muscle mass but not to the same effect. Furthermore, Lee et al. demonstrated that patients with larger dorsal muscle group cross-sectional area have improved survival at 1 year and 5 years with a lower rate of complications at 1 year. To strengthen this relationship, they also demonstrated that dorsal muscle group area correlates well with psoas muscle area, the measure used in previous studies [24]. Valero et al. also demonstrated that the presence of sarcopenia was an independent predictor of postoperative complications, although this study did not demonstrate a difference in 30-day and 90-day mortality rates [25]. Finally, there is data that links the presence of sarcopenia with infections of all types [26] in the posttransplant setting but no clear association with rejection rates.

Muscle Function and End-Stage Liver Disease

One of the biggest limitations of muscle mass measurement is the difficulty incorporating it into daily clinical practice, especially in the ambulatory setting. Additionally, it provides a singular variable, however valuable, that does not necessarily fully capture the degree of functional decline in patients with cirrhosis [27]. There is a desire in the transplant community to find a more practical, reliable, and economical measure to provide an accurate risk assessment of patients both on the waitlist and after liver transplant.

In patients with cirrhosis, there are multiple factors that contribute to waitlist outcomes that are not captured in the MELD score such as age, muscle mass, nutritional status, and comorbidities [12]. Using the "eyeball test," a clinician is attempting to assess the patient's global health status in order to withstand stressors while on the waitlist and recover from a major operation. This approach has long been a subjective component of the evaluation of a patient with cirrhosis, especially in the determination of transplant candidacy. This concept has been objectively operationalized as frailty by the FFI and shown to be a more powerful predictor of functional status in the elderly [28]. In liver patients, this functional reserve has been measured by several tools, which aim to include implicit measurements of coordination, neurologic connection, and stamina.

There is a great human and financial burden associated with repeated hospitalizations for patients with cirrhosis, and muscle function seems to play an important role in this pathology. Simpler single-measure tools have independently predicted outcomes in patients with liver disease. On a continuous spectrum, gait speed was shown to be a strong predictor of hospitalizations and hospital costs. With each decrease of 0.1 m/s, length of stay and costs increased [29]. In the same study, grip strength showed a trend toward similar results, however were not significant. The reasons for hospitalizations extended across the spectrum and included ascites, encephalopathy, infections, and GI bleeding, in order. Furthermore, as determined by the FFI, frail patients were more likely to have ascites, explained by increased resting expenditure in these patients [12]. This carries important prognostic information, as patients with cirrhosis with increased decompensating events and hospitalizations have a higher risk of mortality.

By a variety of measures, both muscle function and frailty have been associated with mortality in liver transplant candidates. The 6MWT, as its name suggests, is a simple test, with the ability to evaluate a host of coordinated body functions and reflect daily physical activities. Carey et al. demonstrated that the 6MWT significantly predicts mortality, with a 52% reduction in mortality with every 100 meter increase from baseline distance [30]. This finding is not terribly surprising as subjectively, patients with cirrhosis suffer from fatigue, deconditioning, and decreased physical ability. However, the ability to define this decline can assist transplant physicians with a tool to identify increased risk of waitlist mortality. Tapper et al. examined the predictive ability of additional frailty metrics and found that an ADL score of <12 (out of 15) and an intermediate Braden score were associated with increased mortality, discharge after transplantation to a rehabilitation hospital, and increased hospital length of stay (Braden score only). When comparing odds ratios, the MELD score had lower OR per unit increase as compared to low ADL score or intermediate Braden score [31]. Additionally, this study demonstrated that patients scoring in the frail range of these measures were associated with HE-related decompensations. These studies underscore the broad applicability of these measures and ease of use in both the ambulatory (Carey) and inpatient (Tapper) settings.

The most recent effort in the assessment of frailty and muscle function has been to develop a composite score to be used in patients with cirrhosis. Initially, as defined by the FFI, frail patients had higher rates of complications of liver disease, including ascites and HE, correlating with previous research [12]. More importantly, frail patients had higher risk of mortality after adjustment for liver disease severity. The key advancement here is that many patients' comorbid conditions and functional decline could now be objectively measured as their liver disease could be. Specifically, the FFI includes subjective components, which the authors argue improves the association of frailty to mortality. The example used is a patient who subjectively is hindered by their liver disease, such that it leads to meeting "frail" criteria, limiting physical activity, and worsening sarcopenia leading to increased risk on the waitlist, that may not be reflected in the MELD score [12]. As with sarcopenia, it was seen that those with a lower MELD score (in this case MELD <18) were seen to have a greater mortality when considered frail. However, the FFI was initially derived in the elderly population. In a seminal study, Lai and colleagues established a specific frailty index for patients with cirrhosis to improve the risk stratification of patients with cirrhosis on the liver transplant waitlist [7]. In this study, gait speed, grip strength, chair stands, balance, low physical activity, ADLs, and IADLs were all associated with waitlist mortality. The final measure consisted of grip strength, chair stands, and balance testing and results in a score across a continuous spectrum defining a patient as robust or frail. This measure, known as the Liver Frailty Index (LFI), enhanced the mortality risk prediction over the MELD-Na score alone, especially in patients who were older and obese and had HE or medical comorbidities [7]. Further analysis of this index demonstrated that frailty is worth about 9 MELD points. Interestingly, increasing LFI scores (indicating pretransplant frailty) were also associated with reduced recovery to robustness posttransplant [32].

Final Thoughts on Muscle Mass or Muscle Function

The spirit of determining reduced muscle mass, or sarcopenia, and loss of physical function, or frailty, are rooted in well-founded principles that these measures have important clinical implications for patients with liver disease awaiting transplantation. Until now, clinical judgment regarding a patient's physical resilience is subjective and at worst not equitable. Both the quantification of muscle mass and characterization of physical function aim to provide objective measurements for a devastating complication of cirrhosis. Both tools have their merits and, depending on the clinical scenario, may be appropriately utilized.

The limitations of quantifying muscle mass include the need for advanced imaging and radiation exposure with CT, appropriate software, expertise in making measurements, as well as the additional time required. It is true that CT and MRI imaging are already widely used for hepatocellular cancer surveillance in patients with cirrhosis, but each image only provides a static evaluation of a potentially dynamic process. One critique of sarcopenia is the timing of when a study is obtained. Is it sufficient to make a determination about a patient's level of sarcopenia if the implication is that this single measure would be used to make a determination about transplant candidacy? Should the determination of muscle mass get reevaluated in patients with a low MELD score the longer they are listed? On the other hand, quantifying muscle mass allows for an objective measure in a patient who for other reasons cannot perform a functional assessment. An instance might be the inpatient transfer patient with acute on chronic liver failure where the question becomes whether that person is physically able to survive liver transplantation. In this instance, the lack of previous ambulatory assessments limits the urgent evaluation. Sarcopenia provides insight on increased morbidity and mortality and provides more objective data to help guide clinical decision making. Sarcopenia also provides an objective endpoint as a research tool. It does not replace clinical judgment but can complement it. Its most useful application may be in the inpatient setting where functional assessments are difficult to obtain or in the initial ambulatory visit to establish a baseline from which progression of decline can be determined for future interventions.

Performance-based testing provides multifaceted information on not only muscle strength or mass but coordinated movements such as balance and cognitive ability. Frailty predicts important outcomes in liver transplantation such as waitlist mortality [33]. There is a level of training involved, but many different providers on a transplant or research team can conduct this type of testing quickly, reliably, and economically. It provides an understanding of a dynamic process as it evolves clinically and can be more readily reassessed than measurements of muscle mass which may or may not parallel a change in the patient's functional status. Measuring physical function can only be performed in patients physically and cognitively able to participate, which in itself is a limitation. Frailty assessments are associated with both pretransplant mortality and posttransplant recovery, suggesting its long-term application. This would be most appropriately used in the outpatient setting, where it can easily be performed and tracked over time to provide prognostic value.

Whether in the research or clinical settings, sarcopenia and frailty may be useful biomarkers to study reduction in physical function and worsened outcomes in patients awaiting liver transplantation. Each has been shown to be linked to morbidity and mortality and is useful in different clinical scenarios. Each requires a certain resource of personnel, equipment, and time. Depending on a center's experience or practices, one may be preferred over the other, and both can provide great insight into the plight of reduced physical function in patients with advanced liver disease.

References

1. Berman K, Tandra S, Forssell K, Vuppalanchi R, Burton JR, Nguyen J, et al. Incidence and predictors of 30-day readmission among patients hospitalized for advanced liver disease. Clin Gastroenterol Hepatol. 2011;9:254–9.
2. Bhanji RA, Carey EJ, Yang L, Watt KD. The long winding road to transplant: how sarcopenia and debility impact morbidity and mortality on the waitlist. Clin Gastroenterol Hepatol. 2017;15:1492–7.

3. Englesbe MJ, Patel SP, He K, Lynch RJ, Schaubel DE, Harbaugh C, et al. Sarcopenia and mortality after liver transplantation. J Am Coll Surg. 2010;211:271–8.
4. Montano-Loza AJ. Skeletal muscle abnormalities and outcomes after liver transplantation. Liver Transpl. 2014;20:1293–5.
5. van VJLA, Levolger S, de BRWF, van RJ, Metselaar HJ, IJzermans JNM. Systematic review and meta-analysis of the impact of computed tomography–assessed skeletal muscle mass on outcome in patients awaiting or undergoing liver transplantation. Am J Transplant. 2016;16:2277–92.
6. Yadav A, Chang Y, Carpenter S, Silva AC, Rakela J, Aqel BA, et al. Relationship between sarcopenia, six-minute walk distance and health-related quality of life in liver transplant candidates. Clin Transpl. 2015;29:134–41.
7. Lai JC, Covinsky KE, Dodge JL, Boscardin WJ, Segev DL, Roberts JP, et al. Development of a novel frailty index to predict mortality in patients with end-stage liver disease. Hepatology. 2017;66:564–74.
8. Cruz-Jentoft AJ, Baeyens JP, Bauer JM, Boirie Y, Cederholm T, Landi F, et al. Sarcopenia: European consensus on definition and diagnosis: report of the European working group on sarcopenia in older people. Age Ageing. 2010;39:412–23.
9. Rolland Y, Czerwinski S, Van Kan GA, Morley JE, Cesari M, Onder G, et al. Sarcopenia: its assessment, etiology, pathogenesis, consequences and future perspectives. J Nutr Health Aging. 2008;12:433–50.
10. Lauretani F, Russo CR, Bandinelli S, Bartali B, Cavazzini C, Di Iorio A, et al. Age-associated changes in skeletal muscles and their effect on mobility: an operational diagnosis of sarcopenia. J Appl Physiol. 2003;95:1851–60.
11. Montano–Loza AJ, Meza–Junco J, CMM P, Lieffers JR, Baracos VE, Bain VG, et al. Muscle wasting is associated with mortality in patients with cirrhosis. Clin Gastroenterol Hepatol. 2012;10:166–173.e1.
12. Lai JC, Feng S, Terrault NA, Lizaola B, Hayssen H, Covinsky K. Frailty predicts waitlist mortality in liver transplant candidates. Am J Transplant. 2014;14:1870–9.
13. Carey EJ, Lai JC, Wang CW, Dasarathy S, Lobach I, Montano-Loza AJ, et al. A multicenter study to define sarcopenia in patients with end-stage liver disease. Liver Transpl. 2017;23:625–33.
14. Merli M, Giusto M, Lucidi C, Giannelli V, Pentassuglio I, Di Gregorio V, et al. Muscle depletion increases the risk of overt and minimal hepatic encephalopathy: results of a prospective study. Metab Brain Dis N Y. 2013;28:281–4.
15. Kalaitzakis E, Olsson R, Henfridsson P, Hugosson I, Bengtsson M, Jalan R, et al. Malnutrition and diabetes mellitus are related to hepatic encephalopathy in patients with liver cirrhosis. Liver Int. 2007;27:1194–201.
16. Merli M, Lucidi C, Giannelli V, Giusto M, Riggio O, Falcone M, et al. Cirrhotic patients are at risk for health care–associated bacterial infections. Clin Gastroenterol Hepatol. 2010;8:979–985.e1.
17. Tandon P, Ney M, Irwin I, Ma MM, Gramlich L, Bain VG, et al. Severe muscle depletion in patients on the liver transplant wait list: Its prevalence and independent prognostic value. Liver Transpl. 2012;18:1209–16.
18. Montano-Loza AJ, Duarte-Rojo A, Meza-Junco J, Baracos VE, Sawyer MB, Pang JXQ, et al. Inclusion of Sarcopenia Within MELD (MELD-Sarcopenia) and the prediction of mortality in patients with cirrhosis. Clin Transl Gastroenterol. 2015;6:e102.
19. Shen W, Punyanitya M, Wang Z, Gallagher D, St.-Onge M-P, Albu J, et al. Total body skeletal muscle and adipose tissue volumes: estimation from a single abdominal cross-sectional image. J Appl Physiol. 2004;97:2333–8.
20. Durand F, Buyse S, Francoz C, Laouénan C, Bruno O, Belghiti J, et al. Prognostic value of muscle atrophy in cirrhosis using psoas muscle thickness on computed tomography. J Hepatol. 2014;60:1151–7.

21. Kaido T, Ogawa K, Fujimoto Y, Ogura Y, Hata K, Ito T, et al. Impact of sarcopenia on survival in patients undergoing living donor liver transplantation. Am J Transplant. 2013;13:1549–56.
22. Hamaguchi Y, Kaido T, Okumura S, Fujimoto Y, Ogawa K, Mori A, et al. Impact of quality as well as quantity of skeletal muscle on outcomes after liver transplantation. Liver Transpl. 2014;20:1413–9.
23. Hamaguchi Y, Kaido T, Okumura S, Kobayashi A, Shirai H, Yagi S, et al. Impact of skeletal muscle mass index, intramuscular adipose tissue content, and visceral to subcutaneous adipose tissue area ratio on early mortality of living donor liver transplantation. Transplantation. 2017;101:565–74.
24. Lee CS, Cron DC, Terjimanian MN, Canvasser LD, Mazurek AA, Vonfoerster E, et al. Dorsal muscle group area and surgical outcomes in liver transplantation. Clin Transpl. 2014;28:1092–8.
25. Valero V, Amini N, Spolverato G, Weiss MJ, Hirose K, Dagher NN, et al. Sarcopenia adversely impacts postoperative complications following resection or transplantation in patients with primary liver tumors. J Gastrointest Surg N Y. 2015;19:272–81.
26. Krell RW, Kaul DR, Martin AR, Englesbe MJ, Sonnenday CJ, Cai S, et al. Association between sarcopenia and the risk of serious infection among adults undergoing liver transplantation. Liver Transpl. 2013;19:1396–402.
27. Englesbe MJ. Quantifying the eyeball test: Sarcopenia, analytic morphomics, and liver transplantation. Liver Transpl. 2012;18:1136–7.
28. Fried LP, Tangen CM, Walston J, Newman AB, Hirsch C, Gottdiener J, et al. Frailty in older adults: evidence for a phenotype. J Gerontol Ser A. 2001;56:M146–57.
29. Dunn MA, Josbeno DA, Tevar AD, Rachakonda V, Ganesh SR, Schmotzer AR, et al. Frailty as tested by gait speed is an independent risk factor for cirrhosis complications that require hospitalization. Am J Gastroenterol. 2016;111:1768.
30. Carey EJ, Steidley DE, Aqel BA, Byrne TJ, Mekeel KL, Rakela J, et al. Six-minute walk distance predicts mortality in liver transplant candidates. Liver Transpl. 2010;16:1373–8.
31. Tapper EB, Finkelstein D, Mittleman MA, Piatkowski G, Lai M. Standard assessments of frailty are validated predictors of mortality in hospitalized patients with cirrhosis. Hepatology. 2015;62:584–90.
32. Lai JC, Segev DL, McCulloch CE, Covinsky KE, Dodge JL, Feng S. Physical frailty after liver transplantation. Am J Transplant [Internet]. 18:1986. [cited 2018 May 9];0. Available from: http://onlinelibrary.wiley.com/doi/abs/10.1111/ajt.14675.
33. Wang CW, Feng S, Covinsky KE, Hayssen H, Zhou L-Q, Yeh BM, et al. A comparison of muscle function, mass, and quality in liver transplant candidates: results from the functional assessment in liver transplantation study. Transplantation. 2016;100:1692–8.

Chapter 10
The Role of Changes in Subcutaneous and Visceral Adiposity, Sarcopenic Obesity, and Myosteatosis/Muscle Quality in Cirrhosis: How to Diagnose It and Its Contribution to Prognosis

Maryam Ebadi and Aldo J. Montano-Loza

Introduction

Body mass index (BMI) has been widely used as a clinically accessible assessment of body composition. However, BMI does not differentiate between the two main body compartments, i.e., muscle and adipose tissue which have different functions. While muscle is mainly responsible for mechanical activity, myokines produced by muscle are involved in regulating metabolism in muscle and other tissues [1]. Adipose tissue is metabolically active tissue involved in fat metabolism and energy homeostasis; it is also involved in regulating glucose metabolism, insulin sensitivity, angiogenesis, appetite, and inflammation by secreting proteins called adipokines [2].

Sex-dependent differences in body composition exist in healthy subjects and patients with cirrhosis, i.e., higher adipose tissue mass (adiposity) in females and greater muscularity in males. However, body composition of patients with cirrhosis is extremely variable with regard to the features of muscle and adipose tissue that confer poor prognosis. Identification of abnormalities in skeletal muscle features, i.e., sarcopenia and myosteatosis (pathological fat accumulation in skeletal muscle), as well as alterations in other aspects of body composition such as visceral adiposity, subcutaneous adiposity, or sarcopenic obesity and their association with outcomes in patients with cirrhosis, has attracted considerable attention in recent years (Table 10.1). Although the link between sarcopenia and poor prognosis in cirrhosis is well established, the prognostic significance of other body composition abnormalities is much less clear. Moreover, little is known about the biological features of these abnormalities and their coincidence in cirrhosis.

M. Ebadi (✉) · A. J. Montano-Loza
Department of Medicine, Division of Gastroenterology and Liver Unit, University of Alberta, Edmonton, AB, Canada
e-mail: ebadi@ualberta.ca; montanol@ualberta.ca

© Springer Nature Switzerland AG 2020
P. Tandon, A. J. Montano-Loza (eds.), *Frailty and Sarcopenia in Cirrhosis*,
https://doi.org/10.1007/978-3-030-26226-6_10

Table 10.1 Summary of studies on CT-determined body composition abnormalities in cirrhosis

Author/year	Study population	Cutoff for body composition abnormality	Major findings
Sarcopenic obesity			
Montano-Loza et al., 2016 [11]	678 patients with cirrhosis evaluated for LT	Sarcopenia: L3 SMI ≤41 cm^2/m^2 for women and ≤53 cm^2/m^2 for men with BMI > =25 and ≤43 cm^2/m^2 Obesity: (BMI > 25 kg/m^2)	Sarcopenic obesity was determined in 20% of the patient population and was associated with mortality MELD, and Child–Pugh scores were higher in patients with sarcopenic obesity
Kobayashi et al., 2017 [30]	465 patients who went through primary hepatectomy for HCC	Sarcopenia: L3 SMI <40.31 cm^2/m^2 for men and 30.88 cm^2/m^2 for women Visceral obesity: Visceral adipose tissue area ≥ 100 cm^2	Sarcopenic obesity was observed in 7% of the population Sarcopenic obesity was a significant predictor of mortality and HCC recurrence
Myosteatosis			
Montano-Loza et al., 2016 [11]	678 patients with cirrhosis evaluated for LT	L3 muscle attenuation <41 HU in patients with a BMI up to 24.9 and <33 in those with a BMI ≥25	Myosteatosis was determined in 52% of patients and was an independent predictor of mortality
Bhanji et al., 2018 [12]	675 patients with cirrhosis evaluated for LT	L3 muscle attenuation <41 HU in patients with a BMI up to 24.9 and < 33 in those with a BMI ≥25	Myosteatosis was identified in 52% of the population and was an independent predictor of both hepatic encephalopathy and mortality
High visceral adiposity			
Terjimanian et al., 2016 [23]	348 liver transplant recipients	Continuous variable (cm^2) Visceral fat area from T12 through L4	Visceral fat area was significantly associated with post-transplant mortality
Montano-Loza et al., 2017 [25]	289 male patients with HCC	L3 VATI ≥65 cm^2/m^2	High visceral adiposity is an independent risk factor for HCC incidence and recurrence after liver transplant in male patients with cirrhosis
Low subcutaneous adiposity			
Ebadi et al., 2018 [21]	221 female patients with cirrhosis	L3 SATI<60 cm^2/m^2	Low SATI was an independent predictor of higher mortality in female patients with cirrhosis Alcohol-induced cirrhosis tended to be higher in patients with low SATI

Body composition can be assessed by an extensive range of indirect and direct modalities such as anthropometry, bioelectrical impedance (BIA), dual-energy X-ray absorptiometry (DEXA), ultrasound (US), magnetic resonance imaging (MRI), and computed tomography (CT). While most of these modalities may be applicable in the general population, some are not appropriate in cirrhosis. A fluid shift which is a common complication in patients with decompensated cirrhosis may influence the accuracy of some of these modalities such as DEXA and BIA.

An objective assessment of body composition features including muscle and adipose tissue mass and radiodensity can be achieved by analyzing a single cross-sectional CT or MRI image. In patients with cirrhosis, cross-sectional imaging is normally requested as part of liver transplantation (LT) assessment and hence is accessible for most patients. Using a single-slide CT image, we can quantify muscle and adipose tissue area and radiodensity by means of tissue attenuation ranges measured in Hounsfield units (HU) (Fig. 10.1). Quantification of body composition parameters provides objective data, which might be applicable for central decisions, such as candidacy for LT. Reproducibility, sensitivity, and specificity of these techniques to capture longitudinal changes in body composition are important considerations to predict patients' long-term outcomes.

Given the association between body composition abnormalities and worse outcomes in patients with cirrhosis, early identification is critical to facilitate proper interventions in order to reverse body composition abnormalities in these patients. Moreover, evaluating the prevalence and clinical impact of body composition abnormalities on morbidity and mortality in cirrhosis can be used to develop a

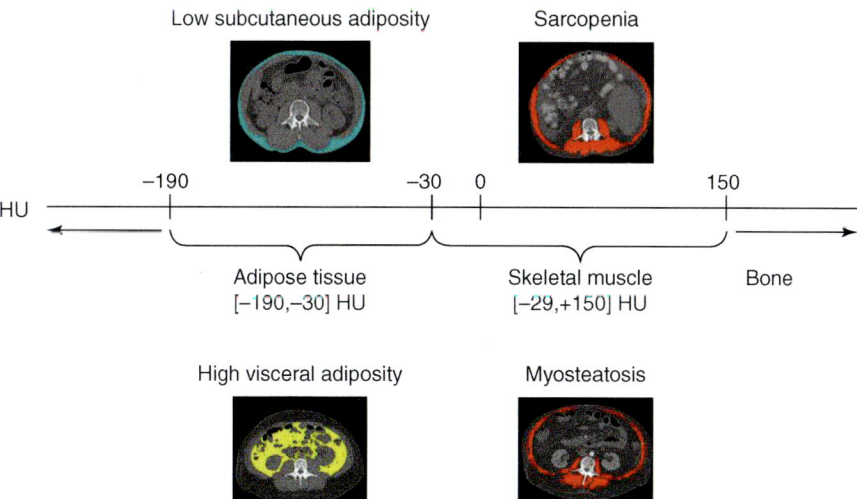

Fig. 10.1 Muscle and adipose tissue quantification for identification of body composition abnormalities. Body composition abnormalities in patients with cirrhosis include sarcopenia, myosteatosis, high visceral adiposity, and low subcutaneous adiposity. These abnormalities can be determined on a single-slice CT image taken at the third lumbar vertebrate, using tissue attenuation ranges measured in Hounsfield Units (HU)

predictive model to work as a clinical tool to estimate the individual mortality risk of patients while waiting for and after LT. Therefore, developing a predictive model to enhance patient selection may help to circumvent futile LT and thus lead to proper advances in the policy for the optimization of the organ allocation criteria in the LT setting.

This chapter summarizes current knowledge regarding the various features of body composition in patients with cirrhosis, focusing on the prevalence and consequences of these abnormalities.

Association Between BMI and Outcomes in Patients with Cirrhosis

BMI equal or greater than 25 kg/m^2 and 30 kg/m^2 are, respectively, considered as overweight and obesity, according to the World Health Organization. Insulin resistance; alterations in the production of growth factors; hormones and adipokines including leptin, adiponectin, and inflammatory cytokines such as tumor necrosis factor-α (TNF-α); and interleukin-6 (IL-6) are main characteristics of obesity. The worsened physiologic state in obesity may associate with a rapid progression of chronic liver diseases. Seven to 10% weight loss has been suggested by European associations to improve liver histology and enzymes in nonalcoholic fatty liver [3].

In patients with end-stage liver disease, LT is the decisive management option. Despite higher peri- and postoperative complications in obese LT recipients, controversy remains regarding the prognostic significance of BMI extremes in predicting LT outcomes. Some studies suggested that obesity may be a paradoxical protective feature for mortality after LT in patients with cirrhosis. This contrary association between obesity and mortality, characterized as the "obesity paradox," is well established in patients with various types of chronic diseases.

In one report, longer hospital stay and shorter survival were reported in patients at the extremes of BMI (BMI < 18.5 kg/m^2 or a BMI > 40 kg/m^2). Nevertheless, LT in severely obese patients with the lower MELD score ($\leq$22) significantly improved the survival of patients suggesting allocation of additional MELD points to severely obese patients [4]. Complications such as hepatic artery and portal vein thrombosis were the main reasons for elevated mortality rate in obese patients (BMI > 35 kg/m^2) undergoing LT [5]. Given confounding impacts of fluid accumulation on BMI, a modified BMI (conventional BMI $*$ serum albumin level) was suggested to predict outcomes after LT. Contrary to conventional BMI, the modified BMI was not a contraindication for LT [6].

When the impact of BMI on early post-LT outcome was investigated in the context of MELD score, elevated BMI was not associated with higher mortality risk or graft loss. Underweight patients (BMI < 18.5 kg/m^2) had higher risk for mortality and graft loss, especially those with the lower MELD score ($\leq$26), in comparison to normal weight recipients [7]. Overall, these results suggest that in listed obese patients with an advanced liver disease, BMI in conjunction with MELD might be used to prioritize patients for organ allocation.

The present evidence concerning the impact of BMI on outcomes in patients with cirrhosis is not consistent, and part of the discrepancy may be explained by variation between studies in regard to the choice of a reference group and obesity definition (BMI upper-limit values). Besides, one of the major limitations of BMI in predicting outcomes in LT is that it is affected by fluid retention. Therefore, weight loss in malnourished patients may be masked by the accumulation of fluid. It also does not discriminate the composition and abnormalities of the body mass to properly predict the risk of adverse outcomes associated with these abnormalities. Recent application of body composition modalities has demonstrated that obesity masks the presence and progression of sarcopenia (i.e., sarcopenic obesity), and it is also associated with elevated fat infiltration into muscle (i.e., myosteatosis) [8]. Both skeletal muscle abnormalities, i.e., sarcopenia and myosteatosis, are common in patients with cirrhosis. Therefore, the prognostic significance of body composition abnormalities in patients with cirrhosis should be evaluated using precise and unified diagnostic imaging rather than BMI across studies.

The Importance of Myosteatosis in Cirrhosis

Excess accumulation of lipids within skeletal muscle is a pathological phenomenon called myosteatosis. It is reflected by low skeletal muscle radiodensity on CT images and might be a manifestation of muscle loss. Pre-defined HU ranges for demarcating skeletal muscle cross-sectional area and attenuation on CT is −29 HU to 150 HU [9]. Although the cutoff values to define normal and low attenuation muscle have not been standardized, muscle radiodensity of <33 HU in patients with a BMI ≥25 and < 41 in those with a BMI <25 was associated with shorter survival in cancer [10]. Even though myosteatosis may be an extension of obesity, fluid retention in majority of patients with cirrhosis questions the applicability of these BMI-dependent cutoffs in cirrhotic population.

Myosteatosis is relatively poorly characterized in cirrhosis; however, it is emerging as a poor prognostic factor in these patients. Using cutoffs established in oncologic population [10], myosteatosis was identified in 52% of 678 patients with cirrhosis. Presence of myosteatosis was independently associated with worse survival and appeared to denote deterioration in physical condition rather than the severity of the liver disease. Despite longer intensive care unit stay in patients with myosteatosis, no significant difference in post-LT complications was reported between patients with and without myosteatosis [11]. In our recent exploration of the association between myosteatosis and overt hepatic encephalopathy (HE) in patients with cirrhosis, frequency of myosteatosis was higher in patients with HE compared to the patients without (70% vs. 45%, $p < 0.001$); both sarcopenia and myosteatosis were independent predictors of HE [12].

Although myosteatosis has been defined as an excess accumulation of lipids within skeletal muscle, the composition of lipids seems to play more important role in pathology of muscle rather than the total amount of lipids per se [13]. Comprehensive evaluation of muscle transcriptome in cancer recognized diabetogenic-like alterations in carbohydrate and lipid metabolism such as impaired lipid metabolism and diminished lipid oxidation as potential pathological mechanisms of myosteatosis [14]. Impaired mitochondrial function and age-related differentiation of muscle stem cells into adipocytes [15] are further probable contributors to myosteatosis. Association between myosteatosis and deficits of physical function has been exhaustively characterized in aging; however, the prognosis of muscle quality in cirrhosis has not been well identified. In summary, poor muscle quality (low attenuation on CTs) was associated with adverse outcomes including mortality and complications such as HE in patients with cirrhosis. While muscle abnormalities such as sarcopenia and myosteatosis constitute important prognostic factors, they are not incorporated in conventional scores for prognosis in cirrhosis, such as the MELD or Child–Pugh scores. This requires further investigation.

Sarcopenic Obesity

Sarcopenia is associated with poor prognosis in various chronic diseases that is ignored in patients with higher BMI. Concordance of these two features, sarcopenia and obesity, called sarcopenic obesity has been gaining attraction in oncology. However, clinical predictors and prognostic significance of sarcopenic obesity in cirrhosis have not been widely investigated. A recent review reported the frequency of 20–35% for sarcopenic obesity in cirrhosis which was significantly associated with mortality [16]. Montano-Loza et al. have profiled this body composition phenotype in patients with cirrhosis as the concurrent presence of sarcopenia and overweight or obesity (BMI > 25 kg/m^2). Sarcopenic obesity was presented in 20% of 678 patients with cirrhosis and was more frequent in male, older patients with higher MELD and lower muscle attenuation when compared to patients without muscle abnormalities [11].

Possible mechanisms for the pathophysiology of sarcopenic obesity in cirrhosis have not been clearly determined. Age-related deterioration in body composition and decreased physical activity, chronic inflammation, and insulin resistance associated with both sarcopenia and elevated visceral obesity might play an important role [16].

Obesity is commonly defined as BMI of ≥ 25 or ≥ 30 kg/m^2; however, its definition varies as defined by BMI, visceral obesity, and ratio of visceral to subcutaneous adipose tissue or whole body fat mass. Moreover, inconsistency in literature regarding the modalities and cutoffs used to define sarcopenia and obesity (visceral) exists and may lead to lack of standardized definition for sarcopenic obesity. Lastly, the accumulation of visceral adipose tissue but not subcutaneous adipose tissue appears to deliberate the majority of obesity complications. Thus, given limitations of using BMI to assess body compartments, prognostic significance of obesity should be evaluated based on adiposity index rather than BMI. Prospective studies are required to improve these definitions in patients with cirrhosis, considering their capability of predicting relevant clinical outcomes.

Prognostic Significance of Adipose Tissue Depots in Cirrhosis

Sex-dependent body composition disparity exists in patients with cirrhosis with females having higher adiposity and males having more skeletal muscle. Body composition discrepancy by sex might be related to differences in fat metabolism, hormonal characteristics, and anatomic location of adipose tissue deposition between male and females [17].

Visceral (VAT) and subcutaneous adipose tissue (SAT) are two main types of adipose tissue with differences in anatomic location, size of adipocytes, lipolytic capacity, insulin response, and adipokine secretion. VAT not only contains insulin-resistant adipocytes that are more responsive to catecholamine-induced lipolysis but also is an active producer of cytokines such as IL-6, TNF-α, and monocyte chemotactic protein 1 (MCP-1) [18]. Elevated lipolysis of VAT, in response to catabolic stimuli, enables direct delivery of free fatty acids to the liver and consequently can cause elevated hepatic triglyceride deposition [19]. SAT is involved in uptake and storage of circulating free fatty acids and triglycerides and also regulates insulin sensitivity, glucose and lipid metabolism, as well as immune response by producing adipokines mainly leptin [18, 20].

Although metabolic differences exist between SAT and VAT, potential differences in their contribution to the outcomes in cirrhosis have not been consistently demonstrated, partially due to the use of modalities with limited applicability and the variability among studies with regard to the time point in cirrhosis trajectory (pre- vs. post-LT) that patients are studied.

Cross-sectional imaging provides the opportunity to precisely quantify two main adipose tissue depots. CT-measured VAT and SAT, calculated as an area at the third lumbar vertebrate (L3) normalized to height and reported as indexes in cm^2/m^2, i.e., visceral adipose tissue index (VATI) and subcutaneous adipose tissue index (SATI), are the most commonly used indicator of body adiposity. Using this techniques, differences in adipose tissue distribution by sex have been characterized by males having more VATI, while SATI was predominant in female patients with cirrhosis [21]. Variability in regional adipose tissue distribution by sex [21] and within each BMI category, as well as different behavior of adipose depots [18, 20], demonstrates the need to understand the prognostic significance of adiposity in cirrhosis by sex and depot.

Controversy remains regarding the association between visceral adiposity and outcomes in patients with cirrhosis as high visceral adiposity is reported to be related to poor survival in patients with hepatocellular carcinoma [22] as well as liver transplant recipients [23], whereas no association between VATI and mortality was observed in neither female nor male patients with cirrhosis evaluated for LT [21, 24]. Visceral adipose tissue has been linked to the higher probability of HCC incidence, recurrence, and outcome. CT-determined high visceral adiposity (VATI > 65 cm^2/m^2) was associated with higher risk of HCC before LT as well as recurrence after LT. However, this association between high VATI and HCC was only observed in male patients. The lack of association between VATI and HCC in female patients might be related to estrogen impact on prioritizing subcutaneous over visceral adipose tissue accumulation in females. Higher deposition of adipose tissue in the visceral region might be associated with chronic inflammatory state which favors neoplastic expansion and clarifies the higher risk for HCC before and after LT. Furthermore, high VATI is associated with insulin resistance, which might affect the risk of HCC [25].

In another large study of 1257 patients with various stages of HCC, among five measured body composition parameters including skeletal muscle index, muscle attenuation, VATI, SATI, and visceral to subcutaneous adipose tissue ratio, the main predictors of survival were sarcopenia, myosteatosis, and visceral adiposity. Interestingly, the prevalence of patients presenting with two or three poor prognostic body composition features was higher in underweight patients compared to normal weight (42% vs. 19%, $P < 0.001$) [22]. However, the use of visceral to subcutaneous adipose ratio as an indicator of visceral obesity was questioned in previous studies as it may lead to the misclassification of patients. This ratio would be similar in people with high adiposity, with large amounts of both VATI and SATI, and in people with low adiposity who have small amounts of both VATI and SATI [22].

CT image-based analysis of body composition in patients with cirrhosis evaluated for LT revealed that subcutaneous adipose tissue but not muscle is an independent predictor of mortality in female patients with cirrhosis. In a recent study of 221 female patients evaluated for liver transplantation, SATI was independently associated with mortality after adjusting for age, alcohol-related cirrhosis, albumin, and MELD [21]. Interestingly, modification of MELD to include SATI showed an excellent discriminative performance for predicting mortality in female patients. This essentially highlights the poor prognostic significance of malnutrition in cirrhosis which has been neglected in the current organ allocation criteria in LT setting. Female patients with low SATI (<60 cm^2/m^2), evaluated or listed for LT, had higher risk of mortality. The clarification for the relationship between SATI and female mortality in cirrhosis has not been clinically recognized. However, severe energy exhaustion triggered by cirrhosis and low serum levels of leptin as an indicator of malnutrition are possible explanations. In addition, estrogen replacement therapy which favors fat accumulation in subcutaneous over visceral depots in females [26] was associated with prolonged survival in patients with HCC [27]. Yet, these results need to be validated in larger prospective, multicentric studies in patients with cirrhosis.

Longitudinal Adipose Tissue Changes in Patients with Cirrhosis

Data on body composition changes in cirrhosis by sex has revealed that depletion of adipose tissue and skeletal muscle is more frequent in female and male patients, respectively [28]. Liver cirrhosis is characterized by a significant reduction in body fat mass [29]; however, the timeline and pattern of loss of adipose tissue depots need to be established using validated body composition assessment tools in cirrhosis.

Assessment of whole body fat mass by triceps skinfold thickness (TSF) in patients with cirrhosis showed that fat loss, described as TSF below the fifth percentile of age- and sex-matched normal population, was more common in females than males [28, 29]. Sever depletion of body fat in female, malnourished hospitalized patients with cirrhosis was independently associated with lower survival rate [28]. Body fat mass assessment by DEXA demonstrated a marked fat loss even in initial stages of liver disease [29] which was defined as total body fat <80% of the 50th percentile of the sex-matched control group. Fat loss augmented with advancing the severity of the liver disease [28, 29]. The metabolic pattern that drives fat loss in female patients with cirrhosis is similar to chronic diseases or starvation, whereas the metabolic pattern of muscle loss in male patients mimics the critical diseases [28].

Cross-sectional body composition assessment at the time of LT evaluation in patients with cirrhosis revealed association between body composition abnormalities and adverse prognosis. However, our understanding of the prognostic value of longitudinal changes in body composition parameters is limited. Result of studies analyzing sequential CT images should be interpreted cautiously as a change between −2% and 2% represents tissue maintenance.

In a retrospective cohort of 136 patients with cirrhosis, skeletal muscle loss occurred in 50% of patients, whereas 33% of patients were experiencing SAT loss with no changes in visceral adipose tissue. The baseline CT in this study was taken as part of the LT evaluation, and the second one was conducted at nearly 1 year later. While no association between mortality and skeletal muscle loss was observed in this study, loss of SAT increased mortality risk by twofold when compared to patients who gained/maintained SAT after adjusting for MELD score and serum albumin [21]. SAT plays an imperative role as a key energy reservoir in the body; consequently, poor prognosis in patients with SAT loss might be related to the exhaustion of body energy reservoirs. Additional understanding of the prognostic significance of sex-specific body composition components, their interaction, as well as longitudinal changes is necessary for a better management of nutritional status of patients with cirrhosis.

Conclusions

Differences in body composition by sex that happen in patients with cirrhosis appear to influence prognosis. This suggests that cirrhotic patients with body composition abnormalities might be underlooked in liver transplant settings, and therefore prioritization of liver transplantation candidates merely based on the MELD score may lead to misclassification of patients. Inclusion of body composition abnormalities within the MELD score demonstrates promise to optimize the organ allocation criteria in the LT setting.

References

1. Trayhurn P, Drevon CA, Eckel J. Secreted proteins from adipose tissue and skeletal muscle – adipokines, myokines and adipose/muscle cross-talk. Arch Physiol Biochem. 2011;117(2):47–56. https://doi.org/10.3109/13813455.2010.535835.
2. Ali AT, Hochfeld WE, Myburgh R, Pepper MS. Adipocyte and adipogenesis. Eur J Cell Biol. 2013;92(6–7):229–36. https://doi.org/10.1016/j.ejcb.2013.06.001.
3. European Association for the Study of the L, European Association for the Study of D, European Association for the Study of O. EASL-EASD-EASO Clinical Practice Guidelines for the management of non-alcoholic fatty liver disease. J Hepatol. 2016;64(6):1388–402. https://doi.org/10.1016/j.jhep.2015.11.004.
4. Dick AA, Spitzer AL, Seifert CF, Deckert A, Carithers RL Jr, Reyes JD, et al. Liver transplantation at the extremes of the body mass index. Liver Transpl. 2009;15(8):968–77. https://doi.org/10.1002/lt.21785.
5. Triguero J, Garcia A, Molina A, San Miguel C, Notario P, Villegas T, et al. Complications associated with liver transplantation in recipients with body mass index >35 kg/m(2): would it be a poor prognosis predictive factor? Transplant Proc. 2015;47(9):2650–2. https://doi.org/10.1016/j.transproceed.2015.10.015.
6. Tanaka T, Renner EL, Selzner N, Therapondos G, Lilly LB. The impact of obesity as determined by modified body mass index on long-term outcome after liver transplantation: Canadian single-center experience. Transplant Proc. 2013;45(6):2288–94. https://doi.org/10.1016/j.transproceed.2012.11.009.
7. Bambha KM, Dodge JL, Gralla J, Sprague D, Biggins SW. Low, rather than high, body mass index confers increased risk for post-liver transplant death and graft loss: risk modulated by model for end-stage liver disease. Liver Transpl. 2015;21(10):1286–94. https://doi.org/10.1002/lt.24188.
8. Goodpaster BH, Theriault R, Watkins SC, Kelley DE. Intramuscular lipid content is increased in obesity and decreased by weight loss. Metabolism. 2000;49(4):467–72.
9. Mitsiopoulos N, Baumgartner RN, Heymsfield SB, Lyons W, Gallagher D, Ross R. Cadaver validation of skeletal muscle measurement by magnetic resonance imaging and computerized tomography. J Appl Physiol. 1998;85(1):115–22. https://doi.org/10.1152/jappl.1998.85.1.115.
10. Martin L, Birdsell L, Macdonald N, Reiman T, Clandinin MT, McCargar LJ, et al. Cancer cachexia in the age of obesity: skeletal muscle depletion is a powerful prognostic factor, independent of body mass index. J Clin Oncol. 2013;31(12):1539–47. https://doi.org/10.1200/JCO.2012.45.2722.
11. Montano-Loza AJ, Angulo P, Meza-Junco J, Prado CM, Sawyer MB, Beaumont C, et al. Sarcopenic obesity and myosteatosis are associated with higher mortality in patients with cirrhosis. J Cachexia Sarcopenia Muscle. 2016;7(2):126–35. https://doi.org/10.1002/jcsm.12039.
12. Bhanji RA, Moctezuma-Velazquez C, Duarte-Rojo A, Ebadi M, Ghosh S, Rose C, et al. Myosteatosis and sarcopenia are associated with hepatic encephalopathy in patients with cirrhosis. Hepatol Int. 2018;12:377. https://doi.org/10.1007/s12072-018-9875-9.
13. Aubrey J, Esfandiari N, Baracos VE, Buteau FA, Frenette J, Putman CT, et al. Measurement of skeletal muscle radiation attenuation and basis of its biological variation. Acta Physiol. 2014;210(3):489–97. https://doi.org/10.1111/apha.12224.

14. Stretch C, Aubin JM, Mickiewicz B, Leugner D, Al-Manasra T, Tobola E, et al. Sarcopenia and myosteatosis are accompanied by distinct biological profiles in patients with pancreatic and periampullary adenocarcinomas. PLoS One. 2018;13(5):e0196235. https://doi.org/10.1371/journal.pone.0196235.

15. Miljkovic I, Zmuda JM. Epidemiology of myosteatosis. Curr Opin Clin Nutr Metab Care. 2010;13(3):260–4. https://doi.org/10.1097/MCO.0b013e328337d826.

16. Eslamparast T, Montano-Loza AJ, Raman M, Tandon P. Sarcopenic obesity in cirrhosis-the confluence of 2 prognostic titans. Liver Int. 2018;38(10):1706–17. https://doi.org/10.1111/liv.13876.

17. Geer EB, Shen W. Gender differences in insulin resistance, body composition, and energy balance. Gend Med. 2009;6(Suppl 1):60–75. https://doi.org/10.1016/j.genm.2009.02.002.

18. Fain JN, Madan AK, Hiler ML, Cheema P, Bahouth SW. Comparison of the release of adipokines by adipose tissue, adipose tissue matrix, and adipocytes from visceral and subcutaneous abdominal adipose tissues of obese humans. Endocrinology. 2004;145(5):2273–82. https://doi.org/10.1210/en.2003-1336.

19. Girard J, Lafontan M. Impact of visceral adipose tissue on liver metabolism and insulin resistance. Part II: visceral adipose tissue production and liver metabolism. Diabetes Metab. 2008;34(5):439–45. https://doi.org/10.1016/j.diabet.2008.04.002.

20. Ebadi M, Baracos VE, Bathe OF, Robinson LE, Mazurak VC. Loss of visceral adipose tissue precedes subcutaneous adipose tissue and associates with n-6 fatty acid content. Clin Nutr. 2016;35(6):1347–53. https://doi.org/10.1016/j.clnu.2016.02.014.

21. Ebadi M, Tandon P, Moctezuma-Velazquez C, Ghosh S, Baracos VE, Mazurak VC, et al. Low subcutaneous adiposity associates with higher mortality in female patients with cirrhosis. J Hepatol. 2018;69(3):608–16. https://doi.org/10.1016/j.jhep.2018.04.015.

22. Fujiwara N, Nakagawa H, Kudo Y, Tateishi R, Taguri M, Watadani T, et al. Sarcopenia, intramuscular fat deposition, and visceral adiposity independently predict the outcomes of hepatocellular carcinoma. J Hepatol. 2015;63(1):131–40. https://doi.org/10.1016/j.jhep.2015.02.031.

23. Terjimanian MN, Harbaugh CM, Hussain A, Olugbade KO Jr, Waits SA, Wang SC, et al. Abdominal adiposity, body composition and survival after liver transplantation. Clin Transpl. 2016;30(3):289–94. https://doi.org/10.1111/ctr.12688.

24. Cruz RJ Jr, Dew MA, Myaskovsky L, Goodpaster B, Fox K, Fontes P, et al. Objective radiologic assessment of body composition in patients with end-stage liver disease: going beyond the BMI. Transplantation. 2013;95(4):617–22. https://doi.org/10.1097/TP.0b013e31827a0f27.

25. Montano-Loza AJ, Mazurak VC, Ebadi M, Meza-Junco J, Sawyer MB, Baracos VE, et al. Visceral adiposity increases risk for hepatocellular carcinoma in male patients with cirrhosis and recurrence after liver transplant. Hepatology. 2018;67(3):914–23. https://doi.org/10.1002/hep.29578.

26. Mattiasson I, Rendell M, Tornquist C, Jeppsson S, Hulthen UL. Effects of estrogen replacement therapy on abdominal fat compartments as related to glucose and lipid metabolism in early postmenopausal women. Horm Metab Res. 2002;34(10):583–8. https://doi.org/10.1055/s-2002-35420.

27. Hassan MM, Botrus G, Abdel-Wahab R, Wolff RA, Li D, Tweardy D, et al. Estrogen replacement reduces risk and increases survival times of women with hepatocellular carcinoma. Clin Gastroenterol Hepatol. 2017;15(11):1791–9. https://doi.org/10.1016/j.cgh.2017.05.036.

28. Alberino F, Gatta A, Amodio P, Merkel C, Di Pascoli L, Boffo G, et al. Nutrition and survival in patients with liver cirrhosis. Nutrition. 2001;17(6):445–50.

29. Figueiredo FA, De Mello Perez R, Kondo M. Effect of liver cirrhosis on body composition: evidence of significant depletion even in mild disease. J Gastroenterol Hepatol. 2005;20(2):209–16. https://doi.org/10.1111/j.1440-1746.2004.03544.x.

30. Kobayashi A, Kaido T, Hamaguchi Y, Okumura S, Shirai H, Yao S, et al. Impact of sarcopenic obesity on outcomes in patients undergoing hepatectomy for hepatocellular carcinoma. Ann Surg. 2017;269:924. https://doi.org/10.1097/SLA.0000000000002555.

Chapter 11
Evidence for the Assessment of Physical Frailty and Sarcopenia in Hospitalized Patients and the Role of Assessing Changes Over Time

Guido Stirnimann

Introduction

Patients with advanced liver cirrhosis require frequent hospitalization, mostly due to cirrhosis-related complications, especially complications of portal hypertension, infections, acute or acute-on-chronic kidney injury, and hepatocellular carcinoma [1].

Importantly, hospitalized patients with cirrhosis also have a high risk for readmission within 30 days ranging from 20 up to 37% [2–4]. As risk factors for readmission, Volk and colleagues identified severity of liver disease (based on MELD score), serum sodium, and number of medications as measures for the complexity of the medical regimen [4]. Furthermore, in patients readmitted within 30 days, 90-day mortality was significantly higher than in patients that were not readmitted within 1 month (26.8% vs 9.8%) [2].

Due to the significant risk for further complications, readmission, and fatal outcome, hospitalized patients with cirrhosis should undergo a careful risk assessment as part of the standard work-up. Based on the individual risk profile, specific measures can be implemented with the final goal of reducing the hospital stay, preventing future complications, and decreasing the overall burden of cirrhosis and its complications.

G. Stirnimann (✉)
Division of Gastroenterology & Liver Unit, University of Alberta Hospital,
Edmonton, AB, Canada

Department of Visceral Surgery and Medicine, University Hospital Inselspital
and University of Bern, Bern, Switzerland
e-mail: guido.stirnimann@dbmr.unibe.ch

© Springer Nature Switzerland AG 2020
P. Tandon, A. J. Montano-Loza (eds.), *Frailty and Sarcopenia in Cirrhosis*,
https://doi.org/10.1007/978-3-030-26226-6_11

Hospitalized Patients with Cirrhosis

General

Hospitalized patients with advanced liver cirrhosis have a significant burden of morbidity and mortality. The risk for further deterioration and for liver-associated complications is increased not only in patients with acute decompensation or acute on chronic liver failure, but also in patients with elective procedures like pre-transplant evaluation. No matter what the reason for the hospitalization is, it facilitates a thorough assessment regarding cirrhosis-associated risk factors and prognosis. Several scores have been developed in the past specifically for hospitalized patients but also more general for patients with cirrhosis.

Pathophysiology of Muscle Breakdown

Due to the decrease in glycogen production and storage, relatively short episodes of fasting, for instance, overnight fasting, lead to an increase in proteolysis and lipolysis, and amino acids from the muscle are used as source of gluconeogenesis to fuel tissues where fatty acid carbon cannot be used [5, 6]. During hospitalization, patients are confronted with additional procedure-related fasting episodes, for instance, during preparation for GI investigations or while on the intensive care unit. This may further accelerate muscle breakdown.

Risk Stratification

CPT and MELD

Conventional prognostic scores commonly used in patients with cirrhosis are the Child-Pugh-Turcotte (CPT) score and the Model for End-Stage Liver Disease (MELD) score, the former including the two subjective parameters: severity of ascites and hepatic encephalopathy. The latter had been developed to predict mortality after transjugular intrahepatic portosystemic shunt (TIPS) placement and then used as an allocation system for deceased donor liver grafts based on the objective laboratory parameters: creatinine, bilirubin, and INR [7]. Later on, the MELD score had been further refined by adding sodium as the fourth parameter. The resulting MELD-Na score is today widely used in the organ allocation process for liver transplants [8, 9]. These scores can be applied during hospitalization as well as in the outpatient setting.

CLIF SOFA

In 2013, Moreau and colleagues introduced the Chronic Liver Failure-Sequential Organ Failure Assessment (CLIF-SOFA) score to better characterize and stratify hospitalized cirrhotic patients with acute decompensation regarding severity of disease and risk of mortality [10]. The CLIF-SOFA score has been developed as an adaptation of the not-cirrhosis-specific Sepsis Organ Failure Assessment (SOFA) score and includes six subscores to assess the liver, kidney, brain, circulation, coagulation, and respiration. Importantly, this score reflects expert opinion and is based on consensus rather than on data and did not lead to a significant improvement of prediction accuracy compared with the MELD and the MELD-Na score [11].

CLIF-C ACLF

In 2014, the CLIF-C ACLF score was published, adding age and white blood cell count to the CLIF-C Organ Failure (CLIF-SOFA) score. This lead to a significant improvement of the prediction of mortality of patients that were hospitalized due to decompensation of cirrhosis as compared with MELD, MELD-Na, and Child-Pugh score [11]. For patients in intensive care units, the Acute Physiology and Chronic Health Evaluation (APACHE) score can be used to predict mortality [12, 13].

However, not all complications of cirrhosis are adequately reflected in the above listed scores that either do not specifically target hospitalized patients (Child-Pugh, MELD, MELD-Na score) or explicitly address subpopulations (i.e., patients with ACLF or ICU patients), and some of these scores are [10–13] technically demanding and require a specific training.

Physical Frailty

How to Assess Physical Frailty

In recent years, physical frailty evolved as a new, important, independent, and potentially modifiable risk factor in patients with advanced chronic liver disease. In hospitalized patients with cirrhosis, frailty has not yet been investigated extensively, but a limited set of frailty assessment tools from other fields of medicine has been validated successfully in this patient population [14]. Tapper et al. investigated three different metrics in the hospital setting (activities of daily living (ADL), Braden scale, and Morse fall scale) that enable a fast and reliable assessment of hospitalized patients with cirrhosis. Although not associated with 30-day hospital readmission, frailty measures were predictive for 90-day mortality, length of hospital stay, and rehabilitation needs [15]. The three tools used for the assessment of physical frailty are described in more detail in the following sections.

Activities of Daily Living (ADL) Score

Activities of daily living is assessed as the self-reported ability to feed, toilet, bath, dress, bathe, and transfer. Each point is rated as "dependent" (1 point), "needs assistance" (2 points), and "independent" (3 points) summing up to a maximum of 15 points [15, 16]. In their study, Tapper et al. found an odds ratio (OR) of 1.83 (95% confidence interval [CI] 1.05–3.20) for 90-day mortality and an OR of 3.78 (95% CI 1.97–7.29) for discharge to a rehabilitation hospital if the ADL score was less than 12 of 15.

Braden Scale

The Braden scale is a measure that is used for the assessment of pressure ulcer risk. It consists of a physical exam and the additional parameters: skin sensory perception, moisture, mobility, activity, nutrition, and friction (ability to hold a comfortable position in a chair and bed). While a score of 23 or more defines no risk for skin lesions, a score of less than 16 is indicative for an increased risk and consequently requires physical and nutritional therapy [15, 17]. For inpatients with decompensated cirrhosis, the OR for discharge to a rehabilitation hospital was 6.23 (95% CI 2.53–15.4) if the Braden scale was <16. In case of an intermediate Braden scale (16–18), an increase in mortality risk was identified (OR 1.62, 95% CI 1.03–2.56).

Morse Fall Scale

The risk to fall can be assessed with the Morse fall scale that includes history of falling, ambulatory aids, intravenous access, gait disturbances, secondary diagnoses, and mental status [15, 18]. However, the Morse fall scale did not predict the mortality risk in hospitalized patients with decompensated cirrhosis.

Sarcopenia

How to Assess Sarcopenia

Another important risk factor in patients with advanced cirrhosis is sarcopenia. The best objective method to assess sarcopenia in cirrhotic patients is based on cross-sectional CT or MR image analysis [19]. Muscularity can be analyzed on abdominal CT or MR scans that have been performed as part of the routine assessment or on single slice images at the respective lumbar level. The need for special image analysis software as well as training to assess the images limits this type of analysis to specialized centers [20].

Sarcopenia Risk Scores

Since sarcopenia is not included in the standard risk assessment tools, new risk scores have been developed. The MELD-sarcopenia score [21] and the MELD-psoas score [22] both take into account the muscularity normalized by height with specific cutoffs for male and female patients. Especially for patients with a MELD score below 20, sarcopenia is an additional risk factor for unfavorable outcome [21]. Although not reflected in the current risk scores, special attention should be given to obese patients with cirrhosis, since sarcopenic obesity and myosteatosis are associated with a higher mortality risk [23].

Treatment of Sarcopenia and Frailty

Ideally, a comprehensive assessment of frailty and sarcopenia is not only used to assess specific risks but also to implement a targeted treatment strategy. If the diagnosis of sarcopenia is confirmed, a nutritional supplementation strategy can be deployed, and in case of frailty, specific physical measures can be implemented. These interventions should address the inhospital period and the time after hospital discharge.

A cornerstone of treatment in patients with frailty and/or sarcopenia is the optimization of nutrition [14]. Daily oral nutritional supplementation (1000 kcal and 34 g of proteins) in patients with alcoholic cirrhosis and treatment with branched-chain amino acids (BCAA) in patients with advanced cirrhosis each have been associated with a reduction in hospital admission rate [24, 25], and BCAA supplementation furthermore lead to an improvement of health-related quality of life [25]. However, oral or enteral nutritional treatment did not affect overall survival in a meta-analysis performed by Ney et al. [26]. The number of trials investigating the effect of physical exercise in mainly compensated cirrhotic patients is still small as is the total number of patients investigated. Although effects on survival and long-term benefit are unclear to date, a positive effect on peak VO2, quadriceps muscle, self-perceived health status, and 6-min walk test could be observed [27–29].

Specific recommendations regarding caloric and protein intake are given in the recently published EASL Clinical Practice Guideline "Nutrition in Chronic Liver Disease" [30]. Daily caloric intake should be at least 35 kcal/kg body weight (BW) in nonobese patients, and the optimal protein intake consists of at least 1.2–1.5 g/kg BW. In sarcopenic obese patients, a moderate hypocaloric diet in combination with a high protein intake of >1.5 g/kg BW is recommended. In decompensated cirrhotic patients, a late evening snack should be added to compensate for catabolic episodes during the night. Prolonged fasting periods in the context of diagnostic or therapeutic procedures and during ICU stays should be avoided whenever possible.

It is important to note that frailty and sarcopenia as well as the associated treatment strategies should be reassessed in a longitudinal way not only during a hospital stay but also in the outpatient setting [31].

Economic Burden

In the USA, the number of hospitalization due to cirrhosis increased from 2001 to 2011 from 350,000 to 650,000 per year, and in parallel, the hospitalization-related costs increased from 5 to 10 billion dollars.

Prevention of Readmissions

Patients with cirrhosis have a high risk for readmission ranging from 20% to 37% [2, 32, 33]. Typical disease-specific complications that require readmission are hepatic encephalopathy, spontaneous bacterial peritonitis, and esophageal variceal bleeding [1].

Due to the high and rising costs that are related to inhospital treatment and especially readmissions of patients with cirrhosis, prevention strategies are important to reduce the economic burden of this patient population. Intervention programs typically require a multidisciplinary approach and should target high-risk patient groups. Readmission reduction programs are not only medically meaningful, but also from a financial point of view [1].

Tapper et al. defined in their review five different strategies to decrease the readmission rate of patients with cirrhosis: (1) interventions should be integrated in the clinical workflow, (2) default options are more powerful than voluntary actions, (3) knowledge improvement should focus on the front line clinicians, (4) process improvements do not always translate into better outcomes, and (5) any successful intervention must include viable alternatives to hospitalization [32].

Future Needs

So far, almost no specific pharmacological treatment of sarcopenia and frailty is available. In male patients with low testosterone, testosterone substitution has demonstrated a positive effect on muscle mass [34]. Ammonia-lowering agents or myostatin antagonists are promising new targets that have to be investigated in more detail in the future [6].

It is important to note that sarcopenia may persist or even progress after liver transplantation and that only a minority of patients show an improvement of sarcopenia posttransplant [35]. Whether an optimal nutrition strategy, ideally in combination with a physical therapy, can improve the long-term and especially the posttransplant outcome regarding sarcopenia and frailty needs to be investigated in future trials.

Conclusion

To date, literature on sarcopenia and frailty assessment in hospitalized patients is still limited. Most techniques and measures used to assess sarcopenia and frailty can be applied in the hospital as well as in the outpatient setting. However, the significance of specific findings may differ significantly in a hospitalized patient, where length of hospital stay, rehabilitation needs after discharge, rehospitalization risk within the next months, and mortality risk are of special interest.

Sarcopenia is ideally assessed as normalized total muscle area or psoas muscle area in CT or MR images at the lumbar level L3; however, a correct assessment requires specific image analysis software and trained personnel. Other assessment techniques like DEXA scan analysis are less precise but easier to perform, do not require special software tools or training, and are associated with less radiation than full CT scans. For the assessment of frailty, clinical scores like the activities of daily living (ADL) score or the Braden scale that have been developed in other medical fields can be used in hospitalized patients with cirrhosis.

Sarcopenia has an impact on survival on the transplant list as well as on the post-transplant evolution. Whether it also affects rehospitalization rates or mortality risk in hospitalized patient with cirrhosis is currently not known. In contrast, frailty measured during hospitalization is associated with an increased risk for rehospitalization and an increased risk for death.

Several measures may help to improve the outcome of hospitalized sarcopenic and frail patients. Optimization of nutrition, if required with enteral tube feeding or parenteral nutrition, the maintenance of a sufficient protein intake, supplementation of vitamin and trace element deficits, and the implementation of specific training to reverse frailty are the most important measures in hospitalized patients with advanced cirrhosis. Whether these interventions effectively lead to less complication, shorter hospital stays, a decreased readmission rate, and a lower mortality risk is currently not fully investigated.

Successful interventions have the potential to improve the medical situation of patients with cirrhosis, to reduce hospital admission and especially readmission rate, and to decrease cirrhosis-related healthcare costs. However, these strategies need further evaluation in future prospective clinical trials.

References

1. Chirapongsathorn S, Talwalkar JA, Kamath PS. Strategies to reduce hospital readmissions. Semin Liver Dis. 2016;36(2):161–6.
2. Berman K, Tandra S, Forssell K, Vuppalanchi R, Burton JR Jr, Nguyen J, et al. Incidence and predictors of 30-day readmission among patients hospitalized for advanced liver disease. Clin Gastroenterol Hepatol. 2011;9(3):254–9.
3. Seraj SM, Campbell EJ, Argyropoulos SK, Wegermann K, Chung RT, Richter JM. Hospital readmissions in decompensated cirrhotics: factors pointing toward a prevention strategy. World J Gastroenterol. 2017;23(37):6868–76.
4. Volk ML, Tocco RS, Bazick J, Rakoski MO, Lok AS. Hospital readmissions among patients with decompensated cirrhosis. Am J Gastroenterol. 2012;107(2):247–52.
5. Petersen KF, Krssak M, Navarro V, Chandramouli V, Hundal R, Schumann WC, et al. Contributions of net hepatic glycogenolysis and gluconeogenesis to glucose production in cirrhosis. Am J Phys. 1999;276(3. Pt 1):E529–35.
6. Dasarathy S, Merli M. Sarcopenia from mechanism to diagnosis and treatment in liver disease. J Hepatol. 2016;65(6):1232–44.
7. Kamath PS, Wiesner RH, Malinchoc M, Kremers W, Therneau TM, Kosberg CL, et al. A model to predict survival in patients with end-stage liver disease. Hepatology. 2001;33(2):464–70.
8. Biggins SW, Kim WR, Terrault NA, Saab S, Balan V, Schiano T, et al. Evidence-based incorporation of serum sodium concentration into MELD. Gastroenterology. 2006;130(6):1652–60.
9. Kim WR, Biggins SW, Kremers WK, Wiesner RH, Kamath PS, Benson JT, et al. Hyponatremia and mortality among patients on the liver-transplant waiting list. N Engl J Med. 2008;359(10):1018–26.
10. Moreau R, Jalan R, Gines P, Pavesi M, Angeli P, Cordoba J, et al. Acute-on-chronic liver failure is a distinct syndrome that develops in patients with acute decompensation of cirrhosis. Gastroenterology. 2013;144(7):1426–37, 37 e1–9.
11. Jalan R, Saliba F, Pavesi M, Amoros A, Moreau R, Gines P, et al. Development and validation of a prognostic score to predict mortality in patients with acute-on-chronic liver failure. J Hepatol. 2014;61(5):1038–47.
12. Knaus WA, Zimmerman JE, Wagner DP, Draper EA, Lawrence DE. APACHE-acute physiology and chronic health evaluation: a physiologically based classification system. Crit Care Med. 1981;9(8):591–7.
13. Knaus WA, Draper EA, Wagner DP, Zimmerman JE. APACHE II: a severity of disease classification system. Crit Care Med. 1985;13(10):818–29.
14. Kok B, Tandon P. Frailty in patients with cirrhosis. Curr Treat Options Gastroenterol. 2018;16(2):215–25.
15. Tapper EB, Finkelstein D, Mittleman MA, Piatkowski G, Lai M. Standard assessments of frailty are validated predictors of mortality in hospitalized patients with cirrhosis. Hepatology. 2015;62(2):584–90.
16. Gobbens RJ, van Assen MA. The prediction of ADL and IADL disability using six physical indicators of frailty: a longitudinal study in the Netherlands. Curr Gerontol Geriatr Res. 2014;2014:358137.
17. Bergstrom N, Braden B, Kemp M, Champagne M, Ruby E. Predicting pressure ulcer risk: a multisite study of the predictive validity of the Braden Scale. Nurs Res. 1998;47(5):261–9.
18. Morse JM, Black C, Oberle K, Donahue P. A prospective study to identify the fall-prone patient. Soc Sci Med. 1989;28(1):81–6.
19. Montano-Loza AJ. Muscle wasting: a nutritional criterion to prioritize patients for liver transplantation. Curr Opin Clin Nutr Metab Care. 2014;17(3):219–25.
20. van Vugt JL, Levolger S, Gharbharan A, Koek M, Niessen WJ, Burger JW, et al. A comparative study of software programmes for cross-sectional skeletal muscle and adipose tissue measurements on abdominal computed tomography scans of rectal cancer patients. J Cachexia Sarcopenia Muscle. 2017;8(2):285–97.

21. Montano-Loza AJ, Duarte-Rojo A, Meza-Junco J, Baracos VE, Sawyer MB, Pang JXQ, et al. Inclusion of sarcopenia within MELD (MELD-sarcopenia) and the prediction of mortality in patients with cirrhosis. Clin Transl Gastroenterol. 2015;6:e102.
22. Durand F, Buyse S, Francoz C, Laouenan C, Bruno O, Belghiti J, et al. Prognostic value of muscle atrophy in cirrhosis using psoas muscle thickness on computed tomography. J Hepatol. 2014;60(6):1151–7.
23. Montano-Loza AJ, Angulo P, Meza-Junco J, Prado CMM, Sawyer MB, Beaumont C, et al. Sarcopenic obesity and myosteatosis are associated with higher mortality in patients with cirrhosis. J Cachexia Sarcopenia Muscle. 2016;7(2):126–35.
24. Hirsch S, Bunout D, de la Maza P, Iturriaga H, Petermann M, Icazar G, et al. Controlled trial on nutrition supplementation in outpatients with symptomatic alcoholic cirrhosis. JPEN J Parenter Enteral Nutr. 1993;17(2):119–24.
25. Marchesini G, Bianchi G, Merli M, Amodio P, Panella C, Loguercio C, et al. Nutritional supplementation with branched-chain amino acids in advanced cirrhosis: a double-blind, randomized trial. Gastroenterology. 2003;124(7):1792–801.
26. Ney M, Vandermeer B, van Zanten SJ, Ma MM, Gramlich L, Tandon P. Meta-analysis: oral or enteral nutritional supplementation in cirrhosis. Aliment Pharmacol Ther. 2013;37(7):672–9.
27. Zenith L, Meena N, Ramadi A, Yavari M, Harvey A, Carbonneau M, et al. Eight weeks of exercise training increases aerobic capacity and muscle mass and reduces fatigue in patients with cirrhosis. Clin Gastroenterol Hepatol. 2014;12(11):1920–6. e2.
28. Roman E, Garcia-Galceran C, Torrades T, Herrera S, Marin A, Donate M, et al. Effects of an exercise programme on functional capacity, body composition and risk of falls in patients with cirrhosis: a randomized clinical trial. PLoS One. 2016;11(3):e0151652.
29. Debette-Gratien M, Tabouret T, Antonini MT, Dalmay F, Carrier P, Legros R, et al. Personalized adapted physical activity before liver transplantation: acceptability and results. Transplantation. 2015;99(1):145–50.
30. European Association for the Study of the Liver. Electronic address eee, European Association for the Study of the L. EASL Clinical Practice Guidelines on nutrition in chronic liver disease. J Hepatol. 2019;70(1).172–93.
31. Tandon P, Raman M, Mourtzakis M, Merli M. A practical approach to nutritional screening and assessment in cirrhosis. Hepatology. 2017;65(3):1044–57.
32. Tapper EB, Volk M. Strategies to reduce 30-day readmissions in patients with cirrhosis. Curr Gastroenterol Rep. 2017;19(1):1.
33. Chirapongsathorn S, Talwalkar JA, Kamath PS. Readmission in cirrhosis: a growing problem. Curr Treat Options Gastroenterol. 2016;14(2):236–46.
34. Sinclair M, Grossmann M, Hoermann R, Angus PW, Gow PJ. Testosterone therapy increases muscle mass in men with cirrhosis and low testosterone: a randomised controlled trial. J Hepatol. 2016;65(5):906–13.
35. Bhanji RA, Takahashi N, Moynagh MR, Narayanan P, Angirekula M, Mara KC, et al. The evolution and impact of sarcopenia pre- and post liver transplantation. Aliment Pharmacol Ther. 2019;49(6):807–13.

Chapter 12
Frailty and Sarcopenia in the Selection of Candidates for Liver Transplantation

Christopher J. Sonnenday

Perhaps the greatest responsibility of transplant hepatologists and surgeons is to evaluate and select appropriate candidates for liver transplantation. Deceased organ donors remain a precious resource of limited supply, and every effort must be made to avoid performing futile transplants in patients without the ability to recover and thrive posttransplant. Furthermore, the candidate pool for liver transplantation is becoming increasingly old, with associated comorbidity and debilitation. The median age at transplant in the USA has risen a decade in the past 15 years and will likely cross 60 in the coming years. Furthermore, the rise of alcohol-related liver disease and NASH-related cirrhosis as the leading indications for liver transplantation in the USA has increased the number of candidates with the significant challenges of malnutrition and associated substance abuse and associated obesity and metabolic syndrome, respectively.

In that context, novel tools for candidate selection are needed, particularly those that reflect global health and physiologic reserve. Accumulating evidence has suggested that frailty and sarcopenia may both serve as useful metrics for candidate selection, but application of these tools in a standardized and validated fashion has been limited. It is important to emphasize that frailty and sarcopenia, while often thought of as similar or interchangeable, are distinct metrics with different clinical implications. Frailty is clearly a functional construct, incorporating measures such as walking speed, grip strength, or chair stands that reflect muscle *function* in addition to muscle *mass*. Furthermore, frailty measures often include subjective measures of the patient experience, such as self-reported exhaustion, which suggest a patient's experience of their global health status may also have an impact on clinical outcomes. Given the functional components, frailty measures have typically been applied only to ambulatory outpatients and may not apply to acutely ill inpatient candidates. Sarcopenia measured by imaging modalities offers objective and

C. J. Sonnenday (✉)
Department of Surgery, University of Michigan, Ann Arbor, MI, USA
e-mail: csonnend@umich.edu

© Springer Nature Switzerland AG 2020
P. Tandon, A. J. Montano-Loza (eds.), *Frailty and Sarcopenia in Cirrhosis*,
https://doi.org/10.1007/978-3-030-26226-6_12

161

reproducible data about muscle mass and quality and therefore may be more broadly applicable across patient populations of varying acuity. However, current sarcopenia tools do not offer a functional component and therefore may not fully reflect an individual patient's clinical presentation. It is best to think of these two metrics as distinct and complementary in the evaluation of candidates for liver transplantation.

Frailty Measures in Transplant Candidate Selection

Measurement

The impact of frailty on outcomes in surgical candidates, acutely ill patients, and even patients with end-stage organ disease is well-established and fits with clinical intuition. However, frailty measurement has suffered from a lack of validated measurement tools, particularly those studied in specific populations. In general, functional assessments of frailty incorporate direct patient assessment, as opposed to other frailty scores derived from administrative data, patient reporting, or subjective clinician grading (Karnofsky Performance Status [KPS], activities of daily living/ instrumental activities of daily living [ADLs/IADLs], clinical frailty score, Braden scale). In liver transplant candidates, a variety of functional measurement tools have been studied including 6-minute walk test, Fried frailty phenotype, the liver frailty index (LFI), short physical performance battery, and cardiopulmonary exercise testing [6]. Of these available tools, the Fried frailty phenotype and the LFI appear to offer the most reliable performance in terms of predictive utility and clinical feasibility. The LFI, as developed and validated by Lai et al., [4] has the additional advantages of minimal subjectivity and faster execution in clinical settings and should be the preferred measurement tool in the liver transplant candidate population.

One challenge particularly relevant to the liver transplant candidate pool is the lack of validated frailty measurement tools in the acutely ill and/or inpatient setting. Acute illness, exacerbated by hepatic encephalopathy and other metabolic derangements, can undermine the ability to produce reliable measurements of frailty such as grip strength, chair stands, or walking speed. In this setting, there may be a greater role for clinician-derived subjective measurement scales such as the Karnofsky Performance Status (KPS) for more acute risk stratification. However, such measures only offer reliable prediction of short-term outcomes (inhospital outcomes, risk for readmission) and may not offer any longitudinal value in the end-stage liver disease population where frequent readmissions and acute decompensation episodes are common. It may be reasonable for individual centers to adopt a battery of tools to assess frailty across different settings and patient populations, such as LFI, KPS, ADLs/IADLs, and 6-minute walk test. There is value in choosing a consistent and parsimonious number of tools to assess frailty, such that providers become familiar with the interpretation of individual values and their changes over time in different patients and clinical scenarios (Table 12.1).

Table 12.1 Select frailty measurement tools in candidates for liver transplantation

Tool	Advantages in liver transplant population	Estimated time for assessment	Populations studied	Criteria for high frailty
Karnofsky Performance Score	Intuitive to clinicians and patients Applicable even to critically ill patients Low cost Fast	<10 seconds	Inpatient Outpatient	0–40
ADLs/IADLs	Patient reported No cost Well-associated with outcomes across patient populations	3–4 minutes	Inpatient Outpatient	Difficulty with ≥2 ADLs
Liver frailty index	Objective, performance based Applicable to outpatient setting Easy to perform	<10 minutes	Outpatient	≥4.5
6-minute walk test	Objective, performance based Continuous scale No specialized equipment	~6 minutes	Outpatient	<250 m

Given the relatively rapid changes in clinical condition that can occur in decompensated cirrhotics, with associated decline in muscle mass and nutrition, it is critical that frailty measurement be repeated at regular intervals. While frailty appears to have more long-term predictive ability as a single snapshot when measured in clinically well elderly outpatients (Fried frailty phenotype), that does not appear to be the case for patients with end-stage organ disease where sarcopenia, inactivity, malnutrition, and cognitive decline can occur much more quickly. Ideally, transplant providers and centers wishing to utilize frailty measurement as part of their candidate evaluation process, and waitlist management, should utilize a single measure (e.g., LFI) repeated at regular intervals (such as quarterly or at regular clinic visits every 3–6 months while on the waitlist). Progressive increase in frailty score should prompt reassessment of the patient's physical activity, diet and nutrition assessment, and associated clinical condition (infection, complications of portal hypertension, encephalopathy, accelerated comorbid conditions, etc.).

Implications of Frailty

A growing number of studies have attempted to correlate frailty, defined by multiple measures and tools, with waitlist and transplant outcomes. While available data to date cannot clearly quantify the risk that patients with high frailty face with transplant, it is clear that frailty contributes in important ways to defining a patient phenotype that is of high risk for adverse outcomes on the waiting list. In that context, it is important to consider frailty as an additional domain of risk assessment among transplant candidates, considered alongside severity of synthetic liver dysfunction and portal hypertension, comorbid disease, surgical history and anatomic anomalies, and psychosocial fitness. Frailty in and of itself should not be the single reason to remove a patient from the waiting list nor does a validated cutoff frailty score exist to prevent patients from being listed for transplant.

The magnitude of effect of increasing frailty on patient outcomes is significant and consistent across frailty metrics. Patients unable to achieve 250 m on a 6-minute walk test face a nearly twofold increase in waitlist mortality. A similar doubling of waitlist mortality is observed for each additional point according to the LFI [5]. Even for the more subjective measures of frailty such as KPS and ADLs/IADLs, patients in the highest risk strata face a mortality risk nearly double those without significant deficits in performance status. The effect of frailty appears to be synergistic with increasing severity of liver disease, as high MELD, high frailty patients suffer high waitlist mortality with even short observation periods (<1 year).

Beyond risk stratification for waitlist and transplant outcomes, perhaps the most impactful use of frailty assessment is to identify patients for remediation or "prehabilitation" protocols to mitigate frailty. Such efforts need to be specific to patient needs, simple such that they are reproducible and feasible for patients, and monitored such that they can be adapted as patient needs change [9]. A possible tiered approach to prehabilitation guided by serial frailty measurement is outlined in Table 12.2. Prehabilitation protocols have demonstrated efficacy and cost-effectiveness in several preoperative settings over relatively short periods of time (4–6 weeks prior to major surgery). Applying prehabilitation protocols, which typically include goal-directed daily physical activity and intensive nutrition support interventions, to the more prolonged needs (months or longer) of a patient waiting for transplant, presents logistical and financial challenges [7]. Furthermore, and perhaps most importantly, experience from other prehabilitation programs suggests that compliance falls off sharply when the immediacy of a surgical interven-

Table 12.2 Prehabilitation schematic guided by frailty assessment

Initial frailty assessment	Prehabilitation program	Frequency of frailty testing and clinical reassessment	Implications for transplant candidacy
Mild	Daily exercise program (cumulative 150 min/week) divided into 2–3 sessions daily	12 weeks	Appropriate liver transplant candidate
Moderate	Home-based or outpatient physical therapy	4–8 weeks	Proceed with liver transplantation if no further increase in frailty
Severe	Consider inpatient rehabilitation	2–4 weeks	Consider liver transplantation only if improvement in frailty

Adapted from Lai et al. [6]

tion is lost. Nevertheless, prehabilitation offers the substantial potential benefits of increased patient engagement, improved waitlist survival, and decreased resource utilization (driven by decreased length of stay and fewer complications) posttransplant. More debilitated patients with higher frailty scores may benefit from more intensive interventions such as outpatient physical therapy or even inpatient rehabilitation. Additional study of prehabilitation strategies is essential to document efficacy of these interventions, which would increase availability of these services to listed patients and facilitate reimbursement for these programs.

Sarcopenia Measures in Transplant Candidate Selection

While multiple studies have associated sarcopenia with adverse health outcomes in retrospective cohorts of patients with cirrhosis, including liver transplant candidates and recipients, experience with prospective use of muscle mass measurement in clinical practice is limited. Primary barriers to clinical use include the lack of a validated, simple, and reproducible technique of measuring muscle mass (including a standardized definition of sarcopenia) and limited understanding of the implications of sarcopenia in clinical practice [2].

Measurement

The vast majority of cohort studies of sarcopenia have utilized retrospective analysis of cross-sectional (typically CT) imaging, with variable techniques of manual or semiautomated measurement of muscle mass. While individual investigators have made these techniques relatively high throughput in a research setting, an efficient clinical tool or process for measuring muscle mass in clinical practice has not been developed. "Single-slice" or abbreviated computed tomography is a technique of obvious appeal, as it is based upon the modality with the most use in published research studies and its widespread availability. Concern is appropriately raised about radiation exposure, but the dose involved in such limited CT scans appears to be less than other commonly used diagnostic modalities (e.g., standard chest X-ray). Furthermore, such limited scans can be done without the need for intravenous contrast exposure. Automation of measurement of muscle mass such that a diagnosis of sarcopenia could be readily made has not been established. Nevertheless, this modality is likely to be the most applicable to clinical practice, as it requires little additional work for the clinician (like ordering an imaging test), is not of undue burden to patients (most patients have experience with CT scans), and minimizes operator error in measurement. Similar research efforts have been attempted using single-slice MRI, which does eliminate the concern of radiation exposure although may be logistically and financially more complicated.

Musculoskeletal ultrasound is an obvious alternative to cross-sectional imaging and has advantages in ease of use, lack of radiation exposure, and applicability in a variety of practice settings. One might envision muscle mass estimation becoming a common clinic-based measurement tool in ambulatory care settings, with the increasing availability of ultrasound in outpatient medical units and increasing provider comfort with basic ultrasound techniques and interpretation. Ultrasound suffers from the obvious limitation of variability in measurement by operator technique. Whether this could be overcome with standardized education modules and protocols (such has occurred with FAST ultrasound in trauma assessment or the nearly universal use of ultrasound-guided central line placement) is not clear.

Other techniques have been utilized in research studies to measure muscle mass, including bioelectrical impedance and measurement of mid-arm muscle circumference, but these techniques have suffered from accuracy and variability. Dual energy X-ray absorptiometry (DXA), which has become the standard of care measurement modality for bone mineral density, may also be used to measure appendicular skeletal muscle mass. This metric, which is adjusted to body size, has been adopted by consensus groups (International Working Group on Sarcopenia and the European Working Group on Sarcopenia in Older People) to define criteria for the determination of sarcopenia. However, these criteria have not been validated in larger data sets and diverse populations.

Defining Sarcopenia

Great heterogeneity in the metric used to define sarcopenia exists among published study cohorts. Total psoas area, psoas density, skeletal muscle index, and other metrics have correlated with adverse health outcomes. Furthermore, studies have varied in their use of a standard definition of sarcopenia defined by threshold values, versus evaluating sarcopenia by percentile among a specific population. The specific definition used for determining sarcopenia is obviously linked to the method of measurement, as not all metrics apply or have been validated across modalities. Among the cirrhotic population, skeletal muscle index measured at the level of the third lumbar vertebrae (L3) has been the most well-validated and correlates strongly with survival. This metric obviously implies the use of CT for determination of sarcopenia.

Implications of Sarcopenia

Retrospective studies have correlated sarcopenia primarily with survival outcomes among patients with cirrhosis, including waitlist and posttransplant mortality among liver transplant patients [1]. As profoundly sarcopenic patients may have markedly diminished waitlist and posttransplant survival, some have proposed the use of muscle mass measurement primarily as a risk stratification tool. For example, the presence of sarcopenia could be considered a relative contraindication to liver transplant listing. Or perhaps more applicable in clinical practice, the absence of sarcopenia in an acutely ill and/or debilitated patient could reassure providers that such an individual could be expected to recover fully with appropriate intervention. Sarcopenia provides an objective measurement of physical fitness that is applicable even to patients that cannot participate in bedside measures of frailty or for whom estimates of performance status may not reflect their overall health status.

Available clinical studies of sarcopenia vary in their estimation of the prevalence of impact of sarcopenia among liver transplant candidates, reflecting the need for standard metrics and validated definitions in this domain. Nevertheless, approximately 25–50% of liver transplant candidates and patients with decompensated cirrhosis appear to have significant sarcopenia. Sarcopenic patients, by any metric, appear to have substantially increased risk of adverse posttransplant outcomes including prolonged length of stay, increased postoperative complications, increased infections, and in some studies diminished posttransplant survival [3, 8]. The effect of sarcopenia appears to persist despite adjustment for age, gender, cause of liver disease, or severity of illness at time of transplant, likely reflecting the utility of sarcopenia as a relatively indelible measure of patient fitness and global health.

A significant limitation of utilizing sarcopenia for risk stratification is the lack of a threshold value of muscle loss that predicts health outcomes that are prohibitive for a particular intervention such as liver transplantation. Thus, measurement of muscle mass might best be utilized to identify patients for prehabilitation programs, as discussed above for frailty. While such programs may be effective in improving short- to intermediate-term parameters such as performance status, nutritional metrics, frailty, and weight loss, even the most vigorous exercise and nutrition programs appear unlikely to address sarcopenia in a time frame such that changes in muscle mass could be detected in clinical practice. Whether sarcopenia can be correlated with other surrogate measures (biomarkers, frailty score, nutritional assessments) utilized in clinical practice that may guide prehabilitation initiatives is an area for future study.

Summary

The improved understanding of frailty and sarcopenia among transplant candidates is an important advance in the field, and ongoing studies seek to refine their measurement and application. Recent consensus conferences have attempted to guide the utilization of both frailty and sarcopenia in the assessment of candidates for liver transplantation. Expert consensus has led to a few critical recommendations that apply to both frailty and sarcopenia as metrics of candidate selection:

(i) The isolated or "one-time" use of a frailty or sarcopenia measure should not be used as the sole criterion upon which to base candidate selection decisions.
(ii) Transplant clinicians and centers should adopt standard approaches to measuring frailty and sarcopenia using validated tools.

(iii) Longitudinal measurement of frailty and sarcopenia is critical to understanding the clinical trajectory of transplant candidates, as these measures are not
static and changes could prompt reconsideration of candidate selection
decisions.

Most importantly, interventions to mitigate frailty and sarcopenia are evolving
and will become important to ensuring optimal waitlist and transplant outcomes in
an aging candidate pool.

References

1. Carey EJ, Lai JC, Wang CW, Dasarathy S, Lobach I, Montano-Loza AJ, et al. A multicenter study
to define sarcopenia in patients with end-stage liver disease. Liver Transpl. 2017;23(5):625–33.
2. Carey EJ, Lai JC, Sonnenday C, Tapper EB, Tandon P, Duarte-Rojo A, et al. A North American
expert opinion statement on sarcopenia in liver transplantation. Hepatology. John Wiley &
Sons, Ltd; 2019.
3. Englesbe MJ, Patel SP, He K, Lynch RJ, Schaubel DE, Harbaugh C, et al. Sarcopenia and
mortality after liver transplantation. J Am Coll Surg. 2010;211(2):271–8.
4. Lai JC, Feng S, Terrault NA, Lizaola B, Hayssen H, Covinsky K. Frailty predicts waitlist mortality in liver transplant candidates. Am J Transplant. 2014;14(8):1870–9.
5. Lai JC, Covinsky KE, McCulloch CE, Feng S. The liver frailty index improves mortality prediction of the subjective clinician assessment in patients with cirrhosis. Am J Gastroenterol.
2018;113(2):235–42.
6. Lai JC, Sonnenday CJ, Tapper EB, Duarte-Rojo A, Dunn MA, Bernal W, et al. Frailty in liver
transplantation: an expert opinion statement from the American Society of Transplantation
Liver and Intestinal Community of Practice. Am J Transplant. John Wiley & Sons, Ltd
(10.1111). 2019;111(12):1776.
7. Mathur S, Janaudis-Ferreira T, Wickerson L, Singer LG, Patcai J, Rozenberg D, et al. Meeting
report: consensus recommendations for a research agenda in exercise in solid organ transplantation. Am J Transplant. John Wiley & Sons, Ltd (10.1111). 2014;14:2235–45.
8. Montano-Loza AJ, Meza-Junco J, Baracos VE, Prado CMM, Ma M, Meeberg G, et al. Severe
muscle depletion predicts postoperative length of stay but is not associated with survival after
liver transplantation. Liver Transpl. 2014;20(6):640–8.
9. Waits SA, Englesbe MJ. Making progress toward frailty remediation in end-stage liver disease.
Transplantation. 2016;100(12):2526.

Chapter 13
Physical Frailty and Sarcopenia in End-Stage Liver Disease: Do They Improve After Liver Transplantation?

Rahima A. Bhanji and Elizabeth J. Carey

Introduction

Malnutrition is a common but devastating complication of end-stage liver disease (ESLD). Sarcopenia, defined as a generalized and progressive loss of muscle mass, strength, and function, is a major consequence of malnutrition [1]. Sarcopenia is seen in up to 60% of patients awaiting liver transplantation (LT) [2] and is associated with increased risk of decompensation, risk of infections, risk of hospitalization, and risk of wait list mortality [3]. Following LT, sarcopenia is associated with increased ICU stay, prolonged ventilation, and increased hospital length of stay (LOS) [4].

Sarcopenia is a key component of frailty, another common complication of cirrhosis. Although initially described in the geriatric literature, there have been an increasing number of studies evaluating frailty in patients with cirrhosis, particularly over their pretransplant course [5]. It has been defined as an increased susceptibility to stressors resulting in adverse outcomes in individuals with a cumulative decline in physiologic reserve [5]. Frailty is present in up to 25% of patients with cirrhosis [5]. Like sarcopenia, it is a poor prognostic indicator associated with increased risk of hospitalization, increased hospital LOS, and increased wait list mortality [5]. There is a paucity of literature on the course and impact of both frailty and sarcopenia following LT.

R. A. Bhanji (✉)
Division of Gastroenterology and Liver Unit, Department of Medicine, University of Alberta, Edmonton, AB, Canada
e-mail: rbhanji@ualberta.ca

E. J. Carey
Division of Gastroenterology and Hepatology, Mayo Clinic, Phoenix, AZ, USA
e-mail: carey.elizabeth@mayo.edu

© Springer Nature Switzerland AG 2020   169
P. Tandon, A. J. Montano-Loza (eds.), *Frailty and Sarcopenia in Cirrhosis*,
https://doi.org/10.1007/978-3-030-26226-6_13

Pathophysiology

The pathophysiology of both entities is complex and includes reduced oral intake, malabsorption, need for alternative energy source and breakdown of protein, systemic inflammation, decreased clearance of ammonia, and hypogonadism [2].

The presence of ascites contributes to early satiety, nausea, and abdominal pain, all of which lead to reduced oral intake. Medications prescribed for control of ascites and prescription of a low salt diet may lead to altered taste and further reduce oral intake.

Systemic inflammation likely contributes to the catabolic state seen in cirrhosis leading to further muscle breakdown with prolonged fasting. Increased ammonia promotes protein breakdown by stimulating myostatin [6] an inhibitor of protein synthesis and regeneration. Myostatin acts by activating the major skeletal muscle proteolytic pathways [6]. Finally, low levels of testosterone lead to reduced inhibition of myostatin [6]. Of note, sarcopenia leads to further physical disability and thus functional decline or frailty [1].

Treatment

Lifestyle changes including exercise and nutritional supplementation have been shown to improve both sarcopenia [7, 8] and frailty [7]. Studies are ongoing with regard to use of myostatin antagonists, hormonal replacement (testosterone or growth hormone), or ammonia-lowering agents for treatment of sarcopenia [9].

As LT leads to cure of ascites, improved ammonia clearance, improvement in hypogonadism, and reduced systemic inflammation, it was naturally thought to reverse both sarcopenia and frailty akin to reversal of symptoms secondary to portal hypertension. However, the few studies that have looked at the course of these entities following transplantation do not demonstrate universal improvement.

Sarcopenia Following Liver Transplantation

There is heterogeneity in the literature with regard to both methods and cutoff values for diagnosing sarcopenia, which makes comparison between studies difficult. The L3 skeletal muscle index (L3SMI) assessed by CT has shown to predict survival in patients with ESLD and is considered by many to be the gold standard for diagnosing sarcopenia [10]. However, studies evaluating changes in muscle mass after LT are limited by the fact that not all patients had subsequent CTs following LT, and for those who had the CTs, these were done at varying times and not as protocol.

Muscle Mass

Previous studies assessing body composition following LT using dual-energy X-ray absorptiometry (DEXA) have generally shown no improvement in body composition following LT. In one study, significant reduction in lean body mass was seen up to 9 months after LT, with nonsignificant increase seen up to 24 months following LT [11]. Another study showed an increase in lean body mass from 2 to 24 months post-LT but only in males [12]. Further, no improvement in body composition was seen in patients who were not in an exercise/nutritional counselling group [13].

A Cleveland Clinic study analyzing 53 patients showed 62% ($n = 33$) had pre-LT sarcopenia [14]. Sarcopenia was diagnosed using CT of the L4 region. CT scans of a control group were used to establish normal muscle mass, and sarcopenia was defined as 5th percentile of age- and sex-specific normalized muscle area. Of these, only 6% ($n = 2$) had resolution of sarcopenia seen on an indication-based post-LT CT done at a mean of 13.1 ± 8.0 months. Of note, 75% (15/22) had de novo sarcopenia. Patients with ascites were more likely to have sarcopenia both pre- and post-LT ($p < 0.05$). Patients with hepatocellular carcinoma (HCC) were more likely to have an increase in psoas muscle area following LT (46% vs. 15%), but tumor volume did not predict post-LT sarcopenia.

In another study, subanalysis of 47 patients with sarcopenia pre-LT and a second CT following transplant was done. Sarcopenia was diagnosed using CT of the L3 region. Follow-up CT was done at a mean of 50 ± 6 months showing resolution of sarcopenia in 13 of the 47 patients (28%) [3].

A Korean study ($n = 145$), using psoas muscle area to diagnose sarcopenia (cutoff 5th percentile of age- and sex-specific normalized muscle area for controls), found 36% of patients had pre-LT sarcopenia. None of these patients had resolution seen on second, indication-based CT done at a mean of 12.3 ± 5.7 months following LT. De novo sarcopenia was diagnosed in 15% (14/93) of patients [15]. Patients with pre-LT sarcopenia were more likely to be males (41% vs. 14%; $p = 0.008$). Patients with post-LT sarcopenia were more likely to be male (91%; $p = 0.003$), had a significantly lower BMI (23 Kg/m^2; $p = 0.015$), and most had pre-LT sarcopenia (79%; $p < 0.001$).

Finally, a study out of University of Pittsburgh including a select group of patients ($n = 40$) without post-LT risk factors for sarcopenia (i.e., ICU readmission, admission for infection, persistent renal failure, hepatic artery thrombosis, ischemic cholangiopathy, alcohol relapse, and recurrent disease (PSC, NAFLD), or HCC) found 55% (22/40) of the patients to have pre-LT sarcopenia [16]. CT SMI was used to diagnose sarcopenia (cutoffs: females < 38.5 cm^2/m^2; males <52.4 cm^2/m^2). Sarcopenia persisted in 45% (10/22) of the patients and resolved in another 55% (12/22) on an indication-based, post-LT CT done at a mean of 20.3 ± 7.4 months. Though these results are not applicable to all patients undergoing LT, it shows, in the absence of risk factors, sarcopenia may improve following LT.

Risk Factors

Not surprisingly, there is some overlap between pre-LT and post-LT risk factors for sarcopenia. Pre-LT risk factors include malnutrition, hypercatabolic state, hyperammonemia, systemic inflammation, hypogonadism, and sedentary lifestyle. Cirrhotic patients have an abnormal fuel metabolism and have an increased energy expenditure (120% of the expected value). Elevated pro-inflammatory and anti-inflammatory cytokine levels in these patients likely contribute to this hypercatabolic state [17]. Thus, an overnight fast in a cirrhotic is comparable to a 72 h fast in a healthy individual [17]. It is likely this hypercatabolic state persists following transplantation and contributes to either persistent or de novo sarcopenia.

The main risk factors for post-LT sarcopenia in addition to persistent hypercatabolic state include immunosuppression, renal failure, hospitalizations, metabolic syndrome, disease recurrence, and lifestyle (Table 13.1).

Immunosuppression use post-LT is an important driver of sarcopenia. Corticosteroids have been shown to impair protein synthesis by increasing proteolysis. Their effect may be mediated by myostatin [8]. In addition, steroid use has been shown to result in myopathy due to muscle fiber atrophy [8]. Calcineurin inhibitors (CNIs) may also contribute to impaired muscle growth as intracellular calcineurin activation regulates the genes involved in skeletal muscle growth, remodeling, and maintenance [18]. CNI use, in animal studies, also showed an increase in myostatin expression [18]. Upregulation of myostatin post-LT may explain persistent and de novo sarcopenia [14]. Tacrolimus can also lead to increased energy expenditure and hypercatabolism [8]. Further, the use of CNIs increases the risk of renal failure and renal impairment, which is a risk factor for sarcopenia. mTOR inhibitors have been shown to induce anabolic resistance and thus contribute to reduced muscle mass [8].

Table 13.1 Risk factors for post-liver transplant sarcopenia

Risk factor	Mechanism
Sedentary lifestyle	Reduced energy expenditure Increased risk of MS
Metabolic syndrome	IR leading to promotion of proteolysis Inhibition of GH/IGF-1 axis Inactivation mTOR
Hypercatabolic state	Increased energy expenditure Increased inflammation (cytokines)
Immunosuppression Corticosteroids Calcineurin inhibitors mTOR inhibitors	Increase proteolysis, muscle fiber atrophy, MS, infections Impairs gene regulation muscle growth, upregulates myostatin, renal failure, MS, infections Anabolic resistance, uninhibited autophagy, protein degradation, MS, infections
Renal failure	Increased inflammation
Disease recurrence	Hypercatabolic state, increased inflammation, upregulation myostatin
Hospitalization	Immobility

MS metabolic syndrome, *IR* insulin resistance, *GH* growth hormone, *IGF-1* insulin growth factor-1

Immunosuppressants also increase the risk of posttransplant infections and sepsis, which lead to increased proteolysis and impaired protein synthesis. In addition, infections likely lead to increased hospitalizations and increased length of stay, which lead to increased inactivity and an increased risk for debility. Immunosuppression use also contributes to the risk for metabolic syndrome, which is associated with an increased risk for sarcopenia [9].

Obesity leads to decreased secretion of adipokines, which promotes insulin resistance (IR). IR further inhibits growth hormone (GH)/insulin growth factor-1 axis, which plays a protective role in muscle loss and in muscle regeneration, by way of lipolysis and increased free fatty acids [9]. Moreover, gluconeogenesis, in a state of IR, further exacerbates proteolysis and leads to muscle depletion. Finally, in the presence of IR, the mTOR pathway becomes inactive and autophagic, or lysosomal degradation of proteins and organelles is uninhibited [9].

As in pre-LT sarcopenia, lifestyle may also play a significant role in the persistence of sarcopenia following transplantation. Many transplant recipients continue to remain sedentary [18] with inactivity leading to reduced energy expenditure and increased risk of obesity and metabolic syndrome.

Consequences of Reduced Muscle Mass

Decreased muscle mass following transplant is associated with a threefold increased risk for diabetes (95% CI [1.01 – 9.38]; $p < 0.05$). Further, there is a trend to increased mortality in patients who continue to have a decrease in muscle mass ($p = 0.08$) [14]. Jeon JH et al. have similarly shown there is a trend to increased mortality in patients with sarcopenia post-LT (80 ± 5.2 mo vs. 92 ± 4.2 mo; $p = 0.069$) and patients with de novo sarcopenia have a significantly increased risk of mortality (HR 10.53; 95% CI [1.37 – 80.9]; $p = 0.024$) [15].

Conclusion

Overall these preliminary results indicate that sarcopenia may not reverse after transplantation. Of note, none of these studies use protocol CTs. Thus, there is likely a bias toward a higher prevalence of sarcopenia as follow-up CTs are more likely to be obtained in sicker patients with complications. Indeed, in absence of intervention (exercise/nutrition), there is no change or continued reduction of muscle mass or even de novo sarcopenia seen in the first couple of years following LT. Moreover, sarcopenia post-LT has been associated with a trend to increased mortality, and de novo sarcopenia has been shown to significantly increase mortality risk. The study by Bergerson et al. however suggests that limiting risk factors leads to improvement in sarcopenia [16]. In their study, there was no diagnosis of de novo sarcopenia and muscle mass improved in 55% of the patients. Thus, identification of this high-risk group of patients is paramount for intervention. Further prospective studies are needed to confirm risk factors and prevalence of sarcopenia and to determine impact of intervention. Studies with long-term follow-up are also needed to determine whether these early changes in muscle mass persist and how they affect the long-term outcomes in this patient population.

Frailty Following Liver Transplantation

Frailty was first recognized as a geriatric syndrome and has only recently been studied in patients with ESLD [19]. Due to lack of a gold standard metric, there is a lot of heterogeneity in the literature with regard to diagnosis of frailty. Many different tools, most developed in older community-dwelling individuals, have been used in patients with cirrhosis (Table 13.2). The key aspects of these tests include assessment for weight loss, physical stamina, and function. Fried Frailty Index (FFI) has been used more frequently in patients with ESLD. However, the FFI includes components that are subjective in nature, and its categorical nature makes this test insensitive to changes that occur over time or that may occur with intervention [20]. In efforts to circumvent this, a new tool, the Liver Frailty Index (LFI), comprised of grip strength, chair stands, and balance testing was evaluated in patients with ESLD awaiting LT [19]. The LFI is performance based and is scored on continuous scale, which makes it more suitable to monitor changes over time.

Frailty

Thus far, only one study has assessed frailty following LT [20]. In this study, 21% of the patients were classified as frail pre-LT ($n = 214$). Females were more likely to be frail (50% in frail group vs. 19% in robust group; $p < 0.01$), but patients with HCC were less likely to be frail when compared to their counterparts (23% in frail group vs. 70% in robust group; $p < 0.01$). Frail patients had a significantly higher MELD score (25 vs. 18; $p < 0.01$). The LFI was used to diagnose frailty with the following cutoffs: "robust" (<3.2), "pre- frail" (between 3.2 and <4.5), and "frail" (≥4.5). Median LFI worsened 3 months following LT with 59% of the patients having a worse score. There was some improvement at 6 months following LT; 41% of the patients had a worse LFI score. At 12 months following LT, there was further improvement with 32% of the patients having a worse score than at pre-LT. Though the median LFI improved at 12 months following LT (3.7 [3.2, 4.3] vs. 3.4 [3.0, 3.9]; $p < 0.001$), this improvement was minimally clinically significant.

Other studies in solid organ transplantation, using the FFI to diagnose frailty, have shown significant improvement after transplantation. For instance, following kidney transplantation ¾ of the patients were recategorized from frail to either intermediate-frail or non-frail at a follow-up of 3 months [21]. In another study, all frail patients who received a heart transplant were recategorized to non-frail at the 6-month follow-up [22].

Table 13.2 Tools for diagnosing frailty in patients with ESLD adapted from [7]

Tool	Components	Test results	Advantages and disadvantages
Fried Frailty Index	Unintentional weight loss ($\geq$10 lbs/yr) Jamar hand grip Exhaustion Low activity level Gait speed (per 15 ft)	Frailty score $\geq$3 is abnormal	Has subjective, self-reported components. Categorical score. Limited in individuals with severe HE, ascites, or edema
Liver Frailty Index (LFI)	Grip strength Chair stands Balance testing	Score: <3.2 – non-frail 3.2 – <4.5 -pre- frail $\geq$4.5 – frail	Developed for LT candidates. Performance based, on continuous scale. May be more suitable to monitor changes over time
The 6-minute walk test (6MWT)	Walking distance over 6 min period	> 300 m – normal $\leq$ 300 m – low endurance < 250 m – frail	May be easily accessible in routine clinical care
Gait speed	Usual pace gait speed (5 meters; m/s) Use of assistive devices allowed	1 m/s is normal	Not applicable to patients who are wheelchair bound
Short Physical Performance Battery Protocol (SPPB)	Gait speed balance Timed repeated chair stands	Maximum 4 points/category Score < 9 is abnormal	Quick to complete (takes 2–3 minutes) as an outpatient May be difficult to perform in patients with moderate to severe HE
Activities of daily living (ADL)	Ability to feed, toilet, dress, bathe, and transfer	Points: 3 – independent 2 – needs assistance 1 – dependent Score < 12 abnormal	Can be performed by nurses It is subjective as it is self-reported
The Braden Scale	Physical exam and assessment of 6 criteria: skin sensory perception, moisture, activity, mobility, nutrition, and friction (ability to hold a comfortable position in a chair and bed).	Score of 23 – no risk Score of 16 – requires intervention	Can be performed by nurses

Risk Factors

Worsening of the pre-liver transplant LFI by 0.1 unit was associated with significantly reduced odds of being robust at 3 (OR 0.75; $p < .001$), 6 (OR 0.77; $p < .001$), and 12 months (OR 0.90; $p = .001$) [20]. This association remained significant after adjusting for MELD, age, female sex, and diabetes [20]. Similarly, pretransplant frailty was associated with an increased risk for frailty following kidney transplant [21]. In these patients, diabetes mellitus and delayed graft function were also associated with frailty posttransplant [21].

Consequences of Frailty

The presence of frailty pre-LT is significantly associated with a longer transplant length of stay (LOS) compared to non-frail patients (9 vs. 7 days; $P = .004$), and a trend was seen toward increased ICU LOS among the frail versus non-frail patients (3 vs. 2 days; $P = .06$) [20]. Further, frail patients had more hospital days in 3 months following LT (2 vs. 0 days; $P = .03$). Frail patients were noted to have a trend toward increased rates of death overall compared to their non-frail counterparts (11% vs. 4%; $p = .06$) [20]. Similarly, frail patients following heart transplant had a longer ICU stay compared to the non-frail patients and had a significantly lower 12-month survival [22]. In the renal literature, frailty pretransplant is an important risk factor for adverse outcomes including delayed graft function, hospital readmissions, and mortality following kidney transplant [21].

Conclusion

Early literature suggests that frailty improves following transplantation. There is initial worsening of frailty followed by improvement at 1-year posttransplant [20]. Pretransplant frailty is a risk factor for posttransplant frailty [20–22]. The presence of comorbidities such as diabetes, metabolic syndrome, renal impairment, depression, and cognitive impairment leads to a higher risk of persistent frailty posttransplant. This group of patients will likely benefit the most from interventions including prehabilitation and optimization of comorbid conditions. However, further studies are needed to ascertain the course of frailty following LT and its impact on clinical outcomes including hospitalization, hospital LOS, QOL, and patient survival. Long-term follow-up will be invaluable in allowing for a better understanding of the natural history of frailty and its impact on long-term clinical outcomes.

References

1. Cruz-Jentoft AJ, Baeyens JP, Bauer JM, Boirie Y, Cederholm T, Landi F, et al. Sarcopenia: European consensus on definition and diagnosis: report of the European Working Group on Sarcopenia in Older People. Age Ageing. 2010;39(4):412–23.
2. Sinclair M, Gow PJ, Grossmann M, Angus PW. Review article: sarcopenia in cirrhosis – aetiology, implications and potential therapeutic interventions. Aliment Pharmacol Ther. 2016;43(7):765–77.

3. Montano-Loza AJ, Meza-Junco J, Baracos VE, Prado CM, Ma M, Meeberg G, et al. Severe muscle depletion predicts postoperative length of stay but is not associated with survival after liver transplantation. Liver Transpl. 2014;20(6):640–8.
4. Kalafateli M, Mantzoukis K, Choi Yau Y, Mohammad AO, Arora S, Rodrigues S, et al. Malnutrition and sarcopenia predict post-liver transplantation outcomes independently of the Model for End-stage Liver Disease score. J Cachexia Sarcopenia Muscle. 2017;8(1):113–21.
5. Lai JC, Feng S, Terrault NA, Lizaola B, Hayssen H, Covinsky K. Frailty predicts waitlist mortality in liver transplant candidates. Am J Transplant. 2014;14(8):1870–9.
6. Dasarathy S, Merli M. Sarcopenia from mechanism to diagnosis and treatment in liver disease. J Hepatol. 2016;65(6):1232–44.
7. Bhanji RA, Carey EJ, Yang L, Watt KD. The long winding road to transplant: how sarcopenia and debility impact morbidity and mortality on the waitlist. Clin Gastroenterol Hepatol. 2017;15(10):1492.
8. Dasarathy S. Posttransplant sarcopenia: an underrecognized early consequence of liver transplantation. Dig Dis Sci. 2013;58(11):3103–11.
9. Bhanji RA, Narayanan P, Allen AM, Malhi H, Watt KD. Sarcopenia in hiding: the risk and consequence of underestimating muscle dysfunction in nonalcoholic steatohepatitis. Hepatology. 2017;66(6):2055–65.
10. Carey EJ, Lai JC, Wang CW, Dasarathy S, Lobach I, Montano-Loza AJ, et al. A multicenter study to define sarcopenia in patients with end-stage liver disease. Liver Transplant. 2017;23(5):625–33.
11. Hussaini SH, Oldroyd B, Stewart SP, Soo S, Roman F, Smith MA, et al. Effects of orthotopic liver transplantation on body composition. Liver. 1998;18(3):173–9.
12. Krasnoff JB, Vintro AQ, Ascher NL, Bass NM, Dodd MJ, Painter PL. Objective measures of health-related quality of life over 24 months post-liver transplantation. Clin Transpl. 2005;19(1):1–9.
13. Krasnoff JB, Vintro AQ, Ascher NL, Bass NM, Paul SM, Dodd MJ, et al. A randomized trial of exercise and dietary counseling after liver transplantation. Am J Transplant. 2006;6(8):1896–905.
14. Tsien C, Garber A, Narayanan A, Shah SN, Barnes D, Eghtesad B, et al. Post-liver transplantation sarcopenia in cirrhosis: a prospective evaluation. J Gastroenterol Hepatol. 2014;29(6):1250–7.
15. Jeon JY, Wang HJ, Ock SY, Xu W, Lee JD, Lee JH, et al. Newly developed sarcopenia as a prognostic factor for survival in patients who underwent liver transplantation. PLoS One. 2015;10(11):e0143966.
16. Bergerson JT, Lee JG, Furlan A, Sourianarayanane A, Fetzer DT, Tevar AD, et al. Liver transplantation arrests and reverses muscle wasting. Clin Transpl. 2015;29(3):216–21.
17. Bhanji RA, Carey EJ, Watt KD. Review article: maximising quality of life while aspiring for quantity of life in end-stage liver disease. Aliment Pharmacol Ther. 2017;46(1):16–25.
18. Kallwitz ER. Sarcopenia and liver transplant: the relevance of too little muscle mass. World J Gastroenterol. 2015;21(39):10982–93.
19. Lai JC, Covinsky KE, Dodge JL, Boscardin WJ, Segev DL, Roberts JP, et al. Development of a novel frailty index to predict mortality in patients with end-stage liver disease. Hepatology. 2017;66(2):564–74.
20. Lai JC, Segev DL, McCulloch CE, Covinsky KE, Dodge JL, Feng S. Physical frailty after liver transplantation. Am J Transplant. 2018;18(8):1986–94.
21. McAdams-DeMarco MA, Isaacs K, Darko L, Salter ML, Gupta N, King EA, et al. Changes in frailty after kidney transplantation. J Am Geriatr Soc. 2015;63(10):2152–7.
22. Jha SR, Hannu MK, Newton PJ, Wilhelm K, Hayward CS, Jabbour A, et al. Reversibility of frailty after bridge-to-transplant ventricular assist device implantation or heart transplantation. Transplant Direct. 2017;3(7):e167.

Chapter 14
Measures of Sarcopenia: The Utility of Ultrasound, Bioelectrical Impedance Analysis and Single-Slice Cross-Sectional Imaging

Marina Mourtzakis and Kirsten Elizabeth Bell

The Importance of Body Composition Analysis in Liver Cirrhosis

A number of precise and accurate tools and techniques have evolved to measure the prevalence and implications of sarcopenia in liver cirrhosis; however, the future utility of these tools is contingent on their practicality and feasibility for use in clinical settings. New technologies and novel applications of existing diagnostic equipment are emerging for use in research as well as clinics. For example, computed tomography (CT) imaging and ultrasound can provide complex and progressive information about the composition and distribution of diverse tissues, such as skeletal muscle and adipose tissue. These technologies offer non-invasive strategies to advance our knowledge of the role of body composition in understanding and managing illness and malnutrition [2]. With the enhancement of body composition technologies, we can identify deviations in features of muscle and adipose tissue from normal healthy values and explore how these deviations relate to clinical outcomes [2–7]. Using tools like CT, ultrasound and magnetic resonance imaging (MRI), skeletal muscle can be quantified with a high degree of accuracy and precision; further, these quantifications may be coupled with measurements of muscle quality or integrity, which are representative of the metabolic, physiological and physical function of skeletal muscle [2, 8]. While research has elevated our knowledge of and perspectives on body composition, there is an increasing demand to translate these laboratory-based methods into feasible and practical approaches that assist clinicians in identifying patients who may be at risk of malnutrition [9]. Researchers and clinicians have yet to agree on a single consensus definition of sarcopenia; and numerous skeletal muscle cut-points have been developed and published using both

M. Mourtzakis (✉) · K. E. Bell
Department of Kinesiology, University of Waterloo, Waterloo, ON, Canada
e-mail: mmourtzakis@uwaterloo.ca, kirsten.bell@uwaterloo.ca

© Springer Nature Switzerland AG 2020
P. Tandon, A. J. Montano-Loza (eds.), *Frailty and Sarcopenia in Cirrhosis*,
https://doi.org/10.1007/978-3-030-26226-6_14

diverse populations (e.g. healthy, as well as various clinical populations including cancer and intensive care unit patients) and body composition tools (e.g. CT and DXA). Thus, meticulous attention is needed when reviewing the methodologies used in published studies and interpreting the results of these investigations. In other words, different methods and body composition tools reference different cut-points for identifying individuals with low muscle mass. Classification of liver cirrhosis patients as sarcopenic or non-sarcopenic is essential because low muscularity is associated with numerous clinical complications and deleterious outcomes. Critically, patients who are correctly identified as sarcopenic may benefit from targeted nutrition, exercise and/or pharmacological treatment that is tailored to their specific needs.

Practical Need for Identifying Sarcopenia in Liver Cirrhosis

Low muscularity is associated with serious complications and negative clinical outcomes. More work is needed to accurately identify patients with sarcopenia who are at increased risk of morbidity and mortality. In addition to precision and accuracy, diligence is essential when interpreting results from the literature given that there is no universal consensus definition of sarcopenia. While we need to identify and monitor those at risk of sarcopenia and malnutrition using body composition tools, prudence is fundamental to acquiring and using this data. Clinical personnel who want to incorporate body composition analysis into their practice should consider the following steps:

1. Find and use a protocol that is clearly written and provides sufficient detail about the methodological approach
2. Be vigilant in how you implement and execute the protocol
3. Understand the limitations of your tools and the protocol
4. Interpret your results with caution

Choosing the Right Modality

Currently, weight and, more specifically, body mass index (BMI) are most commonly used in clinic to assess a patient's nutritional status and help clinicians identify patients at risk of malnutrition. Weight (or, more accurately, body mass) is useful in tracking gross changes in total tissue weight (i.e. mass) over time; BMI is weight normalized to height squared (kg/m^2) and is a representation of overall body size. Weight and BMI are cost- and time-efficient methods requiring only access to a scale (for weight) and stadiometer (for height). While weight and BMI are both relatively crude assessment tools, a notable advantage of BMI overweight is that patients can be classified according to World Health Organization standards as underweight (BMI < 18.5 kg/m^2), normal weight (BMI 18.5–24.9 kg/m^2), overweight (BMI 25.0–29.9 kg/m^2) or obese (BMI ≥ 30.0 kg/m^2) for their frame [24].

Although BMI is regularly reported in nutrition and epidemiological studies on healthy and clinical populations, BMI is not capable of distinguishing between different tissues (e.g. differentiating skeletal muscle from adipose tissue), nor does it provide information on the distribution of these distinct tissues within the body; as such, BMI provides only a very limited amount of information on the body composition, and thus nutritional status, of patients. Critically, it is inappropriate to use BMI as a surrogate measure for skeletal muscle mass in clinic or in research, because it has a poor capacity for identifying malnourished or sarcopenic individuals [2, 13, 14]. Baracos and colleagues [14] examined a group of non-small cell lung cancer patients with CT imaging performed at the third lumbar (L3) vertebra and observed that although ~47% were classified as sarcopenic using CT (a direct measure of skeletal muscle mass), only ~7.5% were identified as being underweight according to BMI (BMI < 18.5 kg/m^2). Of particular interest, almost half of the patients in this study were classified as overweight or obese based on BMI, suggesting that a high proportion of patients present with, or are at risk of, sarcopenic obesity. This pattern has also been observed in other studies in cancer [13–16], critical illness [25] and liver cirrhosis [1, 22], where although sarcopenia was noted in as much as 40–71% of patients, only 1–12% were underweight according to BMI [1, 2, 13–16, 22, 25].

Clearly, there are a growing need for clinically friendly equipment to assess body composition in liver cirrhosis and a particular need for tools capable of discriminating between skeletal muscle and adipose tissue with both accuracy and precision. To determine the appropriate tool for body composition analysis, we need to consider (1) the objectives for taking the measures (i.e. classification of the patient as sarcopenic versus monitoring longitudinal changes in muscle or fat mass); (2) the quality of the measurement needed in terms of precision, accuracy and specificity (i.e. identifying whether a measurement of lean tissue rather than muscle is sufficient); and (3) the types of measures of skeletal muscle health that are suitable for addressing the objectives (i.e. characteristics of muscle quantity and muscle quality) (Fig. 14.1).

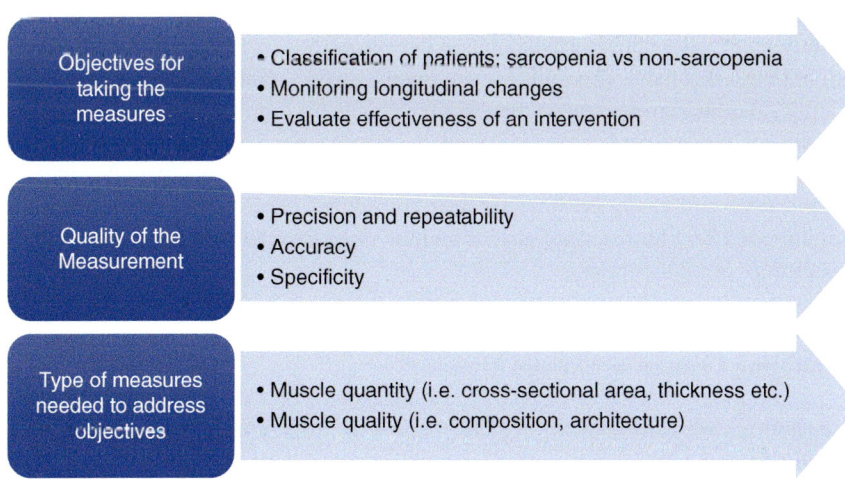

Fig. 14.1 Considerations for choosing the right body composition modality

Objectives for Measuring Skeletal Muscle Health

To select the most appropriate body composition modality for your skeletal muscle assessment, it is important to carefully consider your specific objectives; in other words, 'Why are you taking these measurements?' Consider the following three primary objectives for assessing skeletal muscle health, which are fundamental to most clinical and research investigations:

1. To identify individuals who present with, or who are at risk of developing, low muscle mass (a key component of sarcopenia or cachexia)
2. To monitor changes in skeletal muscle in individuals who are likely to experience muscle atrophy (i.e. critically ill, cancer or liver cirrhosis patients)
3. To evaluate the effectiveness of nutrition/exercise/pharmacological intervention(s) over time

Identifying Individuals at Risk of Low Muscle Mass (with Sarcopenia)

Clinicians and researchers have traditionally used BMI to identify potentially malnourished individuals; however, BMI is a simplistic method that does not distinguish between tissues like skeletal muscle and adipose tissue. Several alternative, more sophisticated modalities have the ability to isolate fat-free mass (BIA, DXA) or even skeletal muscle (ultrasound, CT), and a range of cut-points for identifying sarcopenic patients is available in the literature [12, 13, 15, 22]. Over the last decade, this range has widened, creating some confusion around which cut-points are best to employ in research and in practice.

Two key factors should be considered when selecting cut-points. First, understand the population(s) in which your cut-points of interest were derived. Consider the sex and age distribution of the individuals in this reference population, as well as any details about their clinical or body composition characteristics that may introduce bias when using these cut-points. Second, identify the analytical methods the authors of these papers used to derive the cut-points. For example, some authors will have defined their cut-points for sarcopenia as two standard deviations below a healthy reference group [20], whereas others will have generated their cut-points using a receiver operator curve [12]; the latter approach would be based on a clinical outcome like mortality or a health outcome like a functional test. Given that there is no universal consensus on how we use cut-points, choose the approach in the literature that best fits your population and the objectives for what you are trying to learn from your patient data.

Monitoring Changes in Skeletal Muscle

Longitudinal measurement of skeletal muscle is fundamental to monitoring the magnitude and rate of muscle loss occurring in patients. Acquiring these measures can provide a guide for understanding the nutritional needs of the patient.

In research, there is particular interest in longitudinal evaluation as a foundational measure for comparing any future interventions. However, one needs to consider a few factors regarding their modality of choice. Evaluate the precision, accuracy and specificity of the instrument relative to the changes you will be seeking. If you anticipate relatively small changes compared with the precision of the instrument, then you need to consider whether your skeletal muscle measurements will be confounded by artefact or error. For example, if you expect a 1% change but the error of your instrument is as great as 2% for a single scan, and given that you are comparing two scans for potential changes, you may need to account for error up to 4%. In addition, ensure that you are measuring what you think you are measuring. For example, thickness of muscle using ultrasound will include intramuscular fat; keep this in mind as you interpret your results (further details found in section "Quality of the Measurement: Considering Precision, Accuracy and Specificity").

Evaluating the Effectiveness of Nutrition/Exercise/Pharmacological Interventions

One of the most important reasons for using body composition modalities to measure skeletal muscle mass is to assess the success or failure of a given intervention, the goal of which is to attenuate or prevent muscle loss. However, similar to the objective described above (section "Monitoring Changes in Skeletal Muscle"), awareness of the precision, accuracy and specificity of your instrument is vital and will significantly affect how you interpret your results.

Quality of the Measurement: Considering Precision, Accuracy and Specificity

To reliably identify patients who are at risk of, or who exhibit signs of, sarcopenia, and to reliably monitor changes in features of skeletal muscle and assess the effectiveness of a therapy or intervention, we should evaluate the following parameters: precision, accuracy and specificity of our instruments. These terms are summarized in Table 14.1.

For an in-depth discussion on utilizing body composition tools at the bedside and correctly interpreting your results, please refer to Dr. Carrie Earthman's tutorial [26]. Measures of precision and accuracy are particularly important in determining the ability to measure change longitudinally. Here, 'minimal detectable difference', which infers that a meaningful change in a body tissue needs to exceed the precision of an instrument or method, should be considered. This concept may influence the choice of method one uses to measure skeletal muscle change over time. If you are expecting relatively large changes, then you may use an instrument that is less precise. However, if you are anticipating a relatively small change over time, a highly precise instrument is needed to ensure that the changes measured are not confounded

Table 14.1 Body composition terminology related to interpretation of results

Term	Definition
Precision	The degree of agreement between multiple measurements made by a given instrument/method. This definition may not account for inter- and intra-analyst error, which introduces variability and affects the reproducibility of a measurement
Repeatability	The variability of multiple measures acquired by the same analyst, with the same instrument/method, on the same participant under the same conditions
Reproducibility	The ability to generate the same (similar) multiple measures by different analysts with the same instrument
Inter-analyst measurement	The variability between measurements taken by different analysts using the same instrument/method (i.e. analyst 1 vs. analyst 2)
Intra-analyst measurement	The variability between measurements taken by the same analyst using the same instrument/method (i.e. analyst 1 vs. analyst 1)
Accuracy	The agreement between two measures/methods whereby one of the methods is a reference instrument/method. Does your method measure what it is supposed to be measuring?
Bias	The systematic error in a measures/method relative to the reference method

by instrument or methodological error. To improve specificity, an instrument/method should have the optimal combination of precision (repeatability and reproducibility), inter- and intra-analyst reliability as well as accuracy.

Measuring Skeletal Muscle Health: Muscle Quantity vs. Muscle Quality

Measurements of muscle quantity include – but are not limited to – muscle mass, volume, cross-sectional area and thickness [8]. Conversely, muscle quality refers to the evaluation of features of muscle that influence its metabolic and physical function, such as tissue composition (i.e. fatty infiltration), the presence of myonecrosis or fibrosis, as well as indicators of strength (i.e. pennation angle, fascicle length) [8]. Historically, clinicians and researchers have focused on measurements of muscle quantity alone [8, 13]; however, the combination of measures of muscle quantity and quality may be more clinically valuable. For example, Martin et al. [15] demonstrated that the combination of accelerated weight loss, CT-based low muscle index as well as low muscle attenuation (low muscle quality) were predictive of survival in overweight and obese lung or gastrointestinal cancer patients. On the other hand, ultrasound-based measures of accelerated muscle atrophy are observed in critically ill patients with multi-organ failure compared with those who have single-organ failure, potentially predicting poor prognosis with severity of complications [27]. Features of muscle quality, such as fascicle length and pennation angle, have also been associated with whole body physical function in critically ill patients [28]. Muscle quantity has been extensively evaluated in liver cirrhosis; however, muscle quality using CT imaging has been evaluated to a limited extent, and ultrasound measures of muscle quality in this population are even more limited. When muscle quantity and quality measurements are combined, these may support the definition of sarcopenia, which is based on muscle quantity and function. Thus, exploring these measures in future investigations may help better define sarcopenia. Muscle quantity and muscle quality will be discussed to a greater extent in the sections corresponding to each body composition modality.

Clinically Friendly Modalities: BIA, CT Imaging and Ultrasonography

Despite our growing knowledge of the importance of muscle metabolism and function for positive clinical outcomes, a universal, standardized approach to specifically measure skeletal muscle in a clinically feasible fashion has yet to emerge. We understand that the most practical solutions, such as BMI, do not provide accurate, tissue-specific information. Fortunately, more sophisticated modalities, such as BIA, CT imaging and ultrasonography, are available in clinic and offer important advantages over BMI and skinfold estimates of percent body fat. BIA can efficiently identify changes in fat-free mass, while CT (or MRI) imaging and ultrasound are increasingly used to quantify skeletal muscle and characterize features of this tissue. These modalities are becoming increasingly available in clinic and provide details on the body composition of patients (rather than simply weight and height) that may influence prognosis.

Bioelectrical Impedance Analysis

BIA is the most commonly used body composition tool in clinical settings due to its accessibility and ease of use. The measurements are entirely non-invasive, cost-effective and quick (requiring no more than 15 minutes), making them suitable and safe for longitudinal (i.e. follow-up) assessments. Most BIA instruments are light-weight and portable and therefore feasible for measurements on both inpatients confined to bedrest and ambulatory outpatients. An additional benefit of BIA is that specialized technicians are not required; unlike CT and MRI, anyone may be trained to operate BIA systems. However, counterbalancing these advantages are three important weaknesses. First, although BIA can estimate fat-free mass and % body fat, it does not directly measure muscle or adipose tissue; rather, BIA relies heavily upon validated prediction equations that were developed for specific (often healthy) populations. Second, these prediction equations are greatly influenced by the hydration status of the patient. As such, the accuracy of BIA measurements is significantly reduced by certain characteristics common to clinical populations, such as fluid retention or dehydration. Third, the type of equipment needs to be considered as biases may be introduced based on the arrangement of electrodes (hand-to-hand

Table 14.2 Summary of the merits and limitations of three clinically accessible body composition modalities

	Merits	Limitations
BIA	Quick measurement (approximately 15 min) Cost-effective Non-invasive No medical technician required to operate device (anyone can be trained) Feasible for use at bedside (no burden is placed on patient)	Measurement highly affected by hydration status and fluid shifts Prediction equations specific to population being measured are required, and most equations are only appropriate for use in healthy adults Not accurate in obese populations due to violations of body geometry assumptions and tissue distribution
CT	Highly precise, accurate and direct measurements of skeletal muscle and various adipose tissue depots (subcutaneous adipose tissue, SAT; visceral adipose tissue, VAT; and intramuscular adipose tissue IMAT)	Costly Exposes patient to large doses of radiation Trained medical radiation technologist required to perform scan Not portable May not be feasible or accessible for every patient/institution CSA analysis is time-consuming (approximately 30–40 min per scan)
Ultrasound	Non-invasive Precise, reliable and accurate Directly measures skeletal muscle No medical technician required to operate device (anyone can be trained) Feasible for use at bedside (no burden is placed on patient)	Proper training required to correctly identify landmarks and acquire good quality images Reporting on methods and reliability testing is minimal or lacking No universal protocol Obese and clinical populations may present challenges during landmarking (due to difficulty palpating bony structures), imaging (due to indistinct fascial borders) and analysis (fatty infiltration might artificially inflate muscle thicknesses) No normative data available

vs. foot-to-foot vs. hand-to-foot). Therefore, the practicality of BIA should be carefully weighed against its shortcomings, and caution must be exercised when interpreting body composition measurements performed with BIA in clinical settings, particularly in hospitalized patients. A summary of the merits and limitations of BIA is outlined in Table 14.2.

How Does BIA Work?

BIA involves passing a small electrical current at one or more frequencies through the body to estimate *total body water (TBW)* and body composition. BIA primarily distinguishes between *fat-free mass (FFM)* and fat mass by estimating *TBW*.

The low-voltage current is neither dangerous to nor felt by the patient. Electrolyte-rich tissues, such as blood and muscle, conduct the current easily, whereas fat and bone are poor conductors. BIA instruments measure the change in voltage (i.e. *impedance, Z*) of the current across the body. The two components of impedance, *resistance (R)* and *reactance (X)*, are applied to validated, population-specific prediction equations to estimate TBW and FFM. Certain instruments, such as multi-frequency BIA and bioelectrical impedance spectroscopy, can further distinguish *intracellular water (ICW)* from *extracellular water (ECW)*.

BIA Instruments: What Do They Measure?

The three main categories of instruments are *single-frequency BIA (SF-BIA)*, *multi-frequency BIA (MF-BIA)* and *bioimpedance spectroscopy (BIS)*. The *SF-BIA* utilizes a current of a single frequency (usually 50 kHz), which passes through the water-soluble components of the body [26]. As a result, SF-BIA devices can estimate FFM and TBW, using specific predictive equations. There are three main types of SF-BIA: hand-to-hand, foot-to-foot and hand-to-foot. When applying your patient's data to existing predictive equations, it is important to be mindful of the type and model of BIA system that was used to derive the given equation. Whenever possible, you should attempt to match the BIA system to account for variance in results between instruments.

The *MF-BIA* uses several (usually 2–6) predefined frequencies between 5 and 500 kHz, which pass through the water-soluble components of the body (e.g. muscle and blood) [26]. The use of multiple frequencies permits differentiation between different body water compartments. For example, ECW is predicted from the lower 5 kHz frequency, and TBW is predicted from the higher frequencies. ICW, which represents body cell mass (i.e. metabolically active tissue), can then be calculated by subtracting ECW from TBW.

In contrast to SF-BIA and MF-BIA, *BIS* does not use linear prediction equations. Rather, many currents (range: 50–250 individual currents) across the entire spectrum of frequencies (5–1200 kHz) are passed through the body, and complex modeling is applied to the data to generate estimates of ICW, ECW and FFM [26, 29]. BIS measures both ECW and ICW directly, from the lower and higher ends of the spectrum, respectively.

The raw measures generated by all BIA instruments are *resistance (R)* and *reactance (X)*. The impedance index (height squared/R) is also often reported. Resistance reflects the ability of the current to flow through fluids and tissues; reactance reflects the interaction of the current with interfaces, such as cell membranes. Resistance and/or reactance values are then applied to standard equations from which TBW can be predicted. Some equations estimate FFM, and others estimate TBW (note that dividing by 0.73 will convert TBW to FFM, based on the standard hydration constant of normally hydrated lean tissue). Most prediction equations were derived from, and therefore should be applied exclusively in, healthy adult populations. An example of such an equation is shown here [30]:

$$FFM\ (kg) = -4.104 + 0.518 * (ht^2\ /\ R_{50}) + 0.231 * wt + 0.130 * Xc + 4.229 * sex$$

(Note: ht = height in m; wt = weight in kg; sex values include female = 0; male = 1)

Phase angle (PA) is another raw measure generated by all BIA systems. PA can be calculated from resistance and reactance data collected at 50 kHz using the following equation [31]:

$$PA = arctangent(X\ /\ R) * 180^{\circ}\ /\ \pi$$

PA reflects body cell mass and the integrity of cellular membranes. PA may also be a clinically relevant outcome since low PA values have been independently associated with low fat-free mass, malnutrition and prognosis in liver cirrhosis [37], as well as in a variety of other clinical populations such as cancer [32, 33], HIV [33, 34] and critically ill patients [35]. Normative PA data (mean values and standard deviations) based on healthy reference populations are available in the literature [30, 36–38] and may be used to calculate standardized PA (SPA) [37]:

$$SPA = (observed\ PA - mean\ PA) / SD$$

In cancer patients, SPA values below −1.65 have been shown to indicate malnutrition. Age, sex and BMI all influence PA measurements.

Using BIA with Standardized Protocols

Different institutions and teams have developed standard operating procedures specific to their respective groups, but several essential concepts must be considered when using BIA to minimize measurement artefacts and errors. Some of these considerations may not be possible to implement. However, when a protocol criterion cannot be met, it is essential to document this protocol deviation, as it will affect the interpretation of your results. Below are criteria that we have typically used as a guide to optimize results [26, 39]:

(a) *Environmental temperature*: Choose a testing location with normal ambient temperature (not excessively cool or warm). Temperature may affect conductance of the current, hydration status (e.g. sweat loss with warmer temperatures) or involuntary muscle contraction (e.g. shivering with cooler room temperatures).

(b) *Maintain sufficient distance from electronic or magnetic devices:* Place the instrument on a non-metal surface at least 1 m away from electronic or magnetic devices. If a patient has any metal implants or devices (i.e. a pacemaker), the BIA should *not* be used.

(c) *Calibration*: Ensure that the device is regularly calibrated (according to the manufacturer's recommendations) to ensure reliable and repeatable results.

(d) *Patient preparation:* To minimize variability in hydration status, especially with longitudinal measures, the patient should be fasted for at least 8 hours and should void their bladder immediately prior to beginning the measurement. Take the weight and height of the patient, and instruct them to lay in supine for 5–10 min prior to taking a measurement. This step allows for fluid shifts. Record the exact amount of time the patient lay supine prior to obtaining the measurement, and repeat during any follow-up measurements. Ensure that the patient's arms are separated $\geq 30°$ from the trunk and the legs are separated from each other by approximately 45°. In overweight or obese patients, you may need to place rolled towels/blankets between the limbs and/or trunk in order to achieve full separation of body parts.

(e) *Electrodes and their placement:* The surface area of the skin where the electrodes will be placed should be cleaned with alcohol to ensure optimal conductance of the current through the electrodes. Use electrodes with sufficient surface area (≥ 4 cm^2). Place electrodes at least 5 cm apart (Note: In smaller-framed patients, it may not be possible to separate electrodes by 5 cm. In such cases, record the distance used, and repeat for follow-up assessments).

(f) *Longitudinal measures*: Use same operator and instrument for repeat/longitudinal measurements and even for comparison amongst different patients or with the literature. Try to follow a similar (if not identical) protocol for each longitudinal measure.

Quality of the Measurement

Precision and Repeatability

The consistency of repeat measurements with BIA is very good, with 1–2% variability generally reported in the literature for SF-BIA and MF-BIA instruments [40–42]. The variability of repeat measurements made with BIS instruments is slightly higher (2–3%) due to difficulty obtaining stable measurements at extreme frequencies [43, 44]. Due to its relatively high degree of precision and repeatability, BIA is well suited to reliably detect longitudinal changes in body composition, provided the same device is used (and the above-mentioned conditions are kept constant) for all serial measurements. The minimum detectable change (MDC) for FFM measured by SF-BIA and MF-BIA devices has been reported to be 3–6% [45], and the MDC for TBW measured by BIS is 5–8% [44].

Accuracy and Specificity

Despite its high degree of precision and repeatability, the ability of BIA to measure 'true' values is low to moderate. This is especially true in clinical populations, such as liver cirrhosis patients, who tend to undergo significant changes in body composition and fluid retention as a result of their disease. BIA is generally more accurate in healthy nonobese adults [26, 29]. The accuracy of BIA measurements can be reduced by (1) patient factors such as adiposity, fluid retention, electrolyte status and skin temperature; (2) environmental factors such as ambient temperature and proximity to metal surfaces and electronic devices; (3) human error (e.g. deviations from measurement protocols when measuring height and weight, improper placement of electrodes on body); and (4) equipment error. Additionally, the assumptions underlying the prediction equations introduce a certain amount of error into all BIA measurements. A final limitation is that since BIA measures the ability of an electrical current to travel through water-soluble tissues like blood and muscle, this modality is based on the assumption that the human body is composed of 73% water.

Validations

Despite being commonly employed in clinical populations, only one study [46] has compared predictions made using BIA to an established reference technique, such as multiple dilution (for TBW) or DXA (for FFM). In this study, Simons et al. [46] observed that the impedance index (height squared/R) was a strong predictor of TBW as measured by deuterium dilution in both normal-weight ($r = 0.92$, $r^2 = 0.85$) and underweight ($r = 0.93$, $r^2 = 0.86$) cachectic cancer patients. However, when the BIA predictive equations developed for the normal-weight group were applied to the underweight group, TBW (and therefore FFM) was overestimated by 1.67 L [46]. This example underscores the difficulty of obtaining a true measurement of FFM or TWB using BIA in individuals who are not normally hydrated or who have undergone significant body composition changes as a result of their disease. In contrast to clinical populations, Nickerson et al. [47] recently demonstrated that the agreement between measurements of whole body FFM by SF-BIA and DXA (reference method) was excellent in healthy, normally hydrated men ($r = 0.90$, $r^2 = 0.81$) and women ($r = 0.96$, $r^2 = 0.92$) aged 18–40 years [47]. Of relevance, BIA measurements of arm FFM mass correlated more strongly with DXA compared to leg FFM in women (arm FFM, $r = 0.95$, $r^2 = 0.59$; leg FFM, $r = 0.77$, $r^2 = 0.59$), but not in men (arm FFM, $r = 0.87$, $r^2 = 0.76$; leg FFM, $r = 0.87$, $r^2 = 0.76$).

CT Imaging (with Applications to MRI)

CT and MRI generate highly precise, accurate and specific measurements of body composition [48–51]. These modalities have the capacity to quantify distinct muscle and adipose tissue depots with excellent repeatability. Single-slice scans, usually taken at the level of the third lumbar vertebra (L3), can predict whole body muscle mass [49, 51]. There is a large wave of literature that describes the development of cut-points for identifying individuals with sarcopenia [12, 13, 15, 52] and describes the prevalence of sarcopenia in clinical populations, including cancer [12, 13, 15, 52, 53], critical illness [25, 50] and liver cirrhosis [1, 5, 7, 11, 21, 22]. While CT and MRI scans are costly and may not be feasible for prospective analysis, scans performed for clinical purposes (i.e. diagnostic, prognostic or follow-up) can be retrospectively used for body composition. This unique strategy has been adopted in numerous clinical research settings to better understand sarcopenia in diverse muscle wasting syndromes. However, more clinically friendly protocols are needed to implement the use of these techniques for prospective longitudinal assessments. For illnesses or diseases where CT or MRI scans are frequently performed, this strategy may have practical utility with more clinically friendly protocols especially for identifying and monitoring patients who are at risk of or experiencing muscle atrophy. A summary of the merits and limitations of CT imaging for body composition analysis are detailed in Table 14.2.

Fundamentals of CT Imaging Analysis of Skeletal Muscle

CT scanners use radiation to generate an image of internal structures and organs. As x-rays penetrate the skin, the underlying different tissue types attenuate them to varying degrees. The magnitude of x-ray attenuation is measured by computer software, which creates a pixilated image with distinct tissues identified by density. To accomplish this process, individual pixels are assigned a value based on their attenuation, also referred to as the Hounsfield unit (HU), and these values range across a greyscale spectrum identifying the most to least dense tissues [54–56]. A certain HU range defines each tissue (e.g. the range for skeletal muscle is −29 to +150 HU) [54, 55]. During image analysis, the number of pixels within this assigned range is summed and subsequently multiplied by pixel surface area to calculate the cross-sectional area of skeletal muscle [13, 56]. Conceptually similar techniques are used for MRI, but the majority of studies that describe liver cirrhosis patients have employed CT imaging. While the remainder of this section will focus on CT, many of the points discussed can be applied to MRI [2].

What Can Be Measured?

Cross-sectional area of skeletal muscle (in units of mm^2 or cm^2) is the most common body composition outcome acquired from CT image analysis. To account for differences in individual stature or frame size, many studies normalize their results to height squared (m^2); hence, most papers report or describe sarcopenia or low muscularity as a muscle index (analogous to BMI) where units of measurement are typically presented as cm^2/m^2. The development of this muscle index has also led to the derivation of cut-points for classifying individuals who present with sarcopenia or low muscularity. However, uncertainty exists regarding the significance of these cut-points, how they should be derived and how to apply them in clinical settings (i.e. are specific cut-points needed for specific clinical cohorts).

Numerous CT-derived cut-points for sarcopenia exist; however, there is no universal consensus amongst researchers on (a) the best method with which to derive cut-points or (b) which cut-points should be used in various clinical and healthy populations. The population and methods used to develop a given cut-point have significant implications on its appropriateness for use in clinic. It is therefore important to carefully consider the health status (e.g. healthy adults, liver cirrhosis patients, ICU patients), ethnicity, sex and age of the cohort in which these reference values were derived and validated. For instance, distinct cut-points were developed and tested in a Japanese population [17]; but applying cut-points developed in North American populations to the Japanese group would have increased the reported prevalence of sarcopenia erroneously and substantially. One method to identify distinct cut-points is to use two standard deviations below the mean of a healthy reference group, as per the recommendation of the European Working Group on Sarcopenia in Older People [10]. Another commonly used method to develop and test cut-points is to construct a receiver operator curve against mortality or some other clinical outcome [12, 19]. We need to be exceedingly cautious in our use and interpretation of these cut-points when identifying sarcopenic patients in practice, because of the ethnic and clinical diversity, and differences in sex and age, between our patients and the populations used to generate these cut-points. A comparison of the various statistical approaches to identify cut-points for sarcopenia has yet to be conducted. We must continue to work towards developing a universal standard cut-point that accounts for these key factors so that data is comparable.

Radiodensity, which generally refers to the average x-ray attenuation across the CSA of a given tissue, is emerging as a significant prognostic factor related to CT imaging [14, 15, 23, 57]. It is measured as mean HU (or grey level image, GLI) and represents skeletal muscle density (i.e. the degree to which this tissue is infiltrated with non-muscle tissue like fat). Radiodensity is strongly associated with clinical outcomes in patients with cancer [14, 15, 57] as well as liver cirrhosis [6, 23]. In fact, Martin et al. [15] demonstrated that low muscle mean HU was independently prognostic of survival. They also demonstrated that muscle attenuation may differ in individuals who are overweight or obese based on BMI. Further, they go on to suggest that these individuals may require a different HU classification compared with normal or underweight individuals [15]. Lower attenuation in muscle tissue generally reflects the infiltration of fat, which is less dense and serves to reduce the mean attenuation of the overall tissue.

CT Imaging Protocols

There are two main steps to acquiring and analysing CT images that have been performed retrospectively in a clinical setting: (1) identifying the correct slice to analyse (using bony landmarks) and (2) skeletal muscle image analysis. However, prior to embarking on these steps, consider the following:

(a) *Create a record of pertinent CT image parameters and settings*. There is growing literature on the implications of CT equipment parameters (such as voltage) on skeletal muscle results. The use of contrast agents has emerged as a factor that may affect radiodensity and, in some cases, even the cross-sectional areas of visceral adipose tissue. Cross-sectional areas may be influenced because the threshold ranges that define a given tissue depot, such as visceral adipose tissue, are based on radiodensity of that tissue [58–60]. In addition to these parameters, make note of the scan thickness and the scan number.

(b) *Identify the anatomical landmark that best addresses your objectives.* While several protocols exist in the literature for identifying the correct slice to analyse (whole body and segmental CT scan files normally consist of numerous 3–5 mm slices), the third lumbar vertebra (L3) has consistently been used for landmarking single-slice analysis. The protocol for identifying this site is used widely, resulting in a substantial bank of studies to which healthy and clinical populations can be compared. For patients with liver cirrhosis, the L3 region is commonly scanned for diagnostic and prognostic purposes given the proximity of this region in relation to the liver.

(c) *Identify the muscle groups of interest.* Measuring skeletal muscle cross-sectional area for the entire L3 region (versus the cross-sectional area of a single muscle or group of muscles) generally results in more precise measurements. However, if you are interested in one particular muscle or group of muscles (e.g. the *psoas* or paraspinals), be mindful of the larger relative error associated with measuring these smaller areas. Conceptually, there is some subjective interpretation that occurs by the analyst in terms of whether some pixels are viewed as muscle or fat by the software. If measuring small muscles (i.e. 50 pixels), the misinterpretation of a single pixel will be more profound (i.e. error $= 1/50 = 2\%$) than the misinterpretation of a single pixel in a larger muscle or muscle group (i.e. 100 pixels; thus, error $= 1/100 = 1\%$).

(d) *Determine the level of accuracy and precision needed.* Quantifying the cross-sectional area of the entire L3 region, or even specific muscles within the L3 region, is time-consuming; but this method produces precise and accurate measurements that can be used to assess future longitudinal changes. However, if you simply want to classify patients as presenting with or without sarcopenia, then you may consider a simplified approach using linear measures [61, 62]. This latter approach can be performed with the usual viewing software available in all clinical facilities that house a CT scanner.

Landmarking

The L3 region is the most commonly used bony landmark in studies examining muscle and adipose tissue concurrently. This landmark relates well to both tissues ($r = 0.903$–0.924 for muscle and $r = 0.858$–0.889 for adipose tissue) [49]. If measuring muscle or fat in isolation, then the optimal location for measuring skeletal muscle is 5 cm in the superior direction of the intervertebral space between the fourth and fifth lumbar (L4 and L5, respectively) vertebrae ($r = 0.924$); in contrast, the most optimal site for adipose tissue is 5 cm in the inferior direction of the L4 and L5 intervertebral space ($r = 0.963$) [56]. Consistency in landmarking is vital and permits longitudinal assessment of muscle change [2] and comparisons across populations or clinical sites. We focus on bony landmarks, as these change minimally over time, compared with soft tissues. In addition, the vertebral column exhibits many features that may help identify the L3. For the purposes of this chapter, we will be referring to the L3 region as the landmark of choice.

Skeletal Muscle Imaging Analysis: Cross-Sectional Area and Muscle Indices

Commercialized or open-source software can be used to isolate specific tissues, such as skeletal muscle (Fig. 14.2a, b), using published radiodensity thresholds (−29 to +150 Hounsfield units for skeletal muscle) [2, 54, 55]. Data analysis using this software is semiautomated. Once the HU thresholds are set, the software will identify regions of the scan that reflect this range. However, some manual manipulation is often required to distinguish muscle from different lean tissues, such as skin and certain organs. For example, the liver and muscle have similar threshold ranges, and manual correction may be required if the software highlights pixels that appear to the analyst more likely to be liver. Cross-sectional area muscle indices are calculated by dividing the cross-sectional area of interest (often the total muscle in the L3 region) by height squared (units: cm^2/m^2). Further details provided in section "What Is Measured".

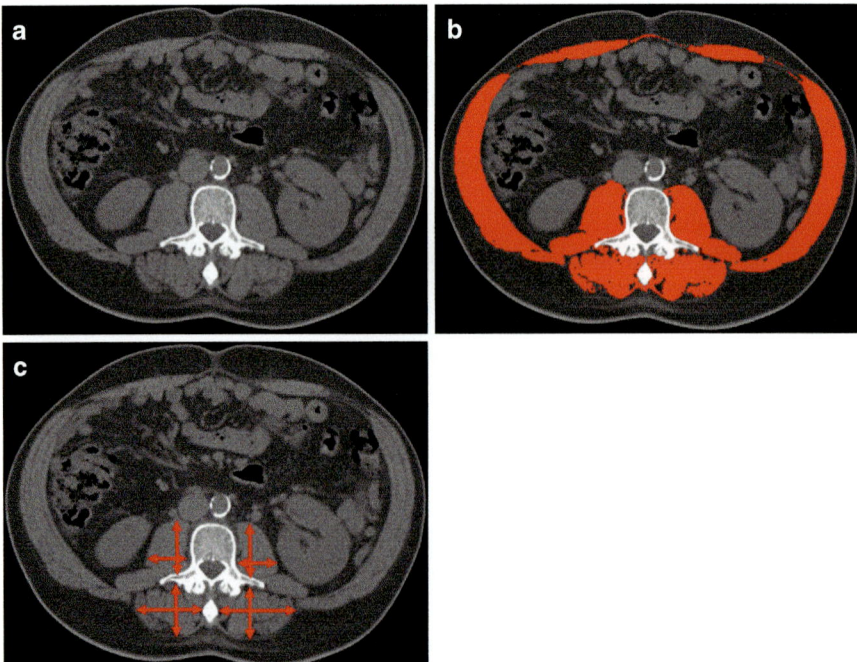

Fig. 14.2 CT image of the third lumbar vertebra (**a**) analyzed for cross-sectional area (**b**) and for linear measures (**c**)

Skeletal Muscle Imaging Analysis: Linear Measures Analysis
and Muscle Indices

One of the major drawbacks associated with using the protocols described in the
previous section (section "Skeletal Muscle Imaging Analysis: Cross-Sectional Area
and Muscle Indices") is the time-consuming nature of the analysis; each scan can
take 30–40 min for a trained analyst to perform. While this method has enormous
utility in research, it is not practical in clinical settings where there are major time
constraints. In cases where precise and specific measures are not imperative for
skeletal muscle imaging analysis, an alternative method is the linear measures
approach [61, 62]. The main purpose of this alternative strategy is to broadly classify the presence or absence of sarcopenia. This technique was developed in critically ill patients [61] and has since been used in colorectal cancer patients [62]. We
refer to the paper by Avrutin et al. [61] for details on implementing this method. In
brief, digital calipers are used to place the longest possible vertical and horizontal
lines on the left and right psoas and paraspinal muscles on the raw CT image taken
at the L3 region (Fig. 14.2c). The products of each muscle (left psoas, right psoas,
left paraspinal, right paraspinal) are calculated with the horizontal and vertical. The
sum of these products is then calculated [61]. There was excellent correlation
between this method and L3 ($r^2 = 0.745$), and the coefficient of variation for inter-
analyst reliability was 2.7% [61].

Quality of the Measurement

Precision and Repeatability

With the solid universal approach to performing CT image analysis at L3 for skeletal muscle, repeatability values are typically <2% for both intra- and inter-analyst
variability [13, 15, 25]. Specifically, in liver cirrhosis, this error is comparable at
~1.4% [18]. However, cross-sectional area is influenced by over hydration [63],
which is important to consider if longitudinal evaluations will occur. At the current
time, there is no singular method to control or manage this. However, BIA can provide total body water, and thus, BIA and CT image analysis may be combined to
better understand potential fluid shifts that may influence results in patients with
liver cirrhosis.

Validations

Single-slice cross-sectional CT images from different regions of the body have been
shown to produce valid, accurate and precise predictions of whole body skeletal
muscle mass in healthy populations [48, 49]. Proper validations can be performed
by comparing single-slice images either with whole body scans [48, 49] or with
specific landmarks in cadavers [51]. However, performing these types of validations

with MRI carries an enormous cost and time burden for the large sample size that would be needed. With CT, whole body scans would also require exposing patients to large doses of radiation. It is rare that the opportunity to explore whole body CT images arises; however, in a study by Halpenny et al. [64], regional muscle volumes were compared against whole body skeletal muscle in patients with melanoma and found to correlate well ($r^2 = 0.82$ for the abdominal region) with healthy participants [48]. Thus, we assume that the L3 relationship that is reported in whole body healthy participants [48, 49] is consistent in most clinical populations.

Ultrasound Imaging

Ultrasound imaging is emerging as a valuable and practical bedside tool that can provide a relatively objective and feasible assessment of muscle health in both inpatients and outpatients. Muscle health is a broad term that encompasses a host of features related to skeletal muscle, including (but not limited to) tissue mass, metabolic function, muscle architecture, physiological regulation, and neural signaling. Body composition modalities, like ultrasound, have the capacity to capture many of these features simultaneously, providing researchers and clinicians with a comprehensive portrait of muscle health. Further, the comparatively holistic assessment of muscle afforded by ultrasound integrates measures of tissue quantity (e.g. muscle thickness) and quality (e.g. fatty/fibrotic infiltration) enhancing our ability to identify potential muscular deficits [8]. Similar to BIA, ultrasound imaging can be performed while the patient is supine, allowing for data acquisition without active participation from the patient. This is particularly beneficial for in- and outpatients who are immobile or who may have reduced mobility. Certain ultrasound-specific muscle characteristics (i.e. fascicle length and pennation angle), when combined with measures of muscle quantity (thickness and cross-sectional area), may constitute a surrogate method with which to evaluate physical function, clinical outcomes or even patient prognosis.

To date, a limited number of studies have used ultrasound to quantify muscle characteristics in liver cirrhosis; it is an area of research that has yet to be explored in an impactful manner for patients with liver cirrhosis. Much of what is presented in this section has been drawn from studies performed in ICU patients and healthy individuals [8]. Future work is needed to measure and compare degradation of muscle quantity and quality during the trajectory of liver cirrhosis, which together may associate with clinical outcomes in these patients. Nonetheless, we have observed that the magnitude of cross-sectional area lost in the *rectus femoris* is associated with degree of organ failure and inflammation in ICU patients [27]. Also, Parry et al. [28] demonstrated that muscle architecture of the quadriceps muscle group was related to measures of patients' strength and physical function at ICU discharge. Given the prevalence of muscle atrophy and poor muscle function in liver cirrhosis, studying muscle health using ultrasound would be worthwhile. A summary of the merits and limitations of using ultrasound imaging for skeletal muscle assessment is presented in Table 14.2.

Fundamentals of Ultrasound Imaging Analysis of Skeletal Muscle

Ultrasound uses high-frequency sound waves (approximately 1–10 MHz) that are generated by the vibrations of an electrically stimulated piezoelectric crystal. The crystal is located within a transducer, and the soundwaves travel through the skin to the underlying tissues. These soundwaves are partially reflected as they travel through various tissues. This reflection is called acoustic impedance, and each tissue returns distinct impedance characteristics to the transducer as an echo, which is subsequently converted to electrical signals that are displayed on a monitor [65]. The strength of the echo depends on a number of factors including (1) the characteristics of the probe selected; (2) the depth of the tissue of interest; (3) the anatomical region of interest; and, importantly, (4) the number of interfaces through which the soundwave must travel through and reflect back [8, 65]. More energy is lost (resulting in an altered or weakened echo signal) when the soundwave is forced to travel larger distances or pass through more interfaces before reaching the tissue of interest. For example, in obese individuals the soundwave must travel through a thick layer of subcutaneous adipose tissue in order to reach the underlying muscle. Echo signals are also weakened if the tissue of interest is sandwiched by soft tissues, as in the case of abdominal muscles, which reside between subcutaneous and visceral adipose tissue. It is essential to carefully consider these factors before attempting to assess muscle quantity and muscle quality using ultrasound; innovative research approaches are emerging to resolve these issues.

What Can Be Measured?

Depending on the muscle of interest, specific anatomical sites are chosen, correctly identified and clearly marked on the skin. One or more image can be acquired at each site. The orientation of the ultrasound probe at each site will determine the type of measurements possible in your images. Muscle thickness, cross-sectional area and echogenicity (an indicator of muscle composition) can be measured when the probe is oriented in the transverse plane (i.e. perpendicular to the muscle fibres), whereas aspects of muscle architecture (e.g. pennation angle, fascicle length) can be measured when the probe is oriented longitudinally (i.e. parallel to the muscle fibres). While other ultrasound-based measures are also possible (e.g. elastography), these measures are often more meaningful for researchers and may not be available on ultrasound machines commonly available in a clinical setting. You may choose to evaluate these measures at a single time point or longitudinally to track muscle health across the trajectory of illness [65, 66].

- *Muscle thickness* of a single muscle or muscle group may be determined. The most common thickness measurement is the combination of the anterior thigh muscles *rectus femoris* and *vastus intermedius*. Thigh muscle thickness measures are generally favoured in research and clinic because they are relatively easy to landmark and analyse, and – notably – they are weight-bearing muscles that are especially prone to muscle atrophy following reduced activity. The probe is placed on the skin in such a manner as to obtain a transverse image of the muscle. Ultrasound systems are typically equipped with digital calipers that permit the on-screen measurement of muscle thickness. Previously developed prediction equations exist to generate estimates of whole body or appendicular lean mass from thickness measurements taken at particular sites [67]. See Fig. 14.3a for a depiction of muscle thickness.
- *Cross-sectional area (CSA)* can only be measured if the entire muscle cross-section is contained within the field of view. This is not always possible, particularly in individuals with larger limbs. If the transverse image you have captured contains the entire muscle, CSA may be measured by (a) tracing the outline of the muscle with the help of an on-screen tool or (b) exporting the saved image for analysis in an open-access software. For CSA assessments, the ultrasound probe should be placed in a similar orientation as for thickness measurements (i.e. in the transverse plane, oriented perpendicular to the muscle fibres). Compared to muscle thickness, CSA may be more sensitive to detecting longitudinal changes in muscle quantity in ICU [28], but this has yet to be established or validated. See Fig. 14.3b for a depiction of the CSA of the *rectus femoris*.
- *Fascicle length* is a physiological measure that evaluates the length of individual muscle fibres. If focusing on the thigh, the muscle typically used for this measure is the *vastus lateralis*. The probe is placed in parallel with the direction of the muscle fibres so as to capture a longitudinal image. Fascicle length is directly related to muscle strength and shortening velocity of the muscle. *Pennation angle*, a related measure of muscle architecture, describes the angle at which the fascicles insert into the deep aponeurosis of the muscle of interest. There is an inverse relationship between pennation angle, force and shortening velocity, which suggests that the greater the angle, the less force is generated by the muscle [68]. See Fig. 14.3c for an illustration of these features.
- In addition to muscle architecture, echogenic properties can also be extracted from ultrasound images and may indicate the deleterious presence of myonecrosis, fatty infiltration and degree of fibrosis [8, 69]. *Echogenicity*, also referred to as *echointensity*, is based on the greyscale of the ultrasound image and is independently associated with reduced strength and physical function [70, 71]. Higher echogenicity values are typically exhibited in patients with myonecrosis [72]. In ultrasound images, lean healthy muscle appears very dark grey (or nearly black), whereas muscle that has a high degree of fatty/fibrotic (i.e. non-muscle tissue) infiltration will appear lighter grey. However, echointensity properties differ somewhat amongst ultrasound systems, making it challenging to compare echointensity measures taken on different devices. Even if the same ultrasound

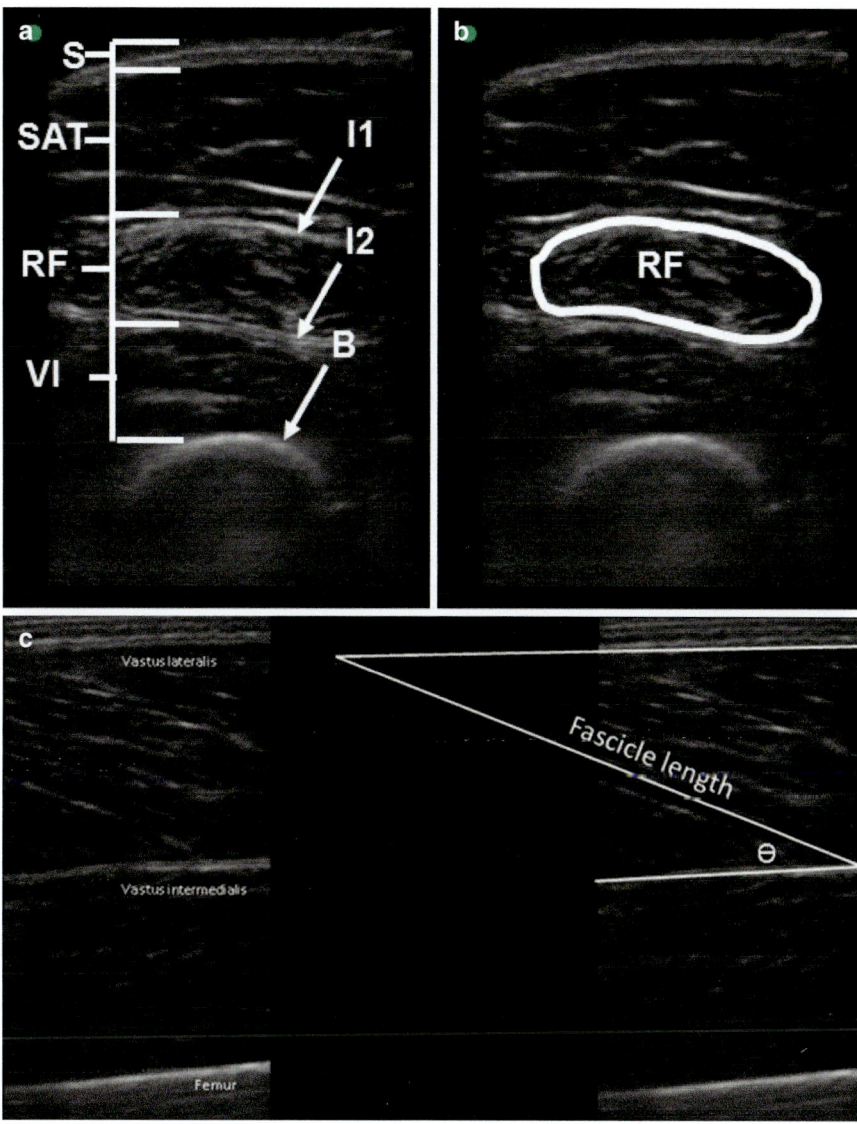

Fig. 14.3 Ultrasound images at the mid-thigh representing muscle thickness (**a**), muscle cross-sectional area (**b**), as well as fascicle length and pennation angle (**c**)

machine/model is used, different analysts and different equipment parameters may generate different results [8]. Texture analysis, which refers to image analysis that is performed by accounting for adjacent pixel intensities, may offer a more normalized approach; but, at this point, texture analysis might not be a clinically feasible option from the perspective of time efficiency [73].

Ultrasound Imaging Protocols

Although several ultrasound imaging protocols have been published, there is currently no universally accepted, standardized protocol for assessing skeletal muscle by ultrasonography [2, 8, 67]. Previously published protocols have each focused on distinct objectives and outcomes, using various anatomical landmarks as well as different skeletal muscle groups [67]. Importantly, few papers have validated existing protocols. Existing protocols range from four to nine anatomical sites that are landmarked and/or imaged either in standing or supine positions. Although it is reasonable to expect that acquiring data from more sites would produce greater accuracy and precision when predicting whole body lean mass, the correlation between five sites using ultrasound against DXA ($r^2 = 0.82$) [74] is comparable to the correlation between nine sites using ultrasound against MRI ($r^2 = 0.94$) [75, 76]. Importantly, the five-site method (four sites on the lower limbs and one site on the upper limb) exhibited an excellent ability to detect individuals with low lean mass using ultrasound images [74]. Importantly, the use of minimal compression (where any pressure of the probe against the skin is avoided as much as possible) agrees better with whole body lean mass compared with maximal compression (where one applies the most possible pressure on the patient's skin) [74]. Interestingly, Ema et al. [77] demonstrated that, at single sites, thickness measurements of the *rectus femoris* obtained using ultrasound varied less than 1% from the cadaveric true thickness. Despite the excellent agreement between ultrasound and other reference methods, no validation studies have been conducted in patients with liver cirrhosis. Given the potential utility and feasibility of using ultrasound in liver cirrhosis, validation studies are urgently needed to develop sarcopenia cut-points and relate these to clinical outcomes.

Quality of the Measurement

Precision and Repeatability

Precision and repeatability with ultrasound is acceptable. For a single anatomical site, Thomaes et al. [78] found that *rectus femoris* muscle thickness varied by ~0.01 cm and produced an intra-class correlation coefficient (ICC) of 0.92 when compared with CT images of the same muscle in coronary artery disease patients. They also indicated limits of agreement of 0.01 cm and a minimal detectable difference of 0.24 cm. Similarly, Seymour et al. [79] compared ultrasound images in healthy adults and COPD patients against CT images of the *rectus femoris* cross-sectional area and found an ICC of $r = 0.88$. Intra- and inter-analyst reliability was 12 mm^2 and 2 mm^2, respectively. On the other hand, Tillquist et al. [80] evaluated 78 healthy individuals across 7 centres with 42 different analysts. Their intra- and inter-analyst correlations were 0.98 and 0.95, respectively; the protocol used here is commonly used in numerous other protocols focused on the quadriceps muscle group. Similar reliability for mid-thigh (ICC = 1.0) was determined by Baldwin et al. [81]. These values are highly dependent on standardization of a protocol. In addition, these reliability values include all components of a protocol: landmarking, data acquisition and image analysis. It is recommended that new reporting standards be implemented in the near future so that one can understand where the limitations in data collection occur. In future studies, consideration might be given to improving repeatability by requiring data analysis to be performed by a single analyst (i.e. one individual does the software analysis for thickness and CSA) despite that multiple analysts may be collecting data. This approach may be favourable and efficient in multisite studies to maintain some consistency across measurements.

Concluding Remarks

Interest in the application of more advanced body composition assessment technologies in various clinical populations continues to grow [2, 29]. Traditionally, BMI has been the predominant tool used in clinic to understand and track changes in nutritional status. Emerging body composition tools, like BIA, CT and ultrasound, are more sophisticated and offer a broad spectrum of data allowing for more accurate identification of individuals with sarcopenia. Additionally, body composition measurements obtained from these alternative technologies relate closely to clinical outcomes and have the potential to greatly impact patient care. BIA has long been clinically feasible, but there are new approaches to provide more useful prognostic data. New methods for muscle assessment using CT images are also emerging that may be more clinically friendly. These newer methods, such as linear measures, may allow for the relatively rapid classification of patients as sarcopenic versus non-sarcopenic using common imaging viewers. Although the linear measures technique requires further investigation and validation, this approach is a promising screening tool for future clinicians. Ultrasound imaging permits in-depth and comprehensive evaluation of muscle quantity and quality – more so than CT imaging and BIA. However, a more standardized and universal method needs to be developed so that results are comparable in the literature and across diverse patient groups and clinics.

The studies referenced in this chapter have been amassed from several disciplines; hence, the findings discussed herein may not translate with perfect fidelity to liver cirrhosis patients. Ergo, caution should be exercised when interpreting data generated from diverse clinical populations. Each clinical cohort experiences distinct disease-specific challenges, and while we can learn much from other illnesses and diseases, factors that influence body composition in distinct groups may not be relevant to liver cirrhosis.

To determine which body composition method is best suited to your clinical assessments, consider what questions you are trying to answer about your patient. Identify the modality(ies) that will provide this information, and then determine the magnitude of precision and accuracy you might require in your clinic. Simply classifying a patient as sarcopenic or non-sarcopenic may not require a highly precise tool (i.e. BIA or ultrasound may suffice); however, if you are interested in quantifying muscle CSA at a given landmark and/or tracking changes in CSA longitudinally, you may require a highly precise measurement (e.g. CT imaging).

Regardless of the modality you choose to implement in clinical practice, appropriate training is essential. In-person training that incorporates a 'hands-on' practical component is optimal. Although written manuals and standard operating procedures can provide a solid foundation in the basics of these technologies, there are many important 'tips and tricks' that can only be gained during in-person training sessions led by individuals with a wealth of experience in assessing skeletal muscle with the specific body composition modality of interest.

Interest in body composition assessment, especially the characterization of skeletal muscle, is growing exponentially. Technologies and analysis techniques are expanding in such ways that provide greater feasibility, time efficiencies and reduced burden on patients. While we have made large strides over the past few decades, new applications of older technologies will improve our ability to identify and treat those who are at risk of malnutrition and, ultimately, prevent or manage sarcopenia in future clinical populations.

References

1. Tandon P, Ney M, Irwin I, Ma MM, Gramlich L, Bain VG, Esfandiari N, Baracos V, Montano-Loza AJ, Myers RP. Severe muscle depletion in patients on the liver transplant wait list—its prevalence and independent prognostic value. Liver Transpl. 2012;18:1209–16.
2. Paris M, Mourtzakis M. Assessment of skeletal muscle mass in critically patients: considerations for the utility of computed tomography imaging and ultrasonography. Curr Opin Clin Nutr Metab Care. 2016;19:125–30.
3. Kang SH, Jeong WK, Baik SK, Cha SH, Kim MY. Impact of sarcopenia on prognostic value of cirrhosis: going beyond the hepatic venous pressure gradient and MELD score. J Cachexia Sarcopenia Muscle. 2018;9(5):860–70.
4. Kalafateli M, Karatzas A, Tsiaoussis G, Koutroumpakis E, Tselekouni P, Koukias N, Konstantakis C, Assimakopoulos S, Gogos C, Thomopoulos K, Kalogeropoulou C, Triantos C. Muscle fat infiltration assessed by total psoas density on computed tomography predicts mortality in cirrhosis. Ann Gastroenterol. 2018;31(4):491–8.
5. Bhanji RA, Moctezuma-Velazquez C, Duarte-Rojo A, Ebadi M, Ghosh S, Rose C, Montano-Loza AJ. Myosteatosis and sarcopenia are associated with hepatic encephalopathy in patients with cirrhosis. Hepatol Int. 2018;12:377–86.
6. Ju S, Choi SM, Park YS, Lee CH, Lee SM, Yoo CG, Kim YW, Han SK, Lee J. Rapid muscle loss negatively impacts survival in critically ill patients with cirrhosis. J Intensive Care Med. In Press:088506661877570. https://doi.org/10.1177/0885066618775706.
7. Van Vugt JLA, Alferink LJM, Buettner S, Gaspersz MP, Bot D, Darwish Murad S, Feshtali S, van Ooijen PMA, Polak WG, Porte RJ, van Hoek B, van den Berg AP, Metselaar HJ, IJzermans JNM. A model including sarcopenia surpasses the MELD score in predicting waiting list mortality in cirrhotic liver transplant candidates: a competing risk analysis in a national cohort. J Hepatol. In Press; https://doi.org/10.1016/j.hep.2017.11.030.
8. Mourtzakis M, Parry S, Connolly B, Puthucheary Z. Skeletal muscle ultrasound in critical care: a tool in need of translation. Ann Am Thorac Soc. 2017;14(10):1495–503.

9. Tandon P, Raman M, Mourtzakis M, Merli M. A practical approach to nutritional screening and assessment in cirrhosis. Hepatology. 2017;65(3):1044–57.
10. Cruz-Jentoft AJ, Baeyens JP, Bauer JM, Boirie Y, Cederholm T, Landi F, Martin FC, Michel JP, Rolland Y, Schneider SM, Topinkova E, Vandewoude M, Zamboni M. Sarcopenia: European consensus on definition and diagnosis. Report of the European Working Group on Sarcopenia in Older People. Age Ageing. 2010;39:412–23.
11. Tandon P, Low G, Mourtzakis M, Zenith L, Myers RP, Abraldes JG, Shaheen AA, Qamar H, Mansoor N, Carbonneau M, Ismond K, Mann S, Alaboudy A, Ma M. A model to identify sarcopenia in patients with cirrhosis. Clin Gastroenterol Hepatol. 2016;14(10):1473–80.
12. Prado CM, Lieffers JR, McCargar LJ, Reiman T, Sawyer MB, Martin L, Baracos VE. Prevalence and clinical implications of sarcopenic obesity in patients with solid tumours of the respiratory and gastrointestinal tracts: a population-based study. Lancet Oncol. 2008;9:629–35.
13. Mourtzakis M, Prado CMM, Lieffers JR, Reiman T, McCargar LJ, Baracos VE. A practical and precise approach to quantification of body composition in cancer patients using computed tomography images acquired during routine care. Appl Physiol Nutr Metab. 2008;33:997–1006.
14. Baracos VE, Reiman T, Mourtzakis M, Gioulbasanis I, Antoun S. Body composition in patients with non-small cell lung cancer: a contemporary view of cancer cachexia with the use of computed tomography image analysis. Am J Clin Nutr. 2010;91(4):1133S–7S.
15. Martin L, Birdsell L, MacDonald N, Reiman T, Clandinin MT, McCargar LJ, Murphy R, Ghosh S, Sawyer MB, Baracos VE. Cancer cachexia in the age of obesity: skeletal muscle depletion is a powerful prognostic factor, independent of body mass index. J Clin Oncol. 2013;31(12):1539–47.
16. Di Sebastiano KM, Yang L, Zbuk K, Wong RK, Chow T, Koff D, Moran GR, Mourtzakis M. Accelerated muscle and adipose tissue loss may predict survival in pancreatic cancer patients: the relationship with diabetes and anaemia. Br J Nutr. 2013;109:302–12.
17. Fujiwara N, Nakagawa H, Kudo Y, Tateishi R, Taguri M, Watadani T, Nakagomi R, Kondo M, Nakatsuka T, Minami T, Sato M, Uchino K, Enooku K, Kondo Y, Asaoka Y, Tanaka Y, Ohtomo K, Shiina S, Koike K. Sarcopenia, intramuscular fat deposition and visceral adiposity independently predict the outcomes of hepatocellular carcinoma. J Hepatol. 2015;63:131–40.
18. Benjamin J, Shasthry V, Kaal CR, Anand L, Bhardwaj A, Pandit V, Arora A, Rajesh S, Pamecha V, Jain V, Kumar G, Loria A, Puri P, Joshi YK, Sarin SK. Characterization of body composition and definition of sarcopenia in patients with alcoholic cirrhosis: a computed tomography based study. Liver Int. 2017;37:1668–74.
19. Montano-Loza AJ. Muscle wasting: a nutritional criterion to prioritize patients for liver transplantation. Curr Opin Clin Nutr Metab Care. 2014;17:219–25.
20. Baumgartner RN, Koehler KM, Gallagher D, Romero L, Heymsfield SB, Ross RR, Garry PJ, Lindeman RD. Epidemiology of sarcopenia among the elderly in New Mexico. Am J Epidemiol. 1998;147:755–63.
21. Hanai T, Shiraki M, Nishimura K, Ohnishi S, Imai K, Suetsugu A, Takai K, Shimizu M, Moriwaki H. Sarcopenia impairs prognosis of patients with liver cirrhosis. Nutrition. 2015;31:193–9.
22. Montano-Loza AJ, Meza-Junco J, Prado CM, Lieffers JR, Baracos VE, Bain VG, Sawyer MB. Muscle wasting is associated with mortality in patients with cirrhosis. Clin Gastroenterol Hepatol. 2012;10:173.
23. Hamaguchi Y, Kaido T, Okumura S, Fujimoto Y, Ogawa K, Mori A, Hammad A, Tamai Y, Inagaki N, Uemoto S. Impact of quality as well as quantity of skeletal muscle on outcomes after liver transplantation. Liver Transpl. 2014;20(11):1413–9.
24. World Health Organization (WHO). Technical report series 894: Obesity: Preventing and managing the global epidemic. Geneva: World Health Organization; 2000.
25. Moisey LL, Mourtzakis M, Cotton BA, Premji T, Heyland DK, Wade CE, Bulger E, Kozar RA. Nutrition and Rehabilitation Investigators Consortium (NUTRIC). Skeletal muscle predicts ventilator-free days, ICU-free days, and mortality in elderly ICU patients. Crit Care. 2013;17:R206.

26. Earthman CP. Body composition tools for assessment of adult malnutrition at the bedside: a tutorial on research considerations and clinical applications. J Parenter Enter Nutr. 2015;39(7):787–822.

27. Puthucheary ZA, Rawal J, McPhail M, Connolly B, Ratnayake G, Chan P, Hopkinson NS, Phadke R, Dew T, Sidhu PS, Velloso C, Seymour J, Agley CC, Selby A, Limb M, Edwards LM, Smith K, Rowlerson A, Rennie MJ, Moxham J, Harridge SD, Hart N, Montgomery HE. Acute skeletal muscle wasting in critical illness. JAMA. 2013;310(15):1591–600.

28. Parry SM, El-Ansary D, Cartwright MS, Sarwal A, Berney S, Koopman R, Annoni R, Puthucheary Z, Gordon IR, Morris PE, Denehy L. Ultrasonography in the intensive care setting can be used to detect changes in the quality and quantity of muscle and is related to muscle strength and function. J Crit Care. 2015;30(5):1151.

29. Teigen LM, Kuchnia AJ, Mourtzakis M, Earthman CP. The use of technology for estimating body composition. Strengths and weaknesses of common modalities in a clinical setting. Nutr Clin Pract. 2017;32(1):20–9.

30. Kyle UG, Genton L, Slosman DO, Pichard C. Fat-free and fat mass percentiles in 5225 healthy subjects aged 15 to 98 years. Nutrition. 2001;17(7–8):534–41.

31. Barbosa-Silva MCG, Barros AJD. Bioelectrical impedance analysis in clinical practice: a new perspective on its use beyond body composition equations. Curr Opin Clin Nutr Metab Care. 2005;8(3):311–7.

32. Gupta D, Lammersfeld CA, Vashi PG, King J, Dahlk SL, Grutsch JF, Lis CG. Bioelectrical impedance phase angle in clinical practice: implications for prognosis in stage IIB and IV non-small cell lung cancer. BMC Cancer. 2009;9:37.

33. Schwenk A, Eschner W, Kremer G, Ward LC. Assessment of intracellular water by whole body bioelectrical impedance and total body potassium in HIV-positive patients. Clin Nutr. 2000;19(2):109–13.

34. Ott M, Fischer H, Polat H, Helm EB, Frenz M, Caspary WF, Lembcke B. Bioelectrical impedance analysis as a predictor of survival in pateints with human immunodeficiency virus infection. J Acquir Immune Defic Syndr Hum Retrovirol. 1995;9(1):20–5.

35. Wirth R, Volkert D, Rösler A, Sieber CC, Bauer JM. Bioelectric impedance phase angle is associated with hospital mortality of geriatric patients. Arch Gerontol Geriatr. 2010;51:290–4.

36. Bosy-Westphal A, Danielzik S, Dorhofer R-P, Later W, Wiese S, Muller M. Phase angle from bioelectrical impedance analysis: population reference values by age, sex, and body mass index. J Parenter Enter Nutr. 2006;30(4):309–16.

37. Barbosa-Silva MCG, Barros AJD, Wang J, Heymsfield SB, Pierson RN. Bioelectrical impedance analysis: population reference values for phase angle by age and sex. Am J Clin Nutr. 2005;82(1):49–52.

38. Dittmar M. Reliability and variability of bioimpedance measures in normal adults: effects of age, gender, and body mass. Am J Phys Anthropol. 2003;122(4):361–70.

39. Moisey L. A comprehensive assessment of nutritional status and factors impacting nutrition recovery in hospitalized, critically ill patients following liberation from mechanical ventilation. UW Space. http://hdl.handle.net/10012/11937.

40. Jensen M, Hermann A, Hessov I, Mosekilde L. Componenets of variance when assessing the reproducibility of body composition measurements using bio-impedance and the Hologic QDR-2000 DXA scanner. Clin Nutr. 1997;16(2):61–5.

41. Kyle UG, Bosaeus I, De Lorenzo AD, Deurenberg P, Elia M, Gomez JM, Heitmann BL, Kent-Smith L, Melchoir JC, Pirlich M, Scharfetter H, Schols AM, Pichard C, Composition of the ESPEN Working Group. Bioelectrical impedance analysis-part I: review of principles and methods. Clin Nutr. 2004;23(5):1226–43.

42. Kushner RF, de Vries PM, Gudivaka R. Use of bioelectrical impedance analysis measurements in the clinical management of patients undergoing dialysis. Am J Clin Nutr. 1996;64(3 Suppl):503S–9S.

43. Earthman CP, Matthie JR, Reid PM, Harper IT, Ravussin E, Howell WH. A comparison of bio-impedance methods for detection of body cell mass change in HIV infection. J Appl Physiol. 2000;88(3):944–56.
44. Moon JR, Stout JR, Smith AE, et al. Reproducibility and validity of bioimpedance spectroscopy for tracking changes in total body water: implications for repeated measurements. Br J Nutr. 2010;104(9):1384–94.
45. Ellis KJ. Human body composition: in vivo methods. Physiol Rev. 2000;80(2):649–80.
46. Simons JP, Schols AM, Westerterp KR, ten Veide GP, Wouters EF. The use of bioelectrical impedance analysis to predict total body water in patients with cancer cachexia. Am J Clin Nutr. 1995;61(4):741–5.
47. Nickerson BS. Agreement between single-frequency bioimpedance analysis and dual-energy x-ray absorptiometry varies based on sex and segmental mass. Nutr Res. 2018;54:33–9.
48. Shen W, Punyanitya M, Wang Z, Gallagher D, St-Onge MP, Albu J, Heymsfield SB, Heshka S. Visceral adipose tissue: relations between single-slice areas and total volume. Am J Clin Nutr. 2004;80(2):271, 278.
49. Shen W, Punyanitya M, Wang Z, Gallagher D, St-Onge MP, Albu J, Heymsfield SB, Heshka S. Total body skeletal muscle and adipose tissue volumes: estimation from a single abdominal cross-sectional image. J Appl Physiol. 2004;97(6):2333–8.
50. Weijs PJM, Looijaard WGPM, Dekker IM, Stapel SN, Girbes AR, Oudemans-van Straaten HM, Beishuizen A. Low skeletal muscle area is a risk factor for mortality in mechanically ventilated critically ill patients. Crit Care. 2014;18:R12.
51. Mitsiopoulos N, Baumgartner RN, Heymsfield SB, Lyons W, Gallagher D, Ross R. Cadaver validation of skeletal muscle measurement by magnetic resonance imaging and computerized tomography. J Appl Physiol. 1998;85(1):115–22.
52. Caan BJ, Meyerhardt JA, Kroenke CH, Alexeeff S, Xiao J, Weltzien E, Feliciano EC, Castillo AL, Quesenberry CP, Kwan ML, Prado CM. Explaining the obesity paradox: the association between body composition and colorectal cancer survival (C-SCANS Study). Cancer Epidemiol Biomark Prev. 2017;26(7):1008–15.
53. Caan BJ, Cespedes Feliciano EM, Prado CM, Alexeeff S, Kroenke CH, Bradshaw P, Quesenberry CP, Weltzien EK, Castillo AL, Olobatuyi TA, Chen WY. Association of muscle and adiposity measured by computed tomography with survival in patients with nonmetastatic breast cancer. JAMA Oncol. 2018;4(6):798–804.
54. Ross R, Janssen I. Computed tomography and magnetic resonance imaging. In: Heymsfield SB, Lohman T, Wang Z, Going S, editors. Human body composition. 2nd ed. Champaign: Human Kinetics; 2005. p. 89–108.
55. Goodpaster GH, Thaete FL, Kelley DE. Composition of skeletal muscle evaluated with computed tomography. Ann N Y Acad Sci. 2000;904:18–24.
56. Prado CMM, Heymsfield SB. Lean tissue imaging: a new era for nutritional assessment and intervention. J Parenter Enter Nutr. 2014;38(8):940–53.
57. Murphy R, Bureyko TF, Milijkovic I, Cauley JA, Satterfield S, Hue TF, Klepin HD, Cummings SR, Newman AB, Harris TB. Association of total adiposity and computed tomographic measures of regional adiposity with incident cancer risk: a prospective population-based study of older adults. Appl Physiol Nutr Metab. 2014;39:687–92.
58. Bae KT. Intravenous contrast medium administration and scan timing at CT: consideration and approaches. Radiology. 2010;256(1):32–61.
59. Van Vugt JLA, Coebergh van den Braak RRJ, Schippers HJW, Veen KM, Levolger S, De Bruin RWF, Koek M, Niessen WJ, IJzermans JNM, Willemsen FEJA. Contrast-enhancement influences skeletal muscle density, but not skeletal muscle mass, measurements on computed tomography. Clin Nutr. 2018;37(5):1707–14.
60. Rollins KE, Javanmard-Emamghissi H, Awwad A, Macdonald IA, Fearon KCH, Lobo DN. Body composition measurement using computed tomography: does the phase of the scan matter? Nutrition. 2017;41:37–44.

61. Avrutin E, Moisey LL, Zhang R, Khattab J, Todd E, Premji T, Kozar R, Heyland DK, Mourtzakis M. Clinically practical approach for screening of low muscularity using electronic linear measures on computed tomography images in critically ill patients. J Parenter Enter Nutr. 2018;42(5):885–91.
62. Cespedes Feliciano EM, Avrutin E, Caan BJ, Boroian A, Mourtzakis M. Screening for low muscularity in colorectal cancer patients: a valid, clinic-friendly approach that predicts mortality. J Cachexia Sarcopenia Muscle. 2018;9(5):898–908.
63. Wells CI, McCall JL, Plank LD. Relationship between total body protein and cross-sectional skeletal muscle area in liver cirrhosis is influenced by overhydration. Liver Transplant. 2019;25:45. https://doi.org/10.1002/lt.25314.
64. Halpenny DF, Goncalves M, Schwitzer E, Golia Pernicka J, Jackson J, Gandelman S, Moskowitz CS, Postow M, Mourtzakis M, Caan B, Jones LW, Plodkowski AJ. Computed tomography-derived assessments of regional muscle volume: validating their use as predictors of whole body muscle volume in cancer patients. Br J Radiol. 2018;91:20180451. https://doi.org/10.1259/bjr.20180451.
65. Gruther W, Benesch T, Zorn C, Paternostro-Sluga T, Quittan M, Fialka-Moser V, Spiss C, Kainberger F, Crevenna R. Muscle wasting in intensive care patients: ultrasound observation of the M. quadriceps femoris muscle layer. J Rehabil Med. 2008;40:185–9.
66. Cartwright MS, Kwayisi G, Griffin LP, Sarwal A, Walker FO, Harris JM, Berry MJ, Chahal PS, Morris PE. Quantitative neuromuscular ultrasound in the intensive care unit. Muscle Nerve. 2013;47:255–9.
67. Mourtzakis M, Wischmeyer P. Bedside ultrasound measurement of skeletal muscle. Curr Opin Clin Nutr Metab Care. 2014;17:389–95.
68. Moreau NG, Simpson KN, Teefey SA, Damiano DL. Muscle architecture predicts maximum strength and is related to activity levels in cerebral palsy. Phys Ther. 2010;90(11):1619–30.
69. Harris-Love MO, Monfaredi R, Ismail C, Blackman MR, Cleary K. Quantitative ultrasound: measurement considerations for the assessment of muscular dystrophy and sarcopenia. Front Aging Neurosci. 2014;6:172.
70. Rech A, Radaelli R, Goltz FR, da Rosa LH, Schneider CD, Pinto RS. Echointensity is negatively associated with functional capacity in older women. Age. 2014;36:9708–16.
71. Wilhelm EN, Rech A, Minozzo F, Radaelli R, Botton CE, Pinto RS. Relationship between quadriceps femoris echo intensity, muscle power, and functional capacity of older men. Age. 2014;36:1113–22.
72. Puthucheary Z, Phadke A, Rawal R, McPhail MJ, Sidhu PS, Rowlerson A, Moxham J, Harridge S, Hart N, Montgomery HE. Qualitative ultrasound in acute critical illness muscle wasting. Crit Care Med. 2015;43:1603–11.
73. Zaidman CM, Holland MR, Hughes MS. Quantitative ultrasound of skeletal muscle: reliable measurements of calibrated muscle backscatter from different ultrasound systems. Ultrasound Med Biol. 2013;38:1618–25.
74. Paris MT, Lafleur B, Dubin JA, Mourtzakis M. Development of a bedside viable ultrasound protocol to quantify appendicular lean tissue mass. J Cachexia Sarcopenia Muscle. 2017;8(5):713–26.
75. Sanada K, Kearns CF, Midorikawa T, Abe T. Prediction and validation of total and regional skeletal muscle mass by ultrasound in Japanese adults. Eur J Appl Physiol. 2006;96:24–31.
76. Takai Y, Ohta M, Akagi R, Kato E, Wakahara T, Kawakami Y, Fukunaga T, Kanehisa H. Applicability of ultrasound muscle thickness measurements for predicting fat-free mass in elderly population. J Nutr Health Aging. 2014;18:579–85.
77. Ema R, Wakahara T, Mogi Y, Miyamoto N, Komatsu T, Kanehisa H, Kawakami Y. In vivo measurement of human rectus femoris architecture by ultrasonography: validity and applicability. Clin Physiol Funct Imaging. 2013;33:267–73.
78. Thomaes T, Thomis M, Onkelinx S, Coudyzer W, Cornelissen V, Vanhees L. Reliability and validity of the ultrasound technique to measure the rectus femoris muscle diameter in older CAD-patients. BMC Med Imaging. 2012;12:7.

79. Seymour JM, Ward K, Sidhu PS, Puthucheary Z, Steier J, Jolley CJ, Rafferty G, Polkey MI, Moxham J. Ultrasound measurement of the rectus femoris cross-sectional area and the relationship with quadriceps strength in COPD. Thorax. 2009;64:418–23.
80. Tillquist M, Kutsogiannis DJ, Wischmeyer PE, Kummerlen C, Leung R, Stollery D, Karvellas CJ, Preiser JC, Bird N, Kozar R, Heyland DK. Bedside ultrasound is a practical and reliable measurement tool for assessing quadriceps muscle layer thickness. JPEN J Parenter Enteral Nutr. 2014;38(7):886–90.
81. Baldwin CE, Paratz JD, Bersten A. Diaphragm and peripheral muscle thickness on ultrasound: intra-rater reliability and variability of a methodology using nonstandard recumbent position. Respirology. 2011;16:1136–43.

Part III
The Future

Chapter 15
Upcoming Pharmacological and Interventional Therapies for the Treatment of Physical Frailty and Sarcopenia

Penelope Hey and Marie Sinclair

Introduction

In recent years there has been a surge in research investigating mechanisms underlying muscle wasting in cirrhosis. The central role of hormonal alterations, ammonia, and myostatin in muscle wasting is now well established. However, despite these gains, few interventional trials have been conducted, and there are as yet no proven therapies that lead to a sustained improvement in muscle mass and strength. All treatments are therefore still considered investigational and require further validation in large-scale randomized controlled trials.

Interventional trials for sarcopenia and frailty have several inherent challenges. These include a lack of consensus on diagnosis, optimal definition of primary and secondary endpoints, and the subjectivity of performance and strength measures. Furthermore, whether reversing sarcopenia in cirrhosis has a meaningful impact on patient outcomes is still yet to be determined. Given the multifactorial nature of sarcopenia in cirrhosis, it is also likely that a unique pattern of alterations in skeletal muscle biology are present in an individual patient with cirrhosis, meaning that specific single pathway interventions may impact each patient to varying degrees.

In this chapter we summarize the available literature for pharmacological and interventional therapies that have been explored in sarcopenia and frailty in both cirrhotic and non-cirrhotic populations (Table 15.1). While some therapies have shown promising results in small clinical trials or pilot studies, there is currently a lack of large randomized trials to support their use.

P. Hey · M. Sinclair (✉)
Department of Gastroenterology and Hepatology, Austin Health, Melbourne, VIC, Australia

The University of Melbourne, Melbourne, VIC, Australia
e-mail: marie.sinclair@austin.org.au

© Springer Nature Switzerland AG 2020   211
P. Tandon, A. J. Montano-Loza (eds.), *Frailty and Sarcopenia in Cirrhosis*,
https://doi.org/10.1007/978-3-030-26226-6_15

Table 15.1 Future interventional therapies for sarcopenia in cirrhosis

Physiological abnormality	Mechanism of muscle loss	Therapeutic target
Testosterone deficiency	Testosterone deficiency common in cirrhosis due to downregulation of the HPA due to systemic inflammation and chronic disease Reduced activation of androgen receptors in muscle cell nuclei and satellite cells	Testosterone replacement[a,b] Selective androgen receptor modulator[a]
Portal hypertension	Malnutrition: Early satiety from ascites, intestinal dysmotility, malabsorption, increased protein losses from paracentesis Hypermetabolism: Promotion of a systemic inflammatory response, increased rates of bacterial translocation and endotoxemia	TIPS[c] Continuous terlipressin infusion[c]
Hyperammonemia	Cataplerosis: Detoxification of ammonia in skeletal muscle depletes TCA cycle of key intermediate resulting in mitochondrial dysfunction and reduced protein synthesis Creation of reactive oxygen species leading to increased autophagy of muscle cells Cellular stress response as seen in amino acid starvation	Rifaximin[d] LOLA[d] BCAA therapy[b]
Growth hormone resistance	Reduced IGF-1 and IGFBP-3: Decreased production due to hepatocyte dysfunction Reduction in GH receptors in hepatocytes IGF-1 inhibits myostatin IGF-1 involved in muscle stem cell proliferation, muscle cell repair, and protein synthesis	Growth hormone replacement[a] IGF-1[b]
Upregulation of myostatin	Elevated ammonia, low IGF-1, follistatin, testosterone upregulates myostatin Myostatin inhibits mTORC1 signaling leading to increased muscle cell autophagy, reduced protein synthesis, and proteasome-mediated proteolysis	Inhibitors of myostatin signaling pathway[a]
Malnutrition	Anorexia: Early satiety, systemic inflammatory response, chronic disease	Ghrelin agonist[a]

HPA hypothalamic-pituitary-gonadal axis, *TIPS* transjugular intrahepatic portosystemic shunt, *TCA* tricarboxylic acid cycle, *LOLA* L-ornithine L-aspartate, *IGF-1* insulin-like growth factor-1, *IGFBP-3* insulin-like growth factor-binding protein-3, *GH* growth hormone, *mTORC* mammalian target of rapamycin complex-1
[a]Evidence in non-cirrhotic populations
[b]Evidence from randomized, placebo-controlled trials in humans
[c]Evidence from non-placebo-controlled human cohort or pilot studies
[d]Evidence from animal models of cirrhosis

Testosterone Therapy

Testosterone Replacement

Low testosterone is frequently observed in cirrhotic men and has been shown to correlate with severity of sarcopenia in this cohort [1, 2]. The cause of low testosterone is multifactorial and poorly understood but likely relates to downregulation of the hypothalamic-pituitary-gonadal axis due to systemic inflammation and chronic disease [3]. In addition to low testosterone, sex hormone-binding globulin is elevated in cirrhosis, leading to a further reduction in free testosterone, with low free testosterone observed in up to 90% of cirrhotics [4].

Signs of low testosterone are common in cirrhosis, including impaired sexual function, low libido, fatigue, osteoporosis, gynecomastia, anemia, and of course muscle wasting. However, the specific contribution of low testosterone to these factors is unclear. Testosterone is a known anabolic hormone, and therefore it is reasonable to expect that returning the level of this hormone to normal physiologic levels should improve muscle mass. However only a small number of trials have investigated the use of testosterone for this purpose with varying methodologies.

In 1960, a study was published in the Lancet that randomized 97 male patients with cirrhosis to either prednisolone 20 mg per day, intramuscular testosterone, or standard therapy on admission to hospital for liver-related disease [5]. Cirrhosis was confirmed by biopsy, but patients were not required to be hypogonadal for study entry. Treatment duration and follow-up were not standardized, and patient attendance was sporadic, making it difficult to compare groups. Patients in both the testosterone and prednisolone arm did appear to have improved morbidity and mortality. Mortality was significantly higher at 55% in the placebo arm compared to 31% in the testosterone arm. However, given the lack of a clear protocol and lack of blinding, these results therefore should be interpreted with caution.

A smaller study was published by Puliyel et al. in 1977 [6] that showed similar but less dramatic results. This study recruited 21 patients with biopsy-proven cirrhosis; however one third of these patients were women. Twelve patients were placed on active therapy with intramuscular testosterone, and nine controls received standard of care. Over only a short period of 4 weeks, albumin and energy levels improved, and edema decreased in the active arm. There was no mortality benefit. Again, the trial was not blinded, patients were not required to be hypogonadal to enter this study, and there was no controlling for baseline confounders. In addition, the very small patient numbers and inclusion of females into a study using male hormones mean that strong conclusions cannot be drawn.

A Cochrane review in 2006 identified trials that examined the use of testosterone in men with alcoholic liver disease [7]. Only five randomized controlled trials were identified that met criteria, which included a total of 499 patients. Overall there was no significant impact on liver histology or mortality and no increase in adverse effects in men on testosterone. The sole positive finding was a significant reduction in gynecomastia. The interpretation of this review is limited by the fact that only two of the five studies recruited men with cirrhosis, with three studies examining acute alcoholic hepatitis, limiting the applicability to chronic liver disease. Furthermore, all studies examined men with alcohol-related liver disease who received counseling regarding alcohol intake during the study period, and thus many ceased alcohol during this time. Alcohol cessation can itself improve survival as well as testosterone levels, potentially confounding results. None of the trials required that men have low testosterone for study entry, which may reduce the expected beneficial effect of testosterone.

Of these two trials included in the Cochrane review, one constitutes the largest published study to date on testosterone therapy in men with cirrhosis [8]. This multicenter trial included 221 men with alcohol-related, biopsy-proven cirrhosis, with 134 randomized to active treatment with oral testosterone 3 times a day and 87 to placebo. The median duration of treatment was 30 months. The findings of this study included increased testosterone and estradiol levels on treatment and an increased testosterone-to-estradiol ratio. There was a significant reduction in gynecomastia and increase in hemoglobin. No difference in liver biochemistry or histology was seen, and there was no mortality benefit. Limitations of this study include failure to randomize by severity of liver disease and use of oral testosterone, which is now considered unsafe, particularly in the context of liver disease. In addition, patients were not required to have low testosterone levels for trial entry, and almost all patients in the placebo group had normal testosterone levels. The median on-trial testosterone level was well above normal with 25% of patients achieving testosterone levels >100 nmol/L, which increases the risk of adverse effects.

The other trial in the Cochrane review included 32 men with alcohol-related cirrhosis who were randomized into 1 of 3 different arms [9]. Patients were not required to have low testosterone levels for trial entry. Arm 1 included nine men on intramuscular testosterone. Arm 2 included 12 men on the synthetic anabolic steroid methenolone. Arm 3 was a placebo arm of 11 patients. Treatment duration was only 1 month. There was no significant difference in mortality, ascites, encephalopathy, hepatocellular carcinoma (HCC) incidence, liver biochemistry, or liver histology. The small numbers meant the trial was underpowered to show any significant differences between patient groups. In addition, the short duration of 1 month may not have been adequate to show any difference if it was present.

In 2011, Yurci et al. published a very small study including only 12 men with cirrhosis of any etiology [10]. This was the first trial to require men to have low testosterone levels for study entry. Testosterone gel was administered to all 12 men for 6 months. At trial completion, muscle strength by hydraulic hand dynamometer had significantly improved, and gynecomastia had reduced. There were no significant adverse events. There was no change in bone mineral density. Unfortunately, there was no control arm, so these results must be interpreted with caution, particularly in the context of such low patient numbers, as this increase in muscle strength may have been due to other factors.

Our group recently published a 12-month randomized placebo-controlled trial of 3-monthly testosterone undecanoate in 101 men with established cirrhosis and low baseline testosterone levels [1]. This was the first study with both, a requirement for cirrhosis and low testosterone at baseline and randomization of patients to appropriate testosterone replacement therapy as compared to placebo. In addition, it remains the only trial to specifically quantify changes in muscle mass on testosterone therapy in this cohort. This study showed a significant improvement in lean mass as measured by dual-energy X-ray absorptiometry (mean adjusted difference) (MAD) in appendicular lean mass of +1.69 kg (CI +0.40; +2.97 kg, $p = 0.021$) and MAD in total lean mass of +4.74 kg (CI +1.75; +7.74 kg, $p = 0.008$). Additional positive benefits observed in this study included a significant increase in bone mass in treated subjects (MAD +0.08 kg, CI +0.01; +0.15 kg, $p = 0.009$) and a reduction in fat mass (MAD −4.34 kg, CI −6.65; −2.04, $p < 0.001$). This remains the only pharmacological therapy for sarcopenia that is supported by randomized controlled data.

Selective Androgen Receptor Modulator

The androgen receptor is expressed in many tissues, and therefore the nonselective effects of testosterone therapy limit its widespread use. Of particular concern is the association with increased cardiovascular risk, clot formation, fluid retention, benign prostatic hypertrophy, and its virilization effects, particularly in women. Selective androgen receptor modulators (SARMs) are a novel class of androgenic drug which provide tissue-specific activation of the androgen receptor. They are an attractive alternative anabolic agent as they are orally active without the systemic effects of testosterone therapy. SARMs have been investigated as a potential therapy for osteoporosis, stress urinary incontinence, and breast cancer with a favorable side effect profile [11].

There is also emerging evidence for their use in muscle wasting disorders. In animal models of glucocorticoid-induced muscle wasting, SARMs were effective at blocking the atrophic effects of dexamethasone on muscle cells [12]. In a phase II clinical trial of cancer-related cachexia, a SARM, enobosarm, improved muscle mass compared to placebo [13]. However, in unpublished data from two phase III clinical trials, results have been inconsistent. In the POWER 1 and 2 clinical trials investigating enobosarm in lung cancer patients, the co-primary endpoints were an improvement in muscle mass and stair climb power. While lean muscle mass improved compared to placebo in the POWER 1 trial, stair climb power did not. In POWER 2, neither endpoint met significance compared to placebo [14]. A phase IIA randomized placebo-controlled trial studied the effects of the SARM, MK-0773, in 170 sarcopenic elderly females [15]. MK-0773 improved lean muscle mass after 6 months of therapy; however, there was no significant increase in performance measures compared to placebo. More research is required to establish the anabolic effects of SARMs. Furthermore, their safety and efficacy are untested in a cirrhotic population.

Reduction in Portal Hypertension

Portal hypertension contributes significantly to malnutrition in cirrhosis. Malnutrition is a major driving factor for muscle depletion and sarcopenia. Ascites, a common complication of portal hypertension, leads to reduced gastric reserve and early satiety. It has also been shown to increase the resting energy expenditure in cirrhosis [16]. Large volume paracentesis for control of ascites is associated with protein losses and may further exacerbate protein malnutrition [17]. Portal hypertension is also thought to contribute to malabsorption through gastric and intestinal dysmotility [18]. Elevated portal pressures also result in gut edema, endotoxemia, and increased rates of bacterial translocation. These factors lead to a systemic inflammatory response and hypermetabolism and are associated with anabolic resistance. Endotoxemia in cirrhosis has been shown to have direct effects on protein breakdown and reduced synthesis in rat models [19]. Therefore, therapies to reduce portal pressures mechanistically might increase muscle mass through improved nutrition and reduced endotoxemia, inflammation, and hypermetabolism.

Continuous Terlipressin Infusion

Terlipressin, a synthetic vasopressin analogue, is a potent splanchnic vasoconstrictor. It is used to decrease portal pressures in acute variceal hemorrhage and in the treatment of hepatorenal syndrome (HRS). Splanchnic vasoconstriction promotes increased relative circulating blood volume and improves renal perfusion. Terlipressin as a treatment for HRS has demonstrated superiority over octreotide and midodrine and similar efficacy to noradrenaline [20, 21]. However, it has failed to gain Food and Drug Administration (FDA) approval in the USA primarily due to issues with trial design. The short half-life of terlipressin has also traditionally limited its use beyond the acute inpatient setting.

Our center has recently published data on the novel use of continuous outpatient terlipressin infusions for the treatment of refractory ascites and HRS as a bridge to transplantation [22–24]. This work identified significant secondary benefits on nutrition and muscle function [25]. After receiving a continuous outpatient terlipressin infusion for HRS or refractory ascites for a median duration of 51 days, 19 patients who had previously been shown to have progressively deteriorating muscle function had a median increase in handgrip strength of 11% [25]. Energy and protein intake also improved significantly across the cohort. There was a significant reduction in large volume paracentesis during therapy without any safety issues identified. Whether improvements in handgrip strength were solely attributable to improved protein and calorie intake remains unclear; however, it is possible that nutrient absorption and bacterial translocation were also improved. Larger clinical trials are clearly required to validate these positive findings.

Transjugular Intrahepatic Portosystemic Shunt (TIPS)

Transjugular intrahepatic portosystemic shunt (TIPS) is a radiological procedure used to decrease portal pressures. TIPS procedures are performed most commonly for secondary prevention or salvage therapy following variceal hemorrhage and for the management of refractory ascites. There is emerging evidence that TIPS may also improve muscle mass. Plauth et al. prospectively examined changes in body composition in 21 patients who underwent TIPS procedure [26]. Over 12 months of post-procedure follow-up, there was a significant increase in body cell mass measured by bioelectrical impedance. Tsien et al. assessed the effect of TIPS on quantitative measures of muscle and fat mass on serial CT scans at the mid-L4 vertebrae [27]. In patients undergoing TIPS, muscle area improved (psoas muscle area; 22.9 ± 0.9 to 25.1 ± 0.9 cm^2, paraspinal muscle area; 54.5 ± 1.3 to 57.9 ± 1.5 cm^2), and visceral fat mass decreased. Seventy-two percent of patients had an increase in muscle mass. Interestingly, patients who demonstrated an improvement in lean muscle mass had improved overall survival compared to patients who had no change in muscle area. While this study was retrospective, this is the only study to our knowledge that suggests that successful treatment of sarcopenia in cirrhotic subjects may lead to improved overall survival.

The mechanisms underlying the changes in body composition following TIPS placement may be similar to terlipressin therapy via the reduction in portal hypertension and subsequent control of ascites. This may improve gut function and nutrient absorption and reduce the hypermetabolic state associated with ascites and endotoxemia. Improved caloric intake following TIPS has been examined with inconsistent results. Plauth et al. reported an increase in mean protein and caloric intake in 21 patients who underwent TIPS [26]; however, two other prospective studies showed no significant change [28, 29]. Hormonal changes have also been explored. These include plasma leptin, IGF-1, IGF-binding protein, growth hormone, glucagon, insulin, and cortisol levels, all of which showed no significant change following TIPS in small prospective studies [30–32]. Nevertheless, in contrast to terlipressin, by creating a direct portosystemic shunt, the TIPS procedure bypasses hepatic metabolism leading to an increase in circulating levels of ammonia. The increase in incidence of hepatic encephalopathy post-TIPS is well documented, yet the changes in muscle mass following TIPS are incongruous with the cellular effects of hyperammonemia. Clearly sarcopenia in cirrhosis is a complex interplay between multiple factors, and the relative impact of portal hypertension as compared to hyperammonemia remains unclear.

Ammonia-Lowering Therapies

Hyperammonemia is a consistent physiological abnormality in cirrhosis. Ammonia is a cytotoxic by-product of amino acid breakdown, glutamate catabolism, and purine turnover. In normal physiological states, it is removed rapidly from the circulation by the liver and detoxified to urea by the urea cycle. Circulating ammonia levels are elevated in cirrhosis due to portosystemic shunting and hepatocyte dysfunction. Skeletal muscle plays a key role in removing excess ammonia from the circulation. As alpha-ketoglutarate (α-KG), a critical intermediate of the tricarboxylic acid (TCA) cycle, is converted to glutamate and then to glutamine, two molecules of ammonia are removed (Fig. 15.1) [33]. Low skeletal muscle mass therefore may result in reduced clearance of ammonia [34, 35]. Conversely, ammonia also acts as a negative regulator of muscle and has been recently recognized as an important factor that promotes muscle depletion in cirrhosis [36].

Ammonia has several effects on muscle. Firstly, it upregulates myostatin. Myostatin impairs protein synthesis and increases autophagy within muscle through inhibition of mammalian target of rapamycin complex-1 (mTORC1) signaling [37–39]. As mentioned, α-KG detoxifies excess ammonia to form glutamine. This reaction depletes the TCA cycle of a key intermediate (cataplerosis), ultimately resulting in mitochondrial dysfunction and reduced ATP synthesis [33]. Branched-chain amino acids (BCAA) contribute essential carbon skeletons used in the TCA cycle, and consumption of these assists in replenishing α-KG. BCAA depletion is therefore common in states of hyperammonemia and may result in reduced muscle synthesis by downregulating activation of the mTOR pathway [40]. The process of

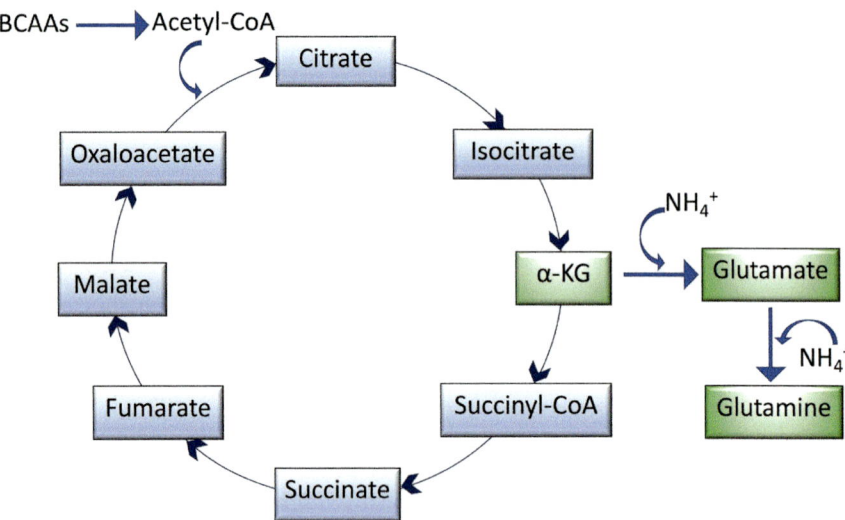

Fig. 15.1 Metabolism of ammonia through the TCA cycle. Ammonia (NH_4^+) detoxification in non-hepatic tissue occurs through the formation of glutamine and glutamate from α-ketoglutarate (α-KG), a key intermediary for the tricarboxylic acid (TCA) cycle. The TCA is critical series of chemical reactions that occurs as part of aerobic respiration to produce ATP for energy. The conversion of glutamate to glutamine is catalyzed by glutamine synthetase which is found in high concentrations in muscle. States of hyperammonemia deplete the TCA cycle of α-KG (cataplerosis), resulting in mitochondrial dysfunction and reduced ATP production, ultimately contributing to muscle loss. Metabolism of branched-chain amino acids (BCAAs) assists in replenishing the TCA cycle of its intermediates through production of acetyl-CoA

ammonia detoxification also releases reactive oxygen species which increase autophagy of skeletal muscle cells. Ammonia also activates the same cellular stress response as seen in amino acid starvation, leading to a further reduction in protein synthesis [36]. Hyperammonemia clearly plays a multifaceted and complex role in muscle depletion in cirrhosis. Therefore, ammonia-lowering therapies may provide a plausible mechanistic, therapeutic target for sarcopenia.

Recently, Kumar et al. explored the impact of ammonia-lowering therapy in portocaval anastomotic (PCA) rat models. Here, hyperammonemia is induced from formation of a direct portosystemic shunt. PCA and control rats were treated with rifaximin and L-ornithine L-aspartate (r-LOLA) for 4 weeks. R-LOLA therapy improved muscle mass, diameter, and grip strength and reduced myostatin and autophagy markers compared to controls [41, 42]. The effects of ammonia-lowering therapies on muscle have not been explored in randomized trials in humans. Borentain et al. reported an increase in psoas muscle area in ten cirrhotic patients treated with rifaximin for hepatic encephalopathy [43]. However, a number of these patients also underwent a TIPS procedure during follow-up which has been shown to increase lean muscle mass and may have confounded results.

Rifaximin, a poorly absorbed antibiotic, is used as a second-line therapy to reduce rates of recurrent hepatic encephalopathy. Recently, there is also evidence to suggest it may improve overall survival and reduce the rates of infectious complications and variceal bleeding in cirrhosis [44]. Through reduction in ammonia-producing colonic bacteria, rifaximin can reduce ammonia absorption from the gut. This is postulated as the key mechanism behind the effects on muscle seen in rat models. However, it may have additional effects on sarcopenia through a reduction in endotoxemia. Small intestinal bacterial overgrowth is common in cirrhosis, and release of endotoxins into the portal venous system worsens portal hypertension. It is associated with increased systemic inflammatory response and anabolic resistance. Rifaximin has been consistently shown to reduce endotoxin levels [45]. Other therapies that lower ammonia and are used for the treatment of hepatic encephalopathy include lactulose, LOLA, and BCAAs. Further research is required to investigate whether these therapies have any role in the prevention and treatment of sarcopenia in cirrhosis.

Growth Hormone

Cirrhosis is a state of acquired growth hormone (GH) resistance. This is associated with reduced levels of insulin-like growth factor-1 (IGF-1), a hormone produced in the liver which mediates the anabolic effects of GH. In cirrhosis, hepatocyte dysfunction and reduced GH receptors account for a reduction in IGF-1 and IGF-binding protein (IGFBP-3). Low serum levels of IGF-1 have been shown to correlate with hepatocyte dysfunction and with higher MELD and Child-Pugh scores [46, 47]. IGF-1 plays a vital role in many paracrine, autocrine, and endocrine functions. It has multimodal effects on muscle. IGF-1 stimulates protein kinase B (PKB/AKT) which upregulates mTOR leading to increased protein synthesis [48, 49]. It also has inhibitory effects on myostatin which acts as a negative regulator of satellite cell proliferation and differentiation [50]. In animal models of aging, GH therapy has been shown to prevent oxidative damage and exerts mitochondrial protection. This leads to reduced muscle cell autophagy and apoptosis [51]. Finally, IGF-1 therapy improved intestinal barrier function in rat models of cirrhosis [52]. This led to reduced rates of bacterial translocation and reduced portal hypertension.

A number of small pilot studies and randomized trials have investigated GH administration in cirrhosis. Donaghy et al. performed the first study investigating the effects of GH administration in adults with cirrhosis. In this pilot study, 20 patients with cirrhosis were given high-dose GH (0.25 IU/kg) for 7 days. Administration of GH resulted in an increase in IGF-I levels and improved nitrogen balance [53]. Wallace et al. investigated the metabolic effects of GH in nine adults with cirrhosis [54]. Compared to placebo, GH increased resting energy expenditure, lipid oxidation, and fasting glucose and insulin.

A randomized controlled trial of 114 patients with cirrhosis investigated the effects of recombinant GH therapy compared to placebo [55]. Baseline data from enrolled patients were compared to that of 15 healthy controls. Patients with cirrhosis had significantly lower serum IGF-1, IGFBP3, and GH levels compared to healthy controls. Following 6 months of intervention, GH therapy resulted in improved IGF-I, IGFBP3, and albumin levels compared to placebo. There was also a marked improvement in 2-week (98.21% vs. 75.86%), 1-month (91.07% vs. 62.07%), 3-month (66.07% vs. 22.41%), and 6-month (55.36% vs. 13.76%) survival in the GH treatment group compared to placebo. This substantial improvement in survival has not been born out in other trials. A thorough comparison of the two treatment groups was not provided to assess whether any other factors, such as severity of liver disease, may have founded these results.

Conchillo et al. (2005) is the only published study that has examined the effects of IGF-I replacement on muscle mass [56]. Eighteen patients with cirrhosis and low levels of IGF-I were randomized to receive daily subcutaneous injection of IGF-1 or a placebo therapy for 4 months. Serum levels of IGF-1 increased as did serum albumin. However, no changes in body composition or muscle mass or strength measures were found. Despite the lack of improvement in sarcopenia parameters, a reduction in resting energy expenditure was noted. This suggests that GH may have a role in reducing the hypermetabolism associated with cirrhosis. The major side effects of GH or IGF-1 administration have been fluid retention [54].

Growth hormone therapies have been researched widely as a therapy for sarcopenia in non-cirrhotic populations. GH levels decline with age making this a potential target for therapy for sarcopenia of aging. Tavares et al. investigated GH therapy in 14 healthy men over the age of 50 years old [57]. Compared to placebo, GH therapy leads to a significant increase in lower limb muscle strength after 6 months of therapy. GH as a therapy for muscle depletion in other chronic disease states has been explored in small trials. Seven patients with chronic obstructive pulmonary disease (COPD) received a high-calorie high-protein diet followed by addition of GH therapy [58]. No significant changes were noted with dietary intervention alone;

however, GH treatment demonstrated an improvement in nitrogen balance and weight gain. Similarly, Burdet et al. randomized 16 underweight patients with COPD to receive GH therapy or placebo [59]. GH improved lean muscle mass, but long-term follow-up failed to demonstrate an improvement in muscle strength or physical performance as measured by the 6-minute walk test (6MWT).

Growth hormone has additional effects on fat distribution and is associated with reduced subcutaneous and visceral fat. Therefore, its use as a therapy for lipodystrophy has been explored in adults with human immunodeficiency virus (HIV) [60]. Lipodystrophy is a side effect of antiretroviral therapy and leads to lipid redistribution and is associated with increased visceral adiposity and metabolic syndrome. HIV-induced cachexia is also common in this population. Improvements in lean body mass have been reported in a number of trials in HIV-infected adults following GH therapy. However, a systematic review of over ten randomized controlled trials found that while GH reduced visceral adiposity and increased subcutaneous fat stores, there was no sustained increase in lean body mass [61].

Ultimately, there is a lack of large-scale clinical trials assessing the effect of GH therapy in sarcopenia in both cirrhotic and non-cirrhotic populations. Currently, a randomized clinical trial investigating the effect of GH on sarcopenia is recruiting (NCT03420144). This aims to be completed by December 2019 and will further clarify the role of GH therapy in this population [62].

Myostatin Inhibition

Myostatin is a signaling protein that inhibits muscle cell growth and differentiation. Upregulation of myostatin is thought to be a key factor driving muscle depletion in many chronic disease states including cirrhosis [63]. Myostatin binds to the activin IIB (ActRIIB) receptor in skeletal muscle. This receptor also binds other ligands including activin A. Activation of ActRIIB stimulates downstream signaling resulting in inhibition of mTORC1. Inhibition of mTORC1 results in increased autophagy, impaired protein synthesis, and proteasome-mediated proteolysis [64].

Myostatin levels are elevated in both muscle and serum of cirrhotic subjects [65]. A recent study also linked elevated serum myostatin to radiological measures of sarcopenia and reduced survival [66]. Circulating ammonia transcriptionally upregulates myostatin. Similarly, key myostatin inhibitors including follistatin, insulin-like growth factor-1 (IGF-1), and testosterone are reduced in cirrhosis [67]. Given the key role of this myokine in muscle regulation, there has been increasing interest into therapies that target myostatin for treatment of sarcopenia in both cirrhotic and non-cirrhotic populations.

The myostatin signaling pathway can be targeted at several different levels (Fig. 15.2). As discussed previously, ammonia reduction may have beneficial effects on skeletal muscle mass through reducing myostatin. Follistatin acts as a potent negative regulator of myostatin by antagonizing ActRIIB. However, it is expressed in many tissues and also plays an important role in gonadal and pituitary function [68].

As such, the systemic effects of follistatin limit its use as a therapeutic agent. Various isoforms have been developed using gene therapy to enable more targeted action as a myostatin antagonist. In rat models and nonhuman primates, adeno-associated virus has been to deliver follistatin via intramuscular injection resulting in an increase in muscle fiber size and improve strength [69]. In limited human studies in Becker's muscular dystrophy, an X-linked recessive dystrophinopathy, intramuscular injection of follistatin into the quadriceps muscle improved distance walked on a 6MWT in four of six patients who received the therapy. Dasarathy et al. have

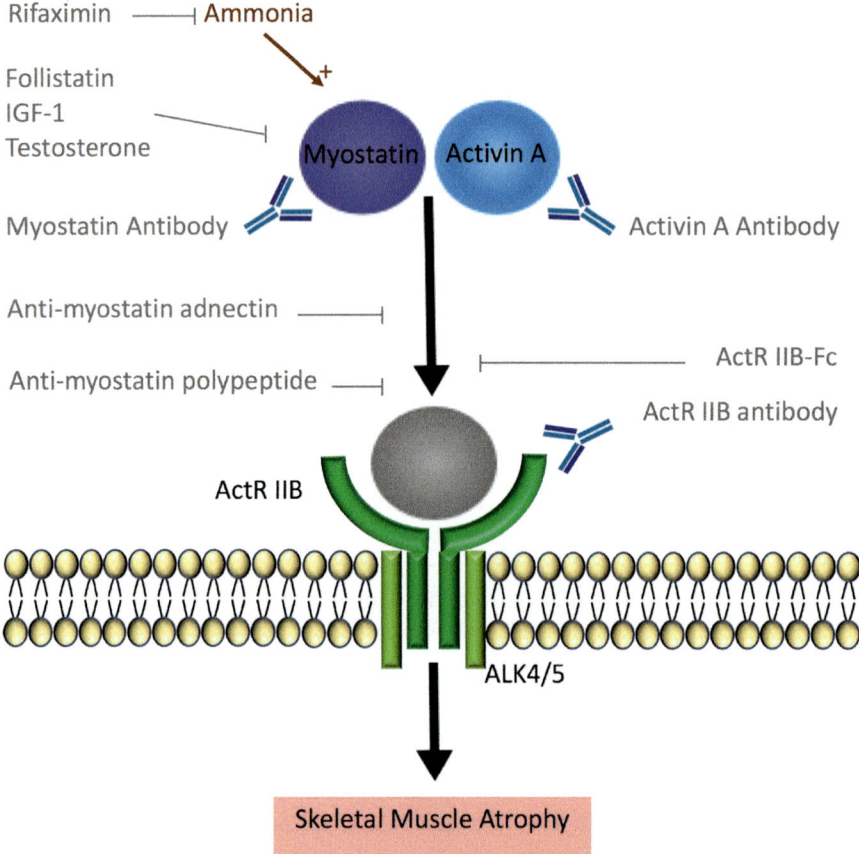

Fig. 15.2 Myostatin signaling pathway and therapeutic targets. Myostatin and activin A bind to the activin IIB receptor (ActR IIB) triggering a cascade of intracellular signaling that leads to alterations of gene transcription and reduced protein synthesis, ultimately leading to skeletal muscle atrophy. Extracellular targets of this pathway have been developed. Rifaximin, an ammonia-lowering therapy, may decrease hyperammonemia-induced upregulation of myostatin. Natural hormones including follistatin, IGF-1, and testosterone inhibit myostatin. Recombinant neutralizing monoclonal antibodies (myostatin antibody, activin A antibody, ActR IIB antibody), combination peptide antibodies (anti-myostatin polypeptide), and a recombinant fusion protein (ActR IIB-Fc) have all been developed to target the extracellular pathway of myostatin

explored the impact of follistatin in PCA rats [37]. PCA rats treated with follistatin demonstrated an increase in grip strength, lean body mass, and synthesis of skeletal muscle protein compared to placebo.

Several synthetic agents and monoclonal antibodies have been developed that target myostatin and its signaling pathway [70]. These have been trialed in a heterogenous group of neuromuscular and chronic diseases with inconsistent clinical results (Table 15.2). At least four monoclonal antibodies that directly target myostatin protein have reached phase II clinical trials [70]. Another two are in clinical development. Landogrozumab (LY2495655) has been the most widely published drug. A phase II clinical trial of landogrozumab in pancreatic cancer-associated cachexia was terminated early due to lack of clinical benefit [71]. Similarly, it failed to meet its primary endpoint of a 2.5% increase in muscle mass compared to placebo in a phase II trial of 400 patients undergoing total hip arthroplasty [72]. However, there were improvements in secondary endpoints in functional measures of muscle strength compared to placebo (<0.0001). In a randomized placebo-controlled trial of landogrozumab in 99 elderly patients with history of falls, the intervention group demonstrated an increase in lean muscle mass and improved physical performance on stair climbing, chair stands, and gait assessments compared to placebo [73]. Stamulumab, another anti-myostatin protein antibody, has discontinued development due to its failure to reach the primary endpoint in the treatment of muscular dystrophies.

Bimagrumab (BYM-338) is a fully human monoclonal antibody against ActR2B and has also been investigated as a therapeutic agent for sarcopenia associated with COPD and pancreatic malignancies. In adult patients with COPD and cachexia, 8 weeks of bimagrumab significantly improved muscle mass but failed to improve physical performance measures including 6MWT [74]. Targeting of the ActRIIB receptor through a recombinant fusion protein, ACE-083, is also under evaluation. ACE-083 has received a fast-tracked designation by the FDA for treatment of facioscapulohumeral muscular dystrophy following promising results in a phase I clinical trial. AMG-745, a peptibody that combines a peptide and myostatin neutralizing antibody, is a novel agent that targets the myostatin signaling pathway. Unfortunately, following promising phase I clinical trial in prostate cancer, it has been discontinued due to failure to meet efficacy endpoints in a phase I/II trial. A number of other phase II clinical trials that inhibit the myostatin pathway are underway, but results are not yet published.

Therapies that inhibit myostatin have the potential to be a powerful intervention in sarcopenia. However, current evidence is limited by small trials that have investigated their effect in a heterogenous group of conditions associated with muscle loss. Most of these trials have only progressed to an early stage of pharmacological testing with fairly limited effectiveness. While myostatin inhibition can result in increased muscle mass, an improvement in functional outcomes is often not achieved. As such, a number of drugs have been discontinued for failing to show improvements in strength or physical performance measures [70]. Larger clinical trials are warranted to define whether myostatin inhibitors will play a role in treatment of muscle wasting disorders in the future. In sarcopenia associated with

Table 15.2 Clinical trials investigating pharmaceutical targets of the myostatin signaling pathway

Name	Mechanism	Population	Phase	Trial design	Evidence
MYO-029/ Stamulumab	Myostatin antibody	Muscular dystrophy	I/II	116 patients randomized to 6 months of placebo, 10 mg/kg or 30 mg/kg of MYO-029	No improvements in muscle strength or function. Development of Myo-029 has since been discontinued
LY-2495655/ Landogrozumab	Myostatin antibody	Elective total hip replacement	II	400 patients randomized to placebo, 35 mg, 105 mg, or 315 mg LY-2495655, administered 4 weekly subcutaneously for 12 weeks	Dose-dependent increases in lean mass were observed compared to placebo but did not meet the primary endpoint of an increase in lean mass of 2.5%
		Elderly (≥75yo) with a recent fall	II	99 patients with a recent fall randomized to placebo or 315 mg LY-2495655 for 20 weeks	Improved appendicular lean body mass, gait speed, chair rise, and stair climbing time compared to placebo. Higher rate of side effects in treatment arm
		Pancreatic cancer	II	116 patients receiving standard of care chemotherapy were randomized to placebo, 100 mg or 300 mg of LY-2495655	300 mg terminated early due to imbalance of death rate. Trial terminated early due to futility following interim analysis. Primary endpoint of improvements in overall survival was not met. No significant difference between muscle volume and functional measures of muscle strength in treatment arm compared to placebo
BYM-338/ Bimagrumab	ActRIIB antibody	Sarcopenic and elderly (≥65yo)	I	40 community dwelling adults randomized to receive IV 30 mg BYM-338 or placebo for 24 weeks	Increased thigh muscle volume, gait speed, and handgrip strength in treatment arm compared to placebo over 16 weeks
		COPD with cachexia	II	67 patients randomized to placebo or 30 mg/kg BYM-338 intravenously for 24 weeks	Increase in thigh muscle volume but no changes in 6MWT. Higher rate of side effects in the treatment arm

| AMG-745/ PINTA 745 | Myostatin peptibody | Prostate cancer on androgen- deprivation therapy | I | Eight subjects randomized to placebo or 0.1 mg/kg, 0.3 mg/kg AMG-745 intravenously for 28 days | 16 weeks of therapy in 8 subjects Increased lean muscle mass compared to placebo with a dose-related increase rates of side effects |
| | | Chronic kidney disease and malnutrition | I/II | 5 patients randomized to placebo or 3 mg/kg or 6 mg/kg PINTA 745 intravenously for 9/12 weeks | Primary endpoint of increased lean body mass as measured on DEXA and secondary endpoint in improvement in physical performance not achieved |

COPD chronic obstructive airways disease, *6MWT* 6-minute walk test, *DEXA* dual-energy X-ray absorptiometry cirrhosis, there is certainly strong evidence that supports the integral role myostatin plays in the development of sarcopenia; however no human trials have been conducted to assess the effectiveness of myostatin inhibition in this population.

Other Therapies

Ghrelin Receptor Agonists

Ghrelin is a hormone that plays a variety of critical roles in nutrition, growth, and metabolism. It is a neuropeptide which stimulates appetite and growth hormone secretion and has additional anti-inflammatory properties [75]. Anorexia is a common symptom of many chronic diseases including cirrhosis and is a major factor that contributes to malnutrition. Fasting ghrelin levels are often normal or slightly elevated in cirrhotic subjects [76]. Lower caloric intake is associated with higher levels of ghrelin. This suggests that cirrhotic patients may be resistant to the appetite stimulant effects of ghrelin. Mechanistically, ghrelin therapy may exert anabolic effects on muscle through improved nutrition, stimulation of growth hormone, and reductions in energy expenditure and systemic inflammation.

Both administration of human ghrelin and an oral selective agonist of the ghrelin/growth hormone secretagogue receptor, anamorelin, have been explored in small studies of non-cirrhotic populations. An open-label pilot study of human ghrelin increased lean body mass, muscle strength, and 6MWT in seven COPD patients with cachexia [77]. In a phase II clinical trial, anamorelin improved muscle mass, handgrip strength, and quality of life compared to placebo in patients with cancer-related cachexia [78]. However, phase III clinical trials (ROMANA 1 and 2) were less promising. A total of 979 patients with lung cancer were treated with anamorelin or placebo. Similar to other sarcopenia trials, lean muscle mass increased in the treatment group, but there was no corresponding improvement in muscle strength or function [79]. The safety and efficacy of ghrelin therapy in cirrhotic subjects have not been explored.

Urocortin II (Corticotropin-Releasing Factor 2 Receptor Agonist)

Corticotropin-releasing factors are a family of peptides that play a critical role in the stress response through regulation of the hypothalamic-pituitary-adrenal axis. The corticotropin-releasing factor 2 receptor (CRF2R) is expressed in skeletal muscle. Urocortin II is a highly selective agonist of CRF2R and expressed within skeletal muscle [80]. Urocortin II has been shown in several animal models of aging and chronic disease states to prevent loss of skeletal muscle mass and function [81, 82]. CRF2R may be a potential target for future clinical trials, but to date, no human studies on efficacy as a treatment for sarcopenia have been conducted.

The Challenges of Clinical Trials for Interventions in Sarcopenia

Interventional trials for sarcopenia and frailty have several inherent challenges. There is no well-validated gold standard for quantifying muscle mass in cirrhosis. There is also still a lack of consensus into its definition. Furthermore, there is emerging evidence that contractile function and muscle mass may not necessarily be linked. While loss of muscle mass and muscle strength likely shares similar underlying pathological mechanisms, improving muscle mass does not necessarily correlate with improvements in muscle strength [42, 79, 83]. Regulatory approval in the USA typically requires therapies for sarcopenia to improve both muscle mass and strength or physical performance. Several therapies for muscle wasting disorders have failed to progress beyond phase II/III clinical trials as they have had difficulty meeting the latter endpoint. Functional parameters are subjective and highly variable and can easily be confounded by other factors. For example, the Fried Frailty index, a measure of muscle strength and performance, loses its survival predictive value during episodes of hepatic encephalopathy [84]. Despite this, performance measures often prove to be more clinically relevant than measures of muscle mass. Regardless, it remains unclear which is the best parameter to use for clinical trials.

The other major challenge is that sarcopenia is a multifactorial process with various competing factors. Whether one therapy alone is enough to arrest or reverse muscle depletion and weakness in this population is unknown. Improved understanding of the different roles each factor plays in sarcopenia of cirrhosis is required to enable more targeted therapy. Alternatively, a combination approach may be required or indeed a personalized approach that addresses the specific deficits in muscle physiology in the individual patient.

Finally, we know that sarcopenia is associated with increased morbidity and mortality. We presume that treating sarcopenia will therefore improve patient health and survival; however, this has never been scientifically proven. This remains a major goal of treatment, and further research is required in the form of large clinical trials using effective anabolic therapy to be able to answer this important question.

References

1. Sinclair M, Grossmann M, Angus PW, Hoermann R, Hey P, Scodellaro T, et al. Low testosterone as a better predictor of mortality than sarcopenia in men with advanced liver disease. J Gastroenterol Hepatol. 2016;31(3):661–7.
2. Moctezuma-Velazquez C, Low G, Mourtzakis M, Ma M, Burak KW, Tandon P, et al. Association between low testosterone levels and sarcopenia in cirrhosis: a cross-sectional study. Ann Hepatol. 2018;17(4):615–23.
3. Jones TH, Kennedy RL. Cytokines and hypothalamic-pituitary function. Cytokine. 1993;5(6):531–8.
4. Grossmann M, Hoermann R, Gani L, Chan I, Cheung A, Gow PJ, et al. Low testosterone levels as an independent predictor of mortality in men with chronic liver disease. Clin Endocrinol. 2012;77(2):323–8.
5. Wells R. Prednisolone and testosterone propionate in cirrhosis of the liver. A controlled trial. Lancet. 1960;2(7166):1416–9.
6. Puliyel MM, Vyas GP, Mehta GS. Testosterone in the management of cirrhosis of the liver – a controlled study. Aust NZ J Med. 1977;7(6):17–30.
7. Rambaldi A, Gluud C. Anabolic-androgenic steroids for alcoholic liver disease. Cochrane Database Syst Rev. 2006(4).
8. Gluud C, Hardt F, Juhl E. Testosterone treatment of men with alcoholic cirrhosis: a double-blind study. Hepatology. 1986;6(5):807–13.
9. Fenster F. The nonefficacy of short-term anabolic steroid therapy in alcoholic liver disease. Ann Intern Med. 1966;65(4):738–44.
10. Yurci A, Yucesoy M, Unluhizarci K, Torun E, Gursoy S, Baskol M, et al. Effects of testosterone gel treatment in hypogonadal men with liver cirrhosis. Clin Res Hepatol Gastroenterol. 2011;35(12):845–54.
11. Bhasin S, Jasuja R. Selective androgen receptor modulators as function promoting therapies. Curr Opin Clin Nutr Metab Care. 2009;12(3):232–40.
12. Jones A, Hwang D-J, Narayanan R, Miller DD, Dalton JT. Effects of a novel selective androgen receptor modulator on dexamethasone-induced and hypogonadism-induced muscle atrophy. Endocrinology. 2010;151(8):3706–19.
13. Crawford J, Prado CMM, Johnston MA, Gralla RJ, Taylor RP, Hancock ML, et al. Study design and rationale for the phase 3 clinical development program of enobosarm, a selective androgen receptor modulator, for the prevention and treatment of muscle wasting in cancer patients (POWER trials). Curr Oncol Rep. 2016;18:37.
14. Crawford J, Dalton JT, Hancock ML, Johnston MA, Steiner M. Results from two Phase 3 randomized trials of enobosarm, selective androgen receptor modulator (SARM), for the prevention and treatment of muscle wasting in NSCLC2013. Eur J Cancer. 2013:S10–S p.
15. Papanicolaou DA, Ather SN, Zhu H, Zhou Y, Lutkiewicz J, Scott BB, et al. A phase IIA randomized, placebo-controlled clinical trial to study the efficacy and safety of the selective androgen receptor modulator (SARM), MK-0773 in female participants with sarcopenia. J Nutr Health Aging. 2013;17(6):533–43. Epub 2013/06/05.
16. Dolz C, Raurich JM, Ibanez J, Obrador A, Marse P, Gaya J. Ascites increases the resting energy expenditure in liver cirrhosis. Gastroenterology. 1991;100(3):738–44.
17. Saunders J, Brian A, Wright M, Stroud M. Malnutrition and nutrition support in patients with liver disease. Front Gastroenterol. 2010;1(2):105–11.
18. Karlsen S, Fynne L, Gronbaek H, Krogh K. Small intestinal transit in patients with liver cirrhosis and portal hypertension: a descriptive study. BMC Gastroenterol. 2012;12:176.
19. Kovarik M, Muthny T, Sispera L, Holecek M. The dose-dependent effects of endotoxin on protein metabolism in two types of rat skeletal muscle. J Physiol Biochem. 2012;68(3):385–95.
20. Papaluca T, Gow P. Terlipressin: current and emerging indications in chronic liver disease. J Gastroenterol Hepatol. 2018;33(3):591–8.

21. Sharma P, Kumar A, Shrama BC, Sarin SK. An open label, pilot, randomized controlled trial of noradrenaline versus terlipressin in the treatment of type 1 hepatorenal syndrome and predictors of response. Am J Gastroenterol. 2008;103(7):1689–97.
22. Gow PJ, Ardalan ZS, Vasudevan A, Testro AG, Ye B, Angus PW. Outpatient terlipressin infusion for the treatment of refractory ascites. Am J Gastroenterol. 2016;111(7):1041–2.
23. Robertson M, Majumdar A, Garrett K, Rumler G, Gow P, Testro A. Continuous outpatient terlipressin infusion for hepatorenal syndrome as a bridge to successful liver transplantation. Hepatology. 2014;60(6):2125–6.
24. Vasudevan A, Ardalan Z, Gow P, Angus P, Testro A. Efficacy of outpatient continuous terlipressin infusions for hepatorenal syndrome. Hepatology. 2016;64(1):316–8.
25. Chapman B, Gow P, Angus P, Sinclair M, Testro A. Outpatient terlipressin infusion increases dietary intake and functional muscle strength in patients awaiting liver transplant. J Hepatol. 2018;68:S726.
26. Plauth M, Schutz T, Buckendahl DP, Kreymann G, Pirlich M, Grungreiff S, et al. Weight gain after transjugular intrahepatic portosystemic shunt is associated with improvement in body composition in malnourished patients with cirrhosis and hypermetabolism. J Hepatol. 2004;40(2):228–33.
27. Tsien C, Shah SN, McCullough AJ, Dasarathy S. Reversal of sarcopenia predicts survival after a transjugular intrahepatic portosystemic stent. Eur J Gastroenterol Hepatol. 2013;25(1):85–93.
28. Allard JP, Chau J, Sandokji K, Blendis LM, Wong F. Effects of ascites resolution after successful TIPS on nutrition in cirrhotic patients with refractory ascites. Am J Gastroenterol. 2001;96(8):2442–7.
29. Montomoli J, Holland-Fischer P, Bianchi G, Gronbaek H, Vilstrup H, Marchesini G, et al. Body composition changes after transjugular intrahepatic portosystemic shunt in patients with cirrhosis. World J Gastroenterol. 2010;16(3):348–53.
30. Nolte W, Wirtz M, Rossbach C, Leonhardt U, Buchwald AB, Scholz KH, et al. TIPS implantation raises leptin levels in patients with liver cirrhosis. Exp Clin Endocrinol Diabetes. 2003;111(7):435–42.
31. Holland-Fischer P, Vilstrup H, Frystyk J, Nielsen DT, Flyvbjerg A, Groonbaek H. The IGF system after insertion of a transjugular intrahepatic porto-systemic shunt in patients with liver cirrhosis. Eur J Endocrinol. 2009;160(6):957–63.
32. Holland-Fischer P, Nielsen MF, Vilstrup H, Nielsen DT, Schmitz O, Gronbaek H. Insulin sensitivity and body composition in cirrhosis: changes after tips. J Hepatol. 2009;1:S80.
33. Dasarathy S, Hatzoglou M. Hyperammonemia and proteostasis in cirrhosis. Curr Opin Clin Nutr Metab Care. 2018;21(1):30–6.
34. Merli M, Giusto M, Lucidi C, Giannelli V, Pentassuglio I, Di Gregorio V, et al. Muscle depletion increases the risk of overt and minimal hepatic encephalopathy: results of a prospective study. Mctab Brain Dis. 2013;28(2):281 4.
35. Bhanji RA, Moctezuma-Velazquez C, Duarte-Rojo A, Ebadi M, Ghosh S, Rose C, et al. Myosteatosis and sarcopenia are associated with hepatic encephalopathy in patients with cirrhosis. Hepatol Int. 2018:1–10.
36. Davuluri G, Krokowski D, Guan BJ, Kumar A, Thapaliya S, Singh D, et al. Metabolic adaptation of skeletal muscle to hyperammonemia drives the beneficial effects of l-leucine in cirrhosis. J Hepatol. 2016;65(5):929–37.
37. Dasarathy S, McCullough AJ, Muc S, Schneyer A, Bennett CD, Dodig M, et al. Sarcopenia associated with portosystemic shunting is reversed by follistatin. J Hepatol. 2011;54(5):915–21.
38. Trendelenburg AU, Meyer A, Rohner D, Boyle J, Hatakeyama S, Glass DJ. Myostatin reduces Akt/TORC1/p70S6K signaling, inhibiting myoblast differentiation and myotube size. Am J Physiol Cell Physiol. 2009;296(6):C1258–70.
39. Davuluri G, Thapaliya S, Kumar A, Have GAT, Welle SL, Engelen M, et al. Hyperammonemia impairs skeletal muscle protein synthesis via a novel Myostatin-ALK5-AMPK dependent mechanism. Hepatology. 2016;64(1 Supplement 1):355A.

40. Matsumura T, Morinaga Y, Fujitani S, Takehana K, Nishitani S, Sonaka I. Oral administration of branched-chain amino acids activates the mTOR signal in cirrhotic rat liver. Hepatol Res. 2005;33(1):27–32.
41. Kumar A, Nascimento ESR, Rennison JH, Allawy A, Van Wagoner DR, Hoppel CL, et al. Ammonia withdrawal reverses impaired skeletal muscle mitochondrial function. Hepatology. 2017;66. S1:1032A.
42. Kumar A, Davuluri G, Silva RNE, Engelen MPKJ, Ten Have GAM, Prayson R, et al. Ammonia lowering reverses sarcopenia of cirrhosis by restoring skeletal muscle proteostasis. Hepatology. 2017;65(6):2045–58.
43. Borentain P, Rouabah K, Allard G, Ressiot E, Gerolami R. Letter: nutritional benefits of rifaximin in cirrhotic patients. Aliment Pharmacol Ther. 2018;47(5):699–700.
44. Kang SH, Lee YB, Lee JH, Nam JY, Chang Y, Cho H, et al. Rifaximin treatment is associated with reduced risk of cirrhotic complications and prolonged overall survival in patients experiencing hepatic encephalopathy. Aliment Pharmacol Ther. 2017;46(9):845–55.
45. Kaji K, Takaya H, Saikawa S, Furukawa M, Sato S, Kawaratani H, et al. Rifaximin ameliorates hepatic encephalopathy and endotoxemia without affecting the gut microbiome diversity. World J Gastroenterol. 2017;23(47):8355–66.
46. Caufriez A, Reding P, Urbain D, Golstein J, Copinschi G. Insulin-like growth factor I: a good indicator of functional hepatocellular capacity in alcoholic liver cirrhosis. J Endocrinol Investig. 1991;14(4):317–21.
47. Khoshnood A, Nasiri Toosi M, Faravash MJ, Esteghamati A, Froutan H, Ghofrani H, et al. A survey of correlation between insulin-like growth factor-I (IGF-I) levels and severity of liver cirrhosis. Hepat Mon. 2013;13(2):e6181.
48. Naranjo JD, Dziki JL, Badylak SF. Regenerative medicine approaches for age-related muscle loss and sarcopenia: a mini-review. Gerontology. 2017;63(6):580–9.
49. Sattler FR. Growth hormone in the aging male. Best Pract Res Clin Endocrinol Metab. 2013;27(4):541–55.
50. Liu W, Thomas SG, Asa SL, Gonzalez-Cadavid N, Bhasin S, Ezzat S. Myostatin is a skeletal muscle target of growth hormone anabolic action. J Clin Endocrinol Metab. 2003;88(11):5490–6.
51. Pérez R, García-Fernández M, Díaz-Sánchez M, Puche JE, Delgado G, Conchillo M, et al. Mitochondrial protection by low doses of insulin-like growth factor- I in experimental cirrhosis. World J Gastroenterol. 2008;14(17):2731–9.
52. Lorenzo-Zúñiga V, Rodríguez-Ortigosa CM, Bartolí R, Martínez-Chantar ML, Martínez-Peralta L, Pardo A, et al. Insulin-like growth factor I improves intestinal barrier function in cirrhotic rats. Gut. 2006;55(9):1306–12.
53. Donaghy A, Ross R, Wicks C, Hughes SC, Holly J, Gimson A, et al. Growth hormone therapy in patients with cirrhosis: a pilot study of efficacy and safety. Gastroenterology. 1997;113(5):1617–22.
54. Wallace JD, Abbott-Johnson WJ, Crawford DHG, Barnard R, Potter JM, Cuneo RC. GH treatment in adults with chronic liver disease: a randomized, double-blind, placebo-controlled, cross-over study. J Clin Endocrinol Metab. 2002;87(6):2751–9.
55. Li N, Zhou L, Zhang B, Dong P, Lin W, Wang H, et al. Recombinant human growth hormone increases albumin and prolongs survival in patients with chronic liver failure: a pilot open, randomized, and controlled clinical trial. Dig Liver Dis. 2008;40(7):554–9.
56. Conchillo M, de Knegt RJ, Payeras M, Quiroga J, Sangro B, Herrero JI, et al. Insulin-like growth factor I (IGF-I) replacement therapy increases albumin concentration in liver cirrhosis: results of a pilot randomized controlled clinical trial. J Hepatol. 2005;43(4):630–6.
57. Tavares ABW, Micmacher E, Biesek S, Assumpção R, Redorat R, Veloso U, et al. Effects of growth hormone administration on muscle strength in men over 50 years old. Int J Endocrinol. 2013;2013:942030.
58. Pape GS, Friedman M, Underwood LE, Clemmons DR. The effect of growth hormone on weight gain and pulmonary function in patients with chronic obstructive lung disease. Chest. 1991;99(6):1495–500.

59. Burdet L, de Muralt B, Schutz Y, Pichard C, Fitting JW. Administration of growth hormone to underweight patients with chronic obstructive pulmonary disease. A prospective, randomized, controlled study. Am J Respir Crit Care Med. 1997;156(6):1800–6.
60. Gelato M, McNurlan M, Freedland E. Role of recombinant human growth hormone in HIV-associated wasting and cachexia: pathophysiology and rationale for treatment. Clin Ther. 2007;29(11):2269–88.
61. Generali JA, Cada DJ. Recombinant human growth hormone: HIV-related lipodystrophy. Hosp Pharm. 2014;49(5):432–4.
62. Available from: https://clinicaltrials.gov/ct2/show/NCT03420144.
63. Dasarathy S. Myostatin and beyond in cirrhosis: all roads lead to sarcopenia. J Cachexia Sarcopenia Muscle. 2017;8(6):864–9. Epub 2017/11/24.
64. Dasarathy S, Merli M. Sarcopenia from mechanism to diagnosis and treatment in liver disease. J Hepatol. 2016;65(6):1232–44.
65. Garcia PS, Cabbabe A, Kambadur R, Nicholas G, Csete M. Brief-reports: elevated myostatin levels in patients with liver disease: a potential contributor to skeletal muscle wasting. Anesth Analg. 2010;111(3):707–9. Epub 2010/08/06.
66. Nishikawa H, Enomoto H, Ishii A, Iwata Y, Miyamoto Y, Ishii N, et al. Elevated serum myostatin level is associated with worse survival in patients with liver cirrhosis. J Cachexia Sarcopenia Muscle. 2017;8(6):915–25. Epub 2017/06/20.
67. Sinclair M, Gow PJ, Grossmann M, Angus PW. Review article: sarcopenia in cirrhosis – aetiology, implications and potential therapeutic interventions. Aliment Pharmacol Ther. 2016;43(7):765–77.
68. Rodino-Klapac LR, Haidet AM, Kota J, Handy C, Kaspar BK, Mendell JR. Inhibition of myostatin with emphasis on follistatin as a therapy for muscle disease. Muscle Nerve. 2009;39(3):283–96.
69. Kota J, Handy CR, Haidet AM, Montgomery CL, Eagle A, Rodino-Klapac LR, et al. Follistatin gene delivery enhances muscle growth and strength in nonhuman primates. Sci Transl Med. 2009;1(6):6ra15. Epub 2010/04/07.
70. Saitoh M, Ishida J, Ebner N, Anker SD, Springer J, Haehling S. Myostatin inhibitors as pharmacological treatment for muscle wasting and muscular dystrophy. J Cachexia Sarcopenia Muscle. 2017;2(1):1–10.
71. Golan T, Geva R, Richards D, Madhusadan S, Lin B, Wang H, et al. LY2495655, an anti-myostatin antibody, in pancreatic cancer: a randomised, phase 2 trail. J Cachexia Sarcopenia Muscle. 2018;9(5):871–9.
72. Woodhouse L, Gandhi R, Warden SJ, Poiraudeau S, Myers SL, Benson CT, et al. A phase 2 randomized study investigating the efficacy and safety of myostatin antibody LY2495655 versus placebo in older patients undergoing elective total hip arthroplasty. J Frailty Aging. 2016;5(1):62–70.
73. Becker C, Lord SR, Studenski SA, Warden SJ, Fielding RA, Recknor CP, et al. Myostatin antibody (LY2495655) in older weak fallers: a proof-of-concept, randomised, phase 2 trial. Lancet Diabetes Endocrinol. 2015;3(12):948–57.
74. Polkey MI, Praestgaard J, Berwick A, Franssen FME, Singh D, Steiner MC, et al. Activin type II receptor blockade for treatment of muscle depletion in COPD: a randomized trial. Am J Respir Crit Care Med. 2019;199(3):313–20.
75. Marchesini G, Bianchi G, Lucidi P, Villanova N, Zoli M, De Feo P. Plasma ghrelin concentrations, food intake, and anorexia in liver failure. J Clin Endocrinol Metab. 2004;89(5):2136.
76. Tacke F, Brabant G, Kruck E, Horn R, Schöffski P, Hecker H, et al. Ghrelin in chronic liver disease. J Hepatol. 2003;38(4):447–54.
77. Nagaya N, Itoh T, Murakami S, Oya H, Uematsu M, Miyatake K, et al. Treatment of cachexia with ghrelin in patients with COPD. Chest. 2005;128(3):1187–93.
78. Temel JS, Abernethy AP, Currow DC, Friend J, Duus EM, Yan Y, et al. Anamorelin in patients with non-small-cell lung cancer and cachexia (ROMANA 1 and ROMANA 2): results from two randomised, double-blind, phase 3 trials. Lancet Oncol. 2016;17(4):519–31.

79. Anker SD, Coats AJS, Morley JE. Evidence for partial pharmaceutical reversal of the cancer anorexia–cachexia syndrome: the case of anamorelin. J Cachexia Sarcopenia Muscle. 2015;6(4):275–7.

80. Reyes TM, Lewis K, Perrin MH, Kunitake KS, Vaughan J, Arias CA, et al. Urocortin II: a member of the corticotropin-releasing factor (CRF) neuropeptide family that is selectively bound by type 2 CRF receptors. Proc Natl Acad Sci U S A. 2001;98(5):2843–8. Epub 2001/02/28.

81. Hinkle RT, Donnelly E, Cody DB, Bauer MB, Isfort RJ. Urocortin II treatment reduces skeletal muscle mass and function loss during atrophy and increases nonatrophying skeletal muscle mass and function. Endocrinology. 2003;144(11):4939–46.

82. Hinkle RT, Lefever FR, Dolan ET, Reichart DL, Zwolshen JM, Oneill TP, et al. Treatment with a corticotrophin releasing factor 2 receptor agonist modulates skeletal muscle mass and force production in aged and chronically ill animals. BMC Musculoskelet Disord. 2011;12:15.

83. Amthor H, Macharia R, Navarrete R, Schuelke M, Brown SC, Otto A, et al. Lack of myostatin results in excessive muscle growth but impaired force generation. Proc Natl Acad Sci U S A. 2007;104(6):1835–40.

84. Tapper EB, Konerman M, Murphy S, Sonnenday CJ. Hepatic encephalopathy impacts the predictive value of the Fried Frailty Index. Am J Transplant. 2018;18(10):2566–70.

Chapter 16
Should Frailty Include Multidimensional and Dynamic Factors?

Darryl B. Rolfson

At the heart of applied research on frailty is a nagging uneasiness about its meaning and therefore its measurement. This problem has been true right from the start, as frailty was emerging as a meaningful clinical paradigm [1–3], distinct from comorbidity and disability. A narrative emerged that dichotomized frailty either as a clinical syndrome [4], along with pathophysiology and promise for biological markers and treatment, or as a state of "accumulated deficits," aligning it with robust risk modelling and multidimensionality [5, 6]. In publications since then, a lack of consensus on the nature of frailty is commonly cited, and likewise an operational definition [7] remains elusive. This has left clinicians with a dilemma to adopt one of the traditional viewpoints, move forward with a sense of uncertainty about its meaning, or simply ignore it. If clinicians are having such difficulty, then they should not be surprised to learn that their patients are equally unsettled when they hear the term, and commonly assign negative connotations that their clinicians never intended [8, 9].

Were it not for the evidence that frailty, however defined, was common [10, 11] and strongly associated with adverse outcomes [12–15], it would have been discarded long ago as a passing curiosity. Instead, it has been well-described as "the most problematic expression of population aging" [16] and as an emerging public health priority [17] and indeed is estimated to be the most common pattern in the last year of life, exceeding traditional clinical clusters such as single-organ failure, dementia, and cancer [18].

In *Frailty and Sarcopenia*, one of the two traditional conceptual models of frailty, the physical phenotype, has been largely adopted. This syndrome-based model may be well-suited to questions that frame frailty as a disease with its own pathogenesis and prognosis, raising hope for future markers and interventions. However, here I will argue that the reductionist approach is problematic from a clinical perspective.

D. B. Rolfson (✉)
Division of Geriatric Medicine, Department of Medicine, University of Alberta, Edmonton, AB, Canada
e-mail: drolfson@ualberta.ca

© Springer Nature Switzerland AG 2020
P. Tandon, A. J. Montano-Loza (eds.), *Frailty and Sarcopenia in Cirrhosis*,
https://doi.org/10.1007/978-3-030-26226-6_16

The messy whole of frailty, along with its multidimensional and dynamic aspects, is a more authentic construct in clinical practice, as it better approximates the experience of the individual who lives with it. I will build this argument by elaborating first on the various conceptual models, then link these to a family of candidate measures, and provide closing remarks on implementation.

1. *Frailty in nature.* Does frailty exist in the natural world? If so, should we think of it as an observable physical trait such as jaundice, as an illness script such as cirrhosis, or as a state of vulnerability such as the Child-Pugh score [19]? In clinical practice, all three of these entities are meaningful and belong to an interrelated whole.

   One useful way to make sense of a complex entity such as frailty is to distinguish between observable variables (directly observed or measured) and latent variables (inferred from observable variables). In the preceding example, jaundice would be a directly observable variable. By comparison, cirrhosis, as a latent variable, requires a clinician to render and then integrate information from various sources. The diagnosis of cirrhosis becomes a mental construct, framed as an illness script, and based on expert clinical judgment. Illness scripts such as cirrhosis are thought to exist in nature, as are the observable traits such as jaundice that comprise them. Risk modelling tools such as the Child-Pugh score are also latent variables that can apply what we know about a defined population to an individual who has a similar clinical pattern. While a prediction tool is strictly a latent variable, such an entity can be powerful when used in the appropriate setting to model expectations and guide dialogue and decisions.

   Likewise, frailty has been framed as a phenotype with observable characteristics [4, 20], as a clinical syndrome [21, 22] with presumed underlying pathophysiology, and as an exaggerated state of risk [23, 24], with special vulnerability to external variables. There are no hard lines between these definitions, and each part comprises the whole of frailty. Reducing frailty to just one of these frameworks makes it a less authentic representation. Some classify frailty as an emerging "geriatric syndrome" [25, 26], adding it to the pantheon of falls, immobility, polypharmacy, urinary incontinence, delirium, and dementia. It may even prove to have added status as a composite and overarching measure [27], reframing the traditional giants as "frailty syndromes."

   The unique challenge for the taxonomists is that frailty is not univocal: the same word can be used to mean very different things, which happen to be closely related, but cannot be easily teased apart. Slippage in the meaning of a word makes discourse difficult in both research and clinical settings, as has been recognized about frailty for some time [28]. One option is to abandon the term altogether. Another is to work toward greater particularity and consensus on the definition of the term, in order to destigmatize it. The following different conceptual models of frailty illustrate the attempts to do just that.

2. *The physiologic basis of frailty.* A physiological basis for frailty has been theorized for some time [29]. In this view, frailty is a decline in homeostatic

function, strength, and physiologic reserve leading to increased vulnerability and making it distinct from sarcopenia, which is a loss of muscle mass, and function with age [30]. It was with this physiology in mind that the phenotype model was proposed [4], along with a hypothesized "cycle of frailty" [31]. The phenotype, first derived for use in the Cardiovascular Health Study, includes five single point items (weight loss, slow walking speed, low levels of physical activity, subjective exhaustion, and weakness) in which a score of 1–2 is "pre-frail" and 3 or higher is frail. A number of physiologic, molecular, and genetic alterations were proposed to explain the multisystem nature of frailty.

This opened doors to a massive research agenda that has inspired investigation in a diverse array of fields. The expectation is that over time such research would be rewarded with a bridge to biological markers that could be used for diagnostic and therapeutic approaches. Indeed, there are many candidate markers based on an association with frailty including hormones (elevated cortisol, low androgens), low vitamin D, glycoproteins, and molecules that relate to inflammation, endothelial dysfunction, insulin resistance, and oxidative damage. However, thus far, none of these have been proven to be "individually of sufficient diagnostic and prognostic capacity to be valid in clinical settings" [32].

The "frailty phenotype"(FP), as it came to be known, did emerge as the most popular instrument to measure frailty in research settings [33] and offered a viable alternative to chronological age in risk modelling [4, 34–36]. Despite this, it has not found widespread acceptance in clinical settings, possibly, because the criteria are not clinically intuitive and special equipment and training are required to administer the test.

3. *Frailty as an accumulation of deficits.* Almost simultaneously, another approach to understand and measure frailty arose which was designed to include a more broad set of variables that could be drawn from large datasets. In comparison to the FP, which understands frailty as a clinical *syndrome*, the deficit accumulation model, typified by the Frailty Index (FI) [5, 37, 38], frames frailty as a *state* of exaggerated vulnerability that can be constructed from a sufficiently rich clinical database or comprehensive geriatric assessment. According to a standard procedure [39], potential deficits (scored as 0 or 1) were defined as any set of variables that accumulate with age, might theoretically threaten health and independence, and collectively cover several body systems. If the list (or denominator) is at least 30, no greater weight need be assigned to any one variable. The FI is the quotient of actual over potential deficits, scored between 0 and 1.

As with the FP, the validation of the FI was largely based on its theoretical sophistication and its predictive validity. With aging, deficits accumulate with little impact on health or independence due to compensating assets. However, the accumulation is clearly nonlinear, accelerating over time regardless of age, and tends to proceed based on stochastic events such as new chronic diseases and the stable effects of accidents.

Deficit accumulation helps explain the state of silent vulnerability that becomes apparent only under conditions of stress. It is multidimensional and flexible to apply in different research contexts. Risk modelling is clearly established in various populations for outcomes such as mortality, institutionalization, hospitalizations, and other adverse outcomes [40–42] and has been cross-validated in numerous populations internationally.

The original FI does not intuitively align with the way that frontline clinicians gather and analyze clinical information. It is end-loaded, as its calculation requires a pre-defined database of candidate deficits in the population of interest, populated with the particular deficits, absent or present in selected individuals.

An electronic version has been implemented in primary care settings in the United Kingdom [43], and the FI based on comprehensive geriatric assessment (FI-CGA) is also beginning to find more mainstream use as an adjunct to comprehensive geriatric assessment [44, 45]. In one regard, the alignment of the FI with multi-morbidity does resonate with clinicians, in the sense that frailty is the logical extension as multi-morbidity accumulates and functional performance begins to supersede any single disease [46].

4. *The multidimensional expression of frailty.* In a consensus-based process governed by modified Delphi methodology, top experts drawn from both traditions of frailty definition were brought together in 2013 [7], and the level of agreement on a large number of statements regarding frailty was determined. There was broad agreement that frailty is a multidimensional syndrome with decreased reserve and diminished resistance to stressors. Importantly, there was strong agreement that these dimensions should include not only physical performance such as gait speed and mobility but also nutritional status, mental health, and cognition. The group agreed that it is useful to define frailty in clinical settings to allow for prevention and treatment, but could not agree on an operative definition or set of clinical or laboratory biomarkers for this purpose.

Even social vulnerability, sometimes known as "social frailty," is an important dimension of frailty also, but is not always included in its expanding multidimensional definition. Still, social gradients appear to be present for frailty [47], and the correlation with the frailty index is strong in various community-based populations worldwide ([48–50)]. Social vulnerability also influences mortality independent of frailty [51].

5. *Frailty as a functional construct.* Functional status, or the ability to carry out activities of daily living, can be derived from self-report, collateral history and by performance-based measures. Function is right at the interface between the intrinsic capacity of an individual and the surrounding social environment, including stable and unstable variables. Function represents integration and is by nature a multidimensional construct.

The World Health Organization in 2016 affirmed its emphasis on the transition state (declining capacity) between healthy aging (high functioning and stable) and disability (significant losses) [17]. Although the term frailty is not used explicitly, this transition state is clearly being adopted as a surrogate for frailty. If so, then it will be important to be clear on the frailty constructs in relation to healthy aging and disability, recognizing the multidimensional nature of healthy aging and disability [52, 53].

Nonetheless, both the 2013 consensus definition and the WHO model emphasize frailty (or the "transition state") as a public health priority and place functional status as a central feature of its manifestation. The WHO has adopted "intrinsic capacity" as the underlying construct to explain this multidimensional transition, constituting the domains of cognition, locomotion, sensory abilities, psychological status, and "vitality," including hormonal function, energy metabolism, and cardiorespiratory function [54]. It should be emphasized that apart functional status, no unique measure of intrinsic capacity per se has been validated.

6. *The dynamic aspects of frailty.* The notion that frailty is by nature unstable and expressed in functional terms was described quite early in its conceptualization. After stating the important differences between disability and frailty, Campbell defined "unstable disability" as an expression of frailty when function fluctuates markedly with minor external events [55]. This early concept of frailty is a lucid illustration of how the various models of frailty work together. Not only does unstable disability acknowledge frailty as both a state and a syndrome, and capture its functional and the multidimensional manifestations, but it also introduces the important role of external events, or stressors, to distinguish frailty from stable disability.

Recent enthusiasm for clinical research in frailty comes from those clinical specialties that hope to understand its interaction with stress, whether intrinsic or extrinsic. Frailty is of special interest in acute surgical and medical settings where care decisions are being made without accounting for the quiet intrinsic state of frailty. Likewise, frailty may become unmasked in individuals for whom functional status is highly influenced by unstable social factors. The modifiable nature of the physical and social stressors in frailty might make a difference to outcomes such as mortality, institutionalization, quality of life, and functional decline. This has typically motivated a dialogue regarding risk prediction and modification. Risk modelling demonstrated with the FP and FI are not instrument-specific. Similar predictive validity has been demonstrated with frailty measures that are judgment-based, performance-based, functional, and multidimensional [56–60].

Systematic reviews in various populations have shown cross-sectional but independent associations between frailty and adverse outcomes. For example, frailty assessment informs surgical risk for mortality, functional decline, and major adverse cardiac or cerebral events (MACCE) in ways that have not been captured with traditional surgical risk scores. The predictive value was best with those instruments that emphasized mobility, nutrition, and multidimensionality [14].

Likewise, frailty in those undergoing cardiac surgery significantly raised the risk of MACCE, mortality, and functional decline [61]. Cancer patients with frailty have a higher risk of all cause and postoperative mortality and treatment complications [62]. Heart failure patients with frailty were significantly more likely to experience adverse events, hospitalization, and death [63]. In critical care settings, frailty is independently associated with death in the hospital and long term [64].

Taken together, these systematic reviews and a countless other cross-sectional studies establish a strong association between frailty and adverse outcomes, but do not establish causality. We are now in a new era of enquiry, which aims to better establish causality through longitudinal cohorts, and more importantly, determine whether interventions that address frailty or its component dimensions prior to anticipated stress might result in improved outcomes.

7. *Geriatric syndromes.* The dynamic, functional, and multidimensional nature of frailty can perhaps be best illustrated by what is known about the other geriatric syndromes that comprise it. One excellent example of this is delirium, a particular manifestation of "unstable disability," showing what can happen when a particular predisposition (i.e., the state of frailty) and acute precipitants (the stressors) interact. Over 20 years ago, Inouye et al. demonstrated that delirium is caused by both precipitating and predisposing variables [65, 66]. In older adults who live with frailty and functional dependency, illness presentations such as delirium may be more atypical [67], reflecting not only the acute precipitant but the particular systems of vulnerability of the individual. Thus, when the dominant pattern of frailty in a particular individual leans toward cognitive impairment, acute illness may be first manifest as delirium, rather than another geriatric syndrome such as acute immobility. Here, frailty can be visualized as a balance scale in which assets and deficits are perfectly in balance. Minor acute stressors will have an exaggerated impact and will be expressed in functional decline and in illness presentations that reflect the particular constellation of underlying vulnerabilities.

Aside from delirium, other geriatric syndromes that seem to follow the same pattern described by Inouye, in which the predisposing variables rival or exceed the precipitating variables in etiologic importance include falls, immobility, urinary incontinence, and acute nutritional crisis. The precipitants may be anything from acute illness to a stressful intervention such as surgery, or even an acute decline in social supports

8. *Integrating the models.* Frailty is as complex a phenomenon as can be found in clinical care, and the models and measures selected to best describe it are likely quite context-dependent. Here, we might do well to adopt a caution from Werner Heisenberg that "there is a fundamental error in separating the parts from the whole, the mistake of atomizing what should not be atomized. Unity and complementarity constitute reality." [68] A recent comparison of frailty with the Golden Gate Bridge [69] seems to take an integrated conceptualization of frailty in the right direction, capturing the key pillars such as the physical phenotype, the many vertical cables that represent the multidimensional and stochastic aspects, and the external forces that capture its dynamic aspects (see Fig. 16.1, used with permission). If the complexity of frailty warrants such an integrated definition, then surely the many measures that are now available should also be integrated and used in a coordinated way.

"Frailty" constructs	Examples	Frailty and resilience from the perspective of a complex structure (Golden Gate Bridge)	Potential strengths
A. Phenotypic frailty (defined state)	Fried CHS Study Sarcopenic Obesity		Capture existence of a clinically defined and measurable phenotypic state Define risk factos and mechanism, with some specificity for given phenotype Measure treatment effects when a degree of treatment specificity is involved
B. Stochastic frailty (accumulation of deficits)	Rockwood FI Index (e.g. Ficlin, Filab)		Perform prognestication Define cross-cutting risk factors Measure treatment effects when more pleiotropic interventions are studied Measure treatment effects when testing geroscience guided therapeutics
C. Resilience (Measure of homeostasis in face of stressor)	Orthostasis Vaccine Responses Recovery from infection, Surgery, anesthesia, dehydration, bedrest, chemotherapy, trauma or BM transplant	WIND → TRAFFIC TRAFFIC WATER ← →	Identify "hidden" vulnerability Identify resident mechanisms Obtain more individualized risk Design more precise interventions Design earlier Interventions Design Interventions targeting resident mechanisms

Fig. 16.1 Integration of frailty models using the Golden Gate Bridge analogy. The Golden Gate Bridge is presented as a visual metaphor for the complementary contributions made by different conceptual constructs to the integrity and function of a complex system. (**a**) Phenotypic frailty involves the existence of a specific state or phenotype defined by measurable changes involving structures such as a major tower (red) or horizontal cable (red long dash) that perform unique functions and are critical to the existence of the overall system. (**b**) Stochastic frailty is defined as a process whereby the accumulation of deficits involving more redundant structures such as vertical cables (absent or red stippled) increases system vulnerability. (**c**) Resilience evaluates the ability of the system to withstand expected stressors such as bridge traffic, wind, and water currents (red arrows). All of these complementary perspectives must be considered when designing a bridge or providing care for older adults. Each approach has its strengths with regard to specific questions, and further research is needed, but phenotypic frailty is most helpful when focusing on a specific clinical state associated with vulnerability and for measuring the effects of an intervention targeting risk factors or mechanisms that are relatively specific to that condition. The concept of stochastic frailty may be most helpful for individual prognostication and for evaluating interventions that are more pleiotropic or that target shared risk factors or biological mechanisms. (Used with permission from the *Journal of the American Geriatrics Society* [69])

9. *Measurement of frailty.* After several systematic reviews, no single measure of frailty has emerged as superior in terms of diagnostic test accuracy [70] or as an outcome measure [71], and it appears that the "needs of the researchers, clinicians, or policy-makers" will likely continue to govern the choice of instrument [72], at least until there is a more ordered taxonomy of frailty measures and more clear guidance on the most appropriate instruments and cut points for defined purposes, populations, and settings.

To this end, the coordinated use of a range of frailty measures has been proposed in both acute [73] and primary care settings [74]. Important distinguishing characteristics include such things as the need for special equipment, availability of prior clinical assessment, intended use by operators with clinical expertise, administration time, ability to grade severity, ability to define components, and speed of interpretation [75]. Depending on the intended use of the tool, construct validity, diagnostic test accuracy, predictive validity, and sensitivity to change should also factor into instrument selection.

When applying existing evidence in the research design or clinical care, it helps to be clear on the predominant models of frailty, as this will likely guide the selection of the most appropriate set of frailty measures. Table 16.1 compares seven different categories of frailty measures in relation to the six models of frailty.

If the construct of frailty includes multidimensional and dynamic variables, then how and when should frailty measures reflect this? Clinicians in primary and acute care tend to use frailty measures opportunistically, to discover whether the condition is present, to enhance diagnostic reasoning, and to predict future outcomes. Frailty measures in home living and institutional care settings might be applied more systematically and with greater uniformity, based on sound data standards and practices [75].

Regardless, it should become apparent that the simple recognition of frailty is not enough to motivate its use by clinicians or citizens. Frailty case finding, whether at an early state, or when the syndrome becomes more obvious, should be motivate clinicians to better anticipate and recognize the expression of frailty in particular individuals. A multidimensional understanding leads naturally to patient-centered dialogue and decisions, including prevention of further decline, targeted interventions, and mitigation of future triggers for poor outcomes. Early case-finding measures would target individuals in whom the state frailty is not obvious, but might be expressed under dynamic conditions.

A detailed description of the measures is beyond the scope of this chapter, but the measurement categories will be briefly described using relevant examples.

(a) Physical frailty. The frailty phenotype (FP) [4] is the classic measure of the physical aspects of frailty, and it has been anchored to its pathophysiology, making it an attractive research-oriented measure. The FP requires the use of a dynamometer and some training on how each of the five items are administered and scored. It has been extensively validated. The Study of Osteoporotic Fractures (SOF) measure is similar in its design and purpose [76].

(b) Biological makers. We do not yet have valid biological markers or imaging techniques, to inform case finding, diagnosis, or therapy. If this is achieved, one further application might be in the dynamic model, where the changing frailty status of the individual could be monitored.

(c) The frailty index. The electronic frailty index (eFI) [43] operationalizes this model very well and is quickly emerging as a measure that can be used system-wide. Typically, the FI and eFI would include a range of multidimensional and functional candidate deficits. Because these deficits tend to accumulate without resolution, an FI is not likely to have the sensitivity to change needed to reflect dynamic changes. However, these measures can be used in anticipation of upcoming stress to detect the early, quiet state of frailty.

Table 16.1 Alignment of different categories of frailty measures by frailty model

	Categories of frailty measures (with examples)						
	Physical frailty	Biological markers	Frailty index	Judgment-based	Self-report	Performance-based	Multidimensional
	FP, SOF	Blood tests, imaging	eFI	CFS	PRISMA 7, TFI, FRAIL	Gait speed, grip strength	EFS, FI-CGA
Models of frailty							
Physiologic frailty	✓	✓					
Deficit accumulation			✓				
Multidimensional and social frailty			✓	✓			✓
Frailty as function and mobility	✓		✓	✓	✓	✓	✓
Dynamic frailty		✓				✓	
Frailty as geriatric syndromes							✓

✓ indicates good alignment. Measures: *FP* frailty phenotype, *SOF* Study of Osteoporotic Fractures measures, *eFI* electronic frailty index, *CFS* Clinical Frailty Scale, *PRISMA 7* Program of Research on Integration of Services for the Maintenance of Autonomy, *TFI* Tilburg Frailty Indicator, *FRAIL* Fatigue, Resistance, Aerobic, Illnesses, Loss of Weight, *EFS* Edmonton Frail Scale, FI-CGA (Frailty Index based on Comprehensive Geriatric Assessment

(d) Judgment-based measures. The Clinical Frailty Scale [57] requires a prior clinical profile reviewed by a clinician who can confidently judge frailty status based primarily on function and, to a lesser extent, cognition. This measure is very attractive in settings where rapid decisions need to be made, informed by frailty severity. While not explicit in the scale, the user of this scale may well include multidimensional and dynamic aspects in forming their judgment about frailty.

(e) Self-report measures. While there are many examples, three measures to be highlighted here are the PRISMA 7 [77], the Tilburg Frailty Indicator [78], and FRAIL [79]. These questionnaire-based measures are attractive in an office setting where patients can complete it before clinical assessment. The emphasis here is on self-rated function, and the content is less multidimensional.

(f) Performance-based measures such as gait speed [80] and grip strength are useful in early case finding and possibly to track frailty in the short or long term. Measures such as these need to be tested for sensitivity to change to determine their usefulness as outcome measures.

(g) Multidimensional measures. The Edmonton Frail Scale (EFS) and Frailty index based on Comprehensive Geriatric Assessment (FI-CGA) break down the frailty severity into dimensions that are clinically meaningful: geriatric syndromes. The EFS is designed to be used by nonspecialists to motivate further targeted geriatric assessment, while the FI-CGA is designed to translate findings of geriatric assessment into a multidimensional frailty measure. Neither are designed to detect the dynamic aspects of frailty, though the recognition of geriatric syndromes does meaningfully inform the possibility of atypical disease presentations.

10. *Implementation of frailty measures.* The importance of context cannot be overstated when considering how frailty models are adopted and measures implemented. Frailty research must now demonstrate relationships between measures and test how care models influence the lived experience of the citizen through improved policy, practices, and products.

Another crucial step is to reframe frailty from the perspective of the individual. Implementation of frailty measures will be challenging while the issue of labelling prevails among citizens and care providers. With other health conditions that once had a stigma such as cancer, dementia, and depression, a respectful dialogue has become possible, and false or unfair perceptions have been addressed. Using the initial example, a respectful discussion about jaundice, cirrhosis, and Child-Pugh score is commonplace for experts, non-expert providers, citizens, and policy-makers.

A similar engagement is possible with frailty. This will require an expansion in research that examines and compares test characteristics, anticipating the full spectrum of uses and settings. There will be a need for research that tests whether the addition of frailty measures improves care practice and outcomes. We will require mixed methods and qualitative research that seeks to better understand the priorities of citizens, patients, frontline teams, and larger organizations. Safeguards and policy will need to be framed to ensure that frailty measures are used appropriately and in a mutually beneficial way.

If these goals are to be achieved, the narrative must move past the dichotomous view that requires researchers and clinicians to adopt only one model, toward an integrated view that better represents the complex whole with greater authenticity. The family of frailty measures can and should be better integrated as well with an expectation of a suite of improved measures, designed to work harmoniously together. If we hope to shift from knowledge transfer to real implementation, multidimensional and dynamic measures of frailty will need to find their place in that family.

References

 1. Hogan DB, MacKnight C, Bergman H. Models, definitions, and criteria of frailty. Aging Clin Exp Res. 2003;15(3 Suppl):1–29.
 2. Fried LP, Ferrucci L, Darer J, Williamson JD, Anderson G. Untangling the concepts of disability, frailty, and comorbidity: implications for improved targeting and care. J Gerontol A Biol Sci Med Sci. 2004;59(3):255–63.
 3. Rockwood K, Hogan DB, MacKnight C. Conceptualisation and measurement of frailty in elderly people. Drugs Aging. 2000;17(4):295–302.
 4. Fried LP, Tangen CM, Walston J, Newman AB, Hirsch C, Gottdiener J, et al. Frailty in older adults: evidence for a phenotype. J Gerontol A Biol Sci Med Sci. 2001;56(3):M146–56.
 5. Mitnitski AB, Mogilner AJ, MacKnight C, Rockwood K. The mortality rate as a function of accumulated deficits in a frailty index. Mech Ageing Dev. 2002;123(11):1457–60.
 6. Kulminski AM, Ukraintseva SV, Kulminskaya IV, Arbeev KG, Land K, Yashin AI. Cumulative deficits better characterize susceptibility to death in elderly people than phenotypic frailty: lessons from the Cardiovascular Health Study. J Am Geriatr Soc. 2008;56(5):898–903.
 7. Rodríguez-Mañas L, Féart C, Mann G, Viña J, Chatterji S, Chodzko-Zajko W, et al. Searching for an operational definition of frailty: a Delphi method based consensus statement. The frailty operative definition-consensus conference project. J Gerontol A Biol Sci Med Sci. 2013;68(1):62–7.
 8. Buta B, Leder D, Miller R, Schoenborn NL, Green AR, Varadhan R. The use of figurative language to describe frailty in older adults. J Frailty Aging. 2018;7(2):127–33.
 9. Warmoth K, Lang IA, Phoenix C, Abraham C, Andrew MK, Hubbard RE, et al. 'Thinking you're old and frail': a qualitative study of frailty in older adults. Ageing Soc. 2016;36(7):1483–500.
10. Collard RM, Boter H, Schoevers RA, Oude Voshaar RC. Prevalence of frailty in community-dwelling older persons: a systematic review. J Am Geriatr Soc. 2012;60(8):1487–92.
11. Soong J, Poots A, Scott S, Donald K, Woodcock T, Lovett D, et al. Quantifying the prevalence of frailty in English hospitals. BMJ Open. 2015;5(1):e008456.
12. Joosten E, Demuynck M, Detroyer E, Milisen K. Prevalence of frailty and its ability to predict in hospital delirium, falls, and 6-month mortality in hospitalized older patients. BMC Geriatr. 2014;14(1):1.
13. Rockwood K, Howlett SE, MacKnight C, Beattie BL, Bergman H, Hebert R, et al. Prevalence, attributes, and outcomes of fitness and frailty in community-dwelling older adults: report from the Canadian study of health and aging. J Gerontol A Biol Sci Med Sci. 2004;59(12):1310–7.
14. Kim DH, Kim CA, Placide S, Lipsitz LA, Marcantonio ER. Preoperative frailty assessment and outcomes at 6 months or later in older adults undergoing cardiac surgical procedures: a systematic review. Ann Intern Med. 2016;165(9):650–60.

15. Carpenter CR, Shelton E, Fowler S, Suffoletto B, Platts-Mills TF, Rothman RE, et al. Risk factors and screening instruments to predict adverse outcomes for undifferentiated older emergency department patients: a systematic review and meta-analysis. Acad Emerg Med. 2015;22(1):1–21.
16. Clegg A, Young J, Iliffe S, Rikkert MO, Rockwood K. Frailty in elderly people. Lancet (London, England). 2013;381(9868):752–62.
17. Cesari M, Prince M, Thiyagarajan JA, De Carvalho IA, Bernabei R, Chan P, et al. Frailty: an emerging public health priority. J Am Med Dir Assoc. 2016;17(3):188–92.
18. Gill TM, Gahbauer EA, Han L, Allore HG. Trajectories of disability in the last year of life. N Engl J Med. 2010;362(13):1173–80.
19. Pugh RN, Murray-Lyon IM, Dawson JL, Pietroni MC, Williams R. Transection of the oesophagus for bleeding oesophageal varices. Br J Surg. 1973;60(8):646–9.
20. Theou O, Cann L, Blodgett J, Wallace LM, Brothers TD, Rockwood K. Modifications to the frailty phenotype criteria: systematic review of the current literature and investigation of 262 frailty phenotypes in the Survey of Health, Ageing, and Retirement in Europe. Ageing Res Rev. 2015;21:78–94.
21. Lang PO, Michel JP, Zekry D. Frailty syndrome: a transitional state in a dynamic process. Gerontology. 2009;55(5):539–49.
22. Xue QL. The frailty syndrome: definition and natural history. Clin Geriatr Med. 2011;27(1):1–15.
23. Howlett SE, Rockwood MR, Mitnitski A, Rockwood K. Standard laboratory tests to identify older adults at increased risk of death. BMC Med. 2014;12:171.
24. Soong J, Poots AJ, Scott S, Donald K, Bell D. Developing and validating a risk prediction model for acute care based on frailty syndromes. BMJ Open. 2015;5(1):e008457.
25. Ahmed N, Mandel R, Fain MJ. Frailty: an emerging geriatric syndrome. Am J Med. 2007;120(9):748–53.
26. Alexa ID, Ilie AC, Morosanu A, Voica A. Approaching frailty as the new geriatric syndrome. Rev Med Chir Soc Med Nat Iasi. 2013;117(3):680–5.
27. Chen LK, Hwang AC, Liu LK, Lee WJ, Peng LN. Frailty is a geriatric syndrome characterized by multiple impairments: a comprehensive approach is needed. J Frailty Aging. 2016;5(4):208–13.
28. Kaufman SR. The social construction of frailty: an anthropological perspective. J Aging Stud. 1994;8(1):45–58.
29. Fried LP. Conference on the physiologic basis of frailty. April 28, 1992, Baltimore, Maryland, U.S.A. Introduction. Aging (Milano). 1992;4(3):251–2.
30. Keevil VL, Romero-Ortuno R. Ageing well: a review of sarcopenia and frailty. Proc Nutr Soc. 2015;74(4):337–47.
31. Fried LP, Hadley EC, Walston JD, Newman AB, Guralnik JM, Studenski S, et al. From bedside to bench: research agenda for frailty. Sci Aging Knowledge Environ. 2005;2005(31):pe24.
32. Vina J, Tarazona-Santabalbina FJ, Perez-Ros P, Martinez-Arnau FM, Borras C, Olaso-Gonzalez G, et al. Biology of frailty: modulation of ageing genes and its importance to prevent age-associated loss of function. Mol Asp Med. 2016;50:88–108.
33. Bouillon K, Kivimaki M, Hamer M, Sabia S, Fransson EI, Singh-Manoux A, et al. Measures of frailty in population-based studies: an overview. BMC Geriatr. 2013;13(1):64.
34. Lahousse L, Maes B, Ziere G, Loth DW, Verlinden VJ, Zillikens MC, et al. Adverse outcomes of frailty in the elderly: the Rotterdam Study. Eur J Epidemiol. 2014;29(6):419–27.
35. Shamliyan T, Talley KM, Ramakrishnan R, Kane RL. Association of frailty with survival: a systematic literature review. Ageing Res Rev. 2013;12(2):719–36.
36. Kiely DK, Cupples LA, Lipsitz LA. Validation and comparison of two frailty indexes: the MOBILIZE Boston Study. J Am Geriatr Soc. 2009;57(9):1532–9.
37. Jones DM, Song X, Rockwood K. Operationalizing a frailty index from a standardized comprehensive geriatric assessment. J Am Geriatr Soc. 2004;52(11):1929–33.

38. Rockwood K, Mitnitski A. Frailty in relation to the accumulation of deficits. J Gerontol A Biol Sci Med Sci. 2007;62(7):722–7.
39. Searle SD, Mitnitski A, Gahbauer EA, Gill TM, Rockwood K. A standard procedure for creating a frailty index. BMC Geriatr. 2008;8:24.
40. Drubbel I, de Wit NJ, Bleijenberg N, Eijkemans RJ, Schuurmans MJ, Numans ME. Prediction of adverse health outcomes in older people using a frailty index based on routine primary care data. J Gerontol A Biol Sci Med Sci. 2013;68(3):301–8.
41. Hoover M, Rotermann M, Sanmartin C, Bernier J. Validation of an index to estimate the prevalence of frailty among community-dwelling seniors. Health Rep. 2013;24(9):10–7.
42. Jones D, Song X, Mitnitski A, Rockwood K. Evaluation of a frailty index based on a comprehensive geriatric assessment in a population based study of elderly Canadians. Aging Clin Exp Res. 2005;17(6):465–71.
43. Clegg A, Bates C, Young J, Ryan R, Nichols L, Ann Teale E, et al. Development and validation of an electronic frailty index using routine primary care electronic health record data. Age Ageing. 2016;45(3):353–60.
44. Hominick K, McLeod V, Rockwood K. Characteristics of older adults admitted to hospital versus those discharged home, in emergency department patients referred to internal medicine. Can Geriatr J. 2016;19(1):9–14.
45. Theou O, Park GH, Garm A, Song X, Clarke B, Rockwood K. Reversing frailty levels in primary care using the CARES model. Can Geriatr J. 2017;20(3):105–11.
46. Vetrano DL, Palmer K, Marengoni A, Marzetti E, Lattanzio F, Roller-Wirnsberger R, et al. Frailty and multimorbidity: a systematic review and meta-analysis. J Gerontol Biol Sci Med Sci. 2019;74(5):659–66.
47. St John PD, Montgomery PR, Tyas SL. Social position and frailty. Can J Aging. 2013;32(3):250–9.
48. Woo J, Goggins W, Sham A, Ho SC. Social determinants of frailty. Gerontology. 2005;51(6):402–8.
49. Theou O, Brothers TD, Rockwood MR, Haardt D, Mitnitski A, Rockwood K. Exploring the relationship between national economic indicators and relative fitness and frailty in middle-aged and older Europeans. Age Ageing. 2013;42(5):614–9.
50. Peek MK, Howrey BT, Ternent RS, Ray LA, Ottenbacher KJ. Social support, stressors, and frailty among older Mexican American adults. J Gerontol B Psychol Sci Soc Sci. 2012;67(6):755–64.
51. Andrew MK, Keefe JM. Social vulnerability from a social ecology perspective: a cohort study of older adults from the National Population Health Survey of Canada. BMC Geriatr. 2014;14:90.
52. Rolfson D. Successful aging and frailty: a systematic review. Geriatrics (Basel). 2018;3(4):79.
53. Beard JR, Officer A, de Carvalho IA, Sadana R, Pot AM, Michel JP, et al. The World report on ageing and health: a policy framework for healthy ageing. Lancet. 2016;387(10033):2145–54.
54. Cesari M, Araujo de Carvalho I, Amuthavalli Thiyagarajan J, Cooper C, Martin FC, Reginster JY, et al. Evidence for the domains supporting the construct of intrinsic capacity. J Gerontol A Biol Sci Med Sci. 2018;73(12):1653.
55. Campbell AJ, Buchner DM. Unstable disability and the fluctuations of frailty. Age Ageing. 1997;26(4):315–8.
56. Theou O, Brothers TD, Mitnitski A, Rockwood K. Operationalization of frailty using eight commonly used scales and comparison of their ability to predict all-cause mortality. J Am Geriatr Soc. 2013;61(9):1537–51.
57. Rockwood K, Song X, MacKnight C, Bergman H, Hogan DB, McDowell I, et al. A global clinical measure of fitness and frailty in elderly people. CMAJ = journal de l'Association medicale canadienne. 2005;173(5):489–95.
58. Wallis SJ, Wall J, Biram RW, Romero-Ortuno R. Association of the clinical frailty scale with hospital outcomes. QJM. 2015;108(12):943–9.

59. Afilalo J, Eisenberg MJ, Morin JF, Bergman H, Monette J, Noiseux N, et al. Gait speed as an incremental predictor of mortality and major morbidity in elderly patients undergoing cardiac surgery. J Am Coll Cardiol. 2010;56(20):1668–76.
60. Studenski S, Perera S, Patel K, Rosano C, Faulkner K, Inzitari M, et al. Gait speed and survival in older adults. JAMA. 2011;305(1):50–8.
61. Sepehri A, Beggs T, Hassan A, Rigatto C, Shaw-Daigle C, Tangri N, et al. The impact of frailty on outcomes after cardiac surgery: a systematic review. J Thorac Cardiovasc Surg. 2014;148(6):3110–7.
62. Handforth C, Clegg A, Young C, Simpkins S, Seymour MT, Selby PJ, et al. The prevalence and outcomes of frailty in older cancer patients: a systematic review. Ann Oncol. 2015;26(6):1091–101.
63. Jha SR, Ha HS, Hickman LD, Hannu M, Davidson PM, Macdonald PS, et al. Frailty in advanced heart failure: a systematic review. Heart Fail Rev. 2015;20(5):553–60.
64. Muscedere J, Waters B, Varambally A, Bagshaw SM, Boyd JG, Maslove D, et al. The impact of frailty on intensive care unit outcomes: a systematic review and meta-analysis. Intensive Care Med. 2017;43(8):1105–22.
65. Inouye SK, Charpentier PA. Precipitating factors for delirium in hospitalized elderly persons. Predictive model and interrelationship with baseline vulnerability. JAMA. 1996;275(11):852–7.
66. Inouye SK. Delirium in older persons. N Engl J Med. 2006;354(11):1157–65.
67. Jarrett PG, Rockwood K, Carver D, Stolee P, Cosway S. Illness presentation in elderly patients. Arch Intern Med. 1995;155(10):1060–4.
68. Piechocinska B. Physics from wholeness: dynamical totality as a conceptual foundation for physical theories: Acta Universitatis Upsaliensis; 2005.
69. Kuchel GA. Frailty and resilience as outcome measures in clinical trials and geriatric care: are we getting any closer? J Am Geriatr Soc. 2018;66(8):1451–4.
70. Clegg A, Rogers L, Young J. Diagnostic test accuracy of simple instruments for identifying frailty in community-dwelling older people: a systematic review. Age Ageing. 2015;44(1):148–52.
71. de Vries NM, Staal JB, van Ravensberg CD, Hobbelen JS, Olde Rikkert MG, Nijhuis-van der Sanden MW. Outcome instruments to measure frailty: a systematic review. Ageing Res Rev. 2011;10(1):104–14.
72. Sternberg SA, Wershof Schwartz A, Karunananthan S, Bergman H, Mark Clarfield A. The identification of frailty: a systematic literature review. J Am Geriatr Soc. 2011;59(11):2129–38.
73. Hogan DB, Maxwell CJ, Afilalo J, Arora RC, Bagshaw SM, Basran J, et al. A scoping review of frailty and acute care in middle-aged and older individuals with recommendations for future research. Can Geriatr J. 2017;20(1):22–37.
74. Abbasi M, Rolfson D, Khera AS, Dabravolskaj J, Dent E, Xia L. Identification and management of frailty in the primary care setting. CMAJ = journal de l'Association medicale canadienne. 2018;190(38):E1134–e40.
75. Rolfson DB, Heckman GA, Bagshaw SM, Robertson D, Hirdes JP. Implementing frailty measures in the Canadian healthcare system. J Frailty Aging. 2018;7(4):208–16.
76. Cawthon PM, Marshall LM, Michael Y, Dam TT, Ensrud KE, Barrett-Connor E, et al. Frailty in older men: prevalence, progression, and relationship with mortality. J Am Geriatr Soc. 2007;55(8):1216–23.
77. Raîche M, Hébert R, Dubois MF, and the PRISMA partners. User guide for the PRISMA-7 questionnaire to identify elderly people with severe loss of autonomy. In: Integrated service delivery to ensure persons' functional autonomy. Quebec: Edisem. p. 147–65.
78. Gobbens RJ, van Assen MA, Luijkx KG, Wijnen-Sponselee MT, Schols JM. The Tilburg Frailty Indicator: psychometric properties. J Am Med Dir Assoc. 2010;11(5):344–55.
79. Morley JE, Malmstrom TK, Miller DK. A simple frailty questionnaire (FRAIL) predicts outcomes in middle aged African Americans. J Nutr Health Aging. 2012;16(7):601–8.
80. Cesari M. Role of gait speed in the assessment of older patients. JAMA. 2011;305(1):93–4.

Chapter 17
Hepatic Encephalopathy, Sarcopenia, and Frailty

Chantal Bémeur and Christopher F. Rose

Introduction

Hepatic encephalopathy (HE), a complex neuropsychiatric syndrome, and sarcopenia (muscle mass loss) are serious complications observed in as many as 80% of patients with end-stage liver disease (i.e., cirrhosis). The impact of these complications is significant as they affect survival and quality of life and lead to poor outcome following liver transplantation. Chronic liver disease leads to hyperammonemia, which is a major factor in the development of HE. Recent data suggest ammonia acts as a metabolic stressor and impairs other organs (in addition to the brain) including muscle. During the setting of chronic liver disease, the muscle plays a vital compensatory role in detoxifying ammonia as it contains an ammonia-removing enzyme, namely, glutamine synthetase. Accordingly, sarcopenia, which is part of the frailty syndrome, may be an important driver of HE development. The goal of this chapter is to provide an updated description of the interplay between HE, sarcopenia, and physical and cognitive frailty. Firstly, HE will be presented in terms of definition, pathogenesis, and therapeutics. Secondly, sarcopenia and frailty will be tackled with regard to definitions and relevance for cirrhosis and HE. Then, evidence-based recommendations for sarcopenia and frailty in the context of HE will be elaborated. Suggestions to inform future research will conclude the chapter.

C. Bémeur
Département de nutrition, Université de Montréal, and Hepato-Neuro Lab, CRCHUM,
Montreal, QC, Canada
e-mail: chantal.bemeur@umontreal.ca

C. F. Rose (✉)
Département de médecine, Université de Montréal, and Hepato-Neuro Lab, CRCHUM,
Montreal, QC, Canada
e-mail: christopher.rose@umontreal.ca

© Springer Nature Switzerland AG 2020
P. Tandon, A. J. Montano-Loza (eds.), *Frailty and Sarcopenia in Cirrhosis*,
https://doi.org/10.1007/978-3-030-26226-6_17

Hepatic Encephalopathy

HE is a common and debilitating neuropsychiatric complication of liver disease. Characterized by a constellation of symptoms, including cognitive, psychiatric, and motor disturbances, HE can progress to coma and death. HE is classified into two primary forms: overt HE (OHE) and covert HE (CHE). OHE encompasses several clinical signs such as gross disorientation, asterixis, stupor, lethargy, and coma, whereas CHE, in the absence of overt HE, is diagnosed using sensitive neuropsychological and neurophysiological tests [1, 2]. CHE is characterized by decreased concentration, poor memory, reduced speed of information processing, impaired motor abilities, and disturbance in sleep-wake rhythms. Assessment tools for HE are described in Table 17.1. These subclinical abnormalities have a significant impact on patients' health-related quality of life and on their ability to function daily and lead to an increased risk of having a car accident [3]. As many as 80% of patients with chronic liver disease suffer from CHE, and this highly underdiagnosed phenomenon leads to a fourfold increased risk of developing severe HE or OHE [4, 5].

Table 17.1 Assessment tools for HE (Weissenborn et al. 2019)

Tool	Components
Psychometric Hepatic Encephalopathy Score (PHES) 　Number Connection Test (NCT) 　A and B 　Digit symbol test 　Serial dotting test 　Line drawing test	Five paper-pencil tests evaluating cognitive/psychomotor processing speed and visuomotor coordination 　Psychometric measures for the assessment of early HE 　Assesses visuoconstructive abilities 　Assesses visuomotor coordination and speed 　Assesses speed and accuracy
Animal Naming Test (ANT)	Number of animals listed in 60 s
Continuous Reaction Time (CRT)	Relies on repeated registration of the motor reaction time to auditory stimuli
Inhibitory control test	Computerized test of response inhibition and working memory
Stroop test	Evaluates psychomotor speed and cognitive flexibility by the interference between recognition reaction time to a colored field and a written color name
Montreal Cognitive Assessment (MoCA)	Paper-pencil test measuring mild cognitive impairment
Scan test	Computerized test that measures speed and accuracy to perform a digit recognition memory task of increasing complexity
Electroencephalogram (EEG)	Can detect changes in cortical cerebral activity across the spectrum of HE
Critical flicker frequency	Frequency at which a flickering light appears to be flickering to the observer
Repeatable Battery for the Assessment of Neuropsychological Status	Assesses cognition across specific domains including immediate memory, visuospatial/constructional, language, attention, and delayed memory

The prevalence of OHE among patients with chronic liver disease is 30–45%, with a 20% annual risk of developing further episodes of OHE [6]. Furthermore, evidence has demonstrated that repeated bouts of OHE can lead to untreatable CHE, possibly as a result of progressive structural brain damage [7]. Overall, the burden of HE is immense considering its wide-ranging effects on the patients, their families, and society. The economic drain on the healthcare system caused by HE is estimated at as much as 50,000 US dollars per patient annually [8], and, with the increasing prevalence of nonalcoholic steatohepatitis (NASH)-related cirrhosis, it is expected to worsen in the coming years [9].

Pathogenesis

The neuropathology of HE in chronic liver disease reveals primarily morphological changes in astrocytes, including Alzheimer type II astrocytosis [10] and cytotoxic cell swelling, which, consequently, lead to brain edema [11]. This common feature is observed in cirrhotic patients suffering from HE [12], an observation that was also confirmed in cirrhotic rats with minimal HE [13]. However, the pathophysiological consequences of brain edema (astrocyte swelling) in HE remain elusive. The pathological basis of HE is multifactorial, and ammonia is believed to play a pivotal role [14, 15]. Furthermore, since astrocytes are the only cells in the brain capable of clearing ammonia via the enzyme glutamine synthetase, it has been postulated that the accumulation of glutamine in astrocytes subsequent to ammonia detoxification results in increased osmotic forces and swelling. There is ample evidence suggesting that lactate may also be implicated in the pathogenesis of HE [16]. Other factors implicated in the pathophysiology of HE include inflammation and oxidative stress. In fact, hyperammonemia and systemic oxidative stress act synergistically to induce cognitive impairment in HE [13].

Treatments

Currently, treatment for HE is based on strategies aimed at reducing the concentration of circulating blood ammonia, by lowering its production, increasing its removal, or combining the two strategies. One obvious approach is to target the source of ammonia production, with the gut being a primary candidate. Reducing ammonia production in the gut will minimize its absorption into the systemic circulation and hence the brain from high ammonia exposure. However, because interorgan ammonia metabolism is altered during the onset of liver disease [17], additional organs, such as skeletal muscle, become important players in the metabolism of ammonia. Skeletal muscle, which contains the ammonia-removing enzyme glutamine synthetase, makes up approximately 40% of total body mass. Therefore, increasing the capacity of skeletal muscle to remove ammonia is a potential approach for the treatment of HE. The following paragraphs depict different therapeutic approaches for the treatment of HE.

Nonabsorbable disaccharides Nonabsorbable disaccharides, particularly lactulose, have been first-line therapy for patients with chronic liver disease and HE for past decades [18]. Lactulose acts as both osmotic laxative, prebiotic, and gut-acidifying agent. Lactulose is a synthetic disaccharide composed of the monosaccharides fructose and galactose. It remains undigested until it reaches the colon, where it is metabolized by colonic bacteria into acetic acid and lactic acid. These carboxylic acids reduce the intraluminal pH, and the resulting acidification of the colon suppresses the growth of the intestinal urease bacteria (ammoniagenic bacteria), leaving the acid-resistant, nonammoniagenic bacteria. Lactulose also decreases the absorption of ammonia through a cathartic effect, clearing the gut of ammonia before it is systemically absorbed, resulting in increased fecal nitrogen excretion. Lactulose has also been shown to impede the uptake of glutamine by the intestinal wall, thus preventing glutamine from being metabolized into ammonia [19]. Although lactulose is safe and beneficial in the treatment of HE, compliance is often underachieved, given the need to titrate the dose in order to reach two or three semi-soft stools per day. In addition, lactulose treatment has been shown to cause abdominal cramping, bloating, nausea, vomiting, flatulence, and abdominal distension. Furthermore, lactulose treatment affects intestinal absorption, and this may amplify the nutritional deficits in patients with chronic liver disease, leading to a poorer outcome after liver transplantation [20].

Antibiotics Orally administered antimicrobial agents targeting the gut have long been utilized with the primary aim of inhibiting urease-containing bacteria in the colon, thereby decreasing ammonia production and preventing absorption through the gastrointestinal tract. Antibiotics such as neomycin, metronidazole, and vancomycin have all been demonstrated to lower blood ammonia in patients with chronic liver disease [21]. Nonetheless, because of the systemic absorption of these antimicrobial agents, serious adverse effects have been reported, which have limited their widespread use. Rifaximin is an antibiotic, with a broad spectrum of antibacterial activity, that has proven to be efficient in lowering blood ammonia levels in patients with HE by reducing the growth of ammonia-producing bacteria [22]. Rifaximin treatment has resulted in fewer adverse effects and a faster and greater decrease in blood ammonia in comparison with neomycin [23]. Rifaximin was the first ever therapy that was approved by the FDA for the treatment of HE. The conclusive study demonstrated rifaximin reduces the recurrence of HE [24]. In addition, an exploratory data analysis of a phase II/III clinical trials concluded that rifaximin may improve liver and neuropsychological functions through the regulation of the gut microbial consortia in patients with HE [25].

Probiotics Probiotic therapy involves monocultures or mixed cultures of live microorganisms, administered orally to improve the properties of the intestinal microflora. Studies have shown that probiotics are beneficial in the treatment of HE, possibly by modulating intestinal bacteria via the colonization of non-urease bacteria and by lowering blood ammonia concentrations [26]. Moreover, probiotic supplementation in patients with HE has been shown to be very well tolerated, and the compliance rates were excellent [27]. Compared with placebo or no intervention, probiotics improve recovery and may lead to improvements in the development of OHE, quality of life, and plasma ammonia concentrations, but little effect on mortality has been shown [28]. Furthermore, evidence regarding probiotics and HE is considered to be of low quality [28]. Therefore, further studies evaluating the potential role of probiotics in HE are needed.

Benzoate and phenylacetate/phenylbutyrate Sodium benzoate and sodium phenylacetate/phenylbutyrate (prodrug of phenylacetate) are metabolically coupled to glycine and glutamine and thus increase the excretion of these two ammoniagenic amino acids [29]. Specifically, sodium benzoate conjugates with the amino acid glycine to form hippuric acid, which is excreted by the kidneys. Glycine is metabolized through the glycine cleavage system, an enzyme complex that consists of four proteins and generates ammonia as an end product. Sodium benzoate is administered to prevent glycine metabolism and thereby prevent the production of ammonia. In the context of chronic liver disease, sodium benzoate reduces blood ammonia levels and attenuates the symptoms of HE as effectively as lactulose [30]. Sodium phenylbutyrate could be effective in reducing ammonia levels and might be effective in improving neurological status and intensive care unit discharge survival [31]. However, the sodium load associated with these treatments, which could lead to fluid retention and exacerbates ascites, has limited its use in patients with chronic liver disease. Glycerol phenylbutyrate improves the organoleptic properties of sodium phenylbutyrate and is not associated with sodium load. A multicenter, randomized, double-blind, placebo-controlled phase II trial revealed that glycerol phenylacetate decreased the likelihood of hospitalization of cirrhotic patients with recurrent HE when compared with placebo, by lowering ammonia levels [32]. Overall, glycerol phenylbutyrate was considered to be safe among cirrhotic patients with recurrent HE; however, larger randomized trials are needed to further establish the role of glycerol phenylbutyrate in patients with HE.

L-ornithine-L-aspartate (LOLA) LOLA is a mixture of two endogenous amino acids with the capacity to fix ammonia in the form of urea and/or glutamine. Its efficacy for the treatment of HE is a subject of debate. A systematic review and meta-analysis of randomized controlled trials revealed that LOLA appears to improve mental state and lower ammonia in patients with HE or minimal HE [33]. Furthermore, results of randomized controlled trials and meta-analyses provide support for the use of LOLA in the treatment of HE. Nevertheless, future trials should focus on the use of LOLA for prophylaxis [34].

Ornithine phenylacetate (OP) The hypothesis behind the combination of ornithine and phenylacetate is that ornithine stimulates glutamine synthetase, generating glutamine and removing ammonia. Preventing glutamine from being metabolized by glutaminase and thereby regenerating ammonia, glutamine combines with phenyl-acetate to form phenylacetylglutamine which is eliminated in the urine [35]. A phase IIa study including 47 patients with acute liver injury or failure found OP to be safe and well tolerated [36]. Presently, there is no clinical evidence of a significant HE-ameliorating effect despite the fact that OP may have a potential for dose-dependent ammonia lowering [37, 38].

Branched-chain amino acids Cirrhotic patients have an increased whole-body clearance of branched-chain amino acids (BCAA) compared to healthy subjects [39]. This may reflect an increased metabolic demand of BCAA in skeletal muscle where the BCAA are primarily metabolized [40]. This is in contrast to the majority of amino acids, which are metabolized mainly in the liver. BCAA enhance ammonia detoxification in skeletal muscle and thereby reduce plasma ammonia concentration. This leads to the assumption that external replenishment of BCAA further enhances the detoxification of ammonia in muscle. Treatment with BCAA has been shown to lower blood ammonia and improve the mental status of patients with cirrhosis [41]. Moreover, a Cochrane meta-analysis showed that BCAA had beneficial effects on HE and there is evidence to support clinical benefits of BCAA [42].

L-Acetylcarnitine L-Acetylcarnitine, a metabolite produced by the degradation of the essential amino acid lysine, serves as a carrier for short-chain fatty acids across the mitochondrial membrane. Treatment with L-acetylcarnitine (the acetylated form of L-carnitine, known to increase its bioavailability) significantly reduced serum ammonia levels and improved mental status as compared with placebo in cirrhotic patients with HE [43]. However, a Cochrane systematic review analyzed a heterogeneous group of five trials at high risk of bias and with a high risk of random errors conducted by only one research team [44]. The authors rated all evidence as of very low quality due to pitfalls and execution, inconsistency, and small sample sizes. The harms profile of L-acetylcarnitine is presently unclear. Accordingly, further randomized clinical trials to assess L-acetylcarnitine versus placebo are needed.

Acarbose Acarbose, an approved treatment for diabetes, is an inhibitor of α-glucosidase that prevents the conversion of carbohydrates into monosaccharides. Furthermore, it has been demonstrated that acarbose can decrease colonic proteolytic flora and dietary nitrogenous substances. In a double-blind, crossover, randomized study, 107 cirrhotic patients with OHE and type 2 diabetes received acarbose treatment and demonstrated a significant reduction in serum ammonia levels and attenuation of HE [45]. Acarbose is well tolerated and is not associated with serious adverse effects. Additional studies are required to further evaluate the role and mechanism of action of acarbose in the treatment of HE.

Liposome-supported peritoneal dialysis (LSPD) LSPD is a detoxification strategy for the removal of small ionizable molecules like ammonia. It was shown that LSPD outperformed conventional peritoneal dialysis in lowering plasmatic ammonia levels and attenuating brain edema in a rat model of cirrhosis [46]. In addition, LSPD does not trigger any hypersensitive reaction in pigs, a side effect commonly observed upon the injection of colloids in this animal model and in humans. These findings support the development of LSPD for the treatment of hyperammonemia-induced encephalopathy. Further studies are needed.

Engineered bacteria Genetically modified *E. coli* Nissle have been programmed to metabolize ammonia. Orally administered, these engineered bacteria have demonstrated to lower blood ammonia in animals with severe liver injury (thioacetamide-induced) as well as in animals ornithine transcarbamylase-deficient (model of urea cycle disorder) [47]. This interesting ammonia-lowering strategy is heading into a phase II clinical trial.

Fecal microbiota transplant Patients with cirrhosis tend to have a reduced abundance of several potentially beneficial bacterial families and an increased abundance of pathogenic ones [48, 49]. An open-labeled, randomized pilot trial on patients with recurrent HE compared the safety of fecal microbiota transplant (from one donor matched to the dysbiosis in HE) versus no such intervention [50]. As a secondary trial outcome, fecal microbiota transplant was associated with fewer liver-related hospitalizations and improved cognitive function.

Liver transplantation Presently, the ultimate management solution for controlling HE is to replace the diseased liver. Indeed, liver transplantation is the only curative treatment to date that has demonstrated to significantly prolong the lives of patients with chronic liver disease. The number of liver transplantations performed annually in the USA has steadily risen from approximately 1700–6300 over 20 years (from 1988 to 2008) (OPTN.hrsa). Although partially due to an increase in the number of organs available from living and cadaveric donors (owing to efficient distribution and excellent liver transplant programs), an increased liver transplantation rate also reflects a rise in the number of patients with end-stage liver disease that are in need of a new liver. Given its success rate of close to 90% [51], liver transplantation is no longer considered an experimental high-risk procedure, and thus the focus on patient survival has now shifted toward quality of outcome, including neurological status. However, evidence suggest that, even following the implantation of a new liver, persisting neurological complications remain a common problem affecting as many as 47% of liver transplant recipients [52–54]. The mechanisms of action responsible for these neurological complications posttransplantation remain undefined. Nutritional status at the time of liver transplant may be involved [55].

Sarcopenia and Its Relation to HE

Sarcopenia, now formally recognized as a muscle disease of the elderly, has been recently defined operationally based on three criteria: (1) low muscle strength, (2) low muscle quantity or quality, and (3) low physical performance [56]. Sarcopenia has a significant impact on the development of HE, affecting the majority of patients with cirrhosis [57]. Indeed, muscle, due to the fact that it contains the ammonia-removing enzyme glutamine synthetase, compensates for ammonia detoxification in chronic liver disease; therefore sarcopenia hastens the development of HE [58, 59]. As such, cirrhotic patients with reduced muscle mass have higher ammonia levels and risk for HE [60]. Accordingly, a systematic review and meta-analysis revealed that there is a significant association between sarcopenia and HE in cirrhotic patients [61]. Also, as mentioned, HE is caused in part by hyperammonemia, a potent driver of muscle catabolism which leads to weakness and sarcopenia [62, 63]. Hence, amelioration of sarcopenia may improve HE in cirrhotic patients [64].

Since ammonia is diffused and transported across all plasma membranes, hyperammonemia may lead to an influx of ammonia in all organ and tissues. It is known that elevated levels of ammonia are toxic to the brain and cause neurological impairment. However, the deleterious effects of ammonia are not specific to the brain, as the direct effect of increased ammonia can occur in any cell type [65]. Tissues potentially affected by hyperammonemia include, apart from the brain, the muscle, kidney, liver, lung, as well as vasculature [65]. As mentioned, during cirrhosis and HE, muscle may play a compensatory role in ammonia detoxification, emphasizing the crucial role of optimal muscle protein homeostasis. In alcohol-related cirrhosis, it has been demonstrated that direct effects of ethanol are synergistic with increased ammonia uptake in causing dysregulated skeletal muscle proteostasis and signaling perturbations with a more severe sarcopenic phenotype [66]. Several studies on ammonia-induced skeletal muscle loss lay the foundation for prolonged ammonia-lowering therapy to reverse sarcopenia of cirrhosis [63]. Ammonia-lowering therapies, including those discussed in section "Treatments", may result in improvement in skeletal muscle phenotype and function and molecular perturbations of hyperammonemia. Further studies await.

Patients with cirrhosis may develop simultaneous loss of skeletal muscle and gain of adipose tissue, culminating in the condition of sarcopenic obesity, which is seen, among other conditions, in patients with nonalcoholic steatohepatitis (NASH), type 2 diabetes, and alcoholism. Pathophysiology of sarcopenic obesity includes inflammation and/or inactivity-induced muscle catabolism in obese patients. It is important to highlight that there are no accepted diagnostic criteria for sarcopenic obesity to date. In addition, muscle depletion is characterized by both a reduction in muscle size and increased proportion of intermuscular and intramuscular fat-denominated myosteatosis. It has been shown that myosteatosis and sarcopenia are associated with HE in patients with cirrhosis [67]. Muscularity (quality and quantity of muscle mass) assessment with cross-sectional imaging studies has become an attractive index of nutritional status evaluation in cirrhosis, as sarcopenia reflects a chronic detriment in general physical condition, rather than acute severity of the liver disease [68].

An integrated multidimensional approach in order to optimize muscle mass and function is required for effective management of sarcopenia. Physical activity may be a protective factor not only in the prevention but also in the management of sarcopenia. Randomized controlled trials have shown good tolerance of exercise and improved muscle mass following supervised physical training in cirrhotic patients [69–71]. However, the optimal exercise program regarding type (aerobic vs resistance) and frequency in cirrhosis and HE is still unexamined. In addition, more investigations are needed to fully understand the beneficial mechanisms of exercise in cirrhosis and HE, including a safe and appropriate exercise regimen as well as nutritional intervention [72, 73]. Another strategy to optimize muscle mass and function and manage sarcopenia is nutrition. It is important to emphasize that exercise under insufficient nutrient and protein intake could be risky in patient with cirrhosis and HE, given that it could promote further protein catabolism and loss of muscle mass. The first step is to assess nutritional status. Nutritional strategies in order to treat sarcopenia in HE are branched-chain amino acids, nutritional supplementation, high-protein diets, as well as late-evening snacks [72, 74].

Importantly, sarcopenia is part of the frailty complex present in cirrhotic patients, resulting from cumulative declines across multiple physiologic systems.

Physical Frailty and Its Relation to HE

Physical frailty, which lacks a universal definition and a validated scoring system, is commonly known as a multidimensional syndrome of decreased reserve, functional impairment, and resistance to stressors [75]. Specifically, physical frailty is a state of vulnerability and non-resilience with limited reserve capacity in major organ systems, leading to reduced capability to withstand stress such as disease and predisposition to poor outcomes [75]. Physical frailty involves two nutrition-related components, namely, weight loss and sarcopenia [75]. Furthermore, physical frailty is a risk factor for dependence and disability [76].

As covered in other chapters, physical frailty in chronic liver disease is a multidimensional construct that is distinct from liver dysfunction and incorporates endurance, strength, and balance. Functional measures of physical frailty have been associated with lower survival in chronic liver disease [77–79]. Physical frailty is strongly and independently associated with an increased risk of unplanned hospitalization or death in outpatients with cirrhosis. A cirrhotic patient can be physically frail for many reasons, including aging, comorbidities, malnutrition, deconditioning, severe liver failure, and cognitive impairment such as HE. When present, HE likely plays a critical role in the frailty phenotype and the implications of physical frailty among patients with cirrhosis evaluated for liver transplantation [80]. In fact, HE contributes to frailty in two ways: (1) each stage of the spectrum of HE is associated with decreased physical function and (2) HE is associated with sarcopenia. Physical frailty is increasingly recognized as a critical determinant of outcomes in liver transplantation candidates [81]. Some components of the frail phenotype, such as sarcopenia, have been associated with worse outcomes after liver transplantation [82]. These observations suggest specific targets for prehabilitation interventions aimed at reducing physical frailty in chronic liver disease in preparation for liver transplantation [81].

Management approaches to physical frailty include exercise (aerobic, resistance, and prehabilitation program prior to surgery or liver transplantation), nutrition (adequate caloric intake to meet daily requirements, protein supplementation, late night snacks), pharmacological (consider testosterone supplementation in patients with low serum testosterone levels) and cognitive stimulation (cognitive training program including memory, attention, and problem-solving tasks) [83]. Specifically, in cirrhosis and HE, several therapeutic interventions have shown beneficial to improve physical function, including nutrition, BCAA, nocturnal nutrition, moderate exercise, as well as aerobic exercise [84]. Furthermore, technology should play a promising role in terms of therapeutic interventions. For example, the use of fitness trackers such as the Fitbit and smartphone applications provides an avenue to screen for conditions and monitor and individual's progress in physical function and nutritional status. The implementation of these technologies to manage patients with chronic liver disease can be challenging. Ongoing research of their efficacy in patients with cirrhosis is emerging.

In the last decade, physical frailty has consistently been linked to cognitive impairment [85, 86], introducing the concept of cognitive frailty.

Cognitive Frailty or the "Frail" Brain

Cognitive impairment and physical frailty often coexist in older adults [87]. Interestingly, a recent definition of frailty has included physical, cognitive, and psychosocial aspects, maintaining a complex relationships between them [88]. Accordingly, cognitive frailty is defined as the simultaneous presence of physical frailty and mild cognitive impairment in the absence of dementia or preexisting brain disorders [89]. Furthermore, cognitive frailty is conceptually described as a state of reduced cognitive reserve that is different from physiological brain aging and is characterized by potential reversibility. In other words, cognitive frailty is characterized by diminished brain neurophysiological reserves (brain frailty) that is related to both the appearance of neurodegenerative and vascular diseases and also to the appearance of physical frailty.

The concept of cognitive frailty or the frail brain should also be addressed in relation with HE. For example, in the context of alcohol-related liver disease, chronic alcohol use is associated with nutritional deficiencies, dementia, cirrhosis, and decompensating events such as HE. Direct toxicity of alcohol on brain tissue and induction of neuro-inflammation are possible mechanisms for the clinical features of HE associated with alcohol consumption [90, 91]. In addition, the presence of inflammation, as observed in HE and cirrhosis, may confer additional disability risk with regard to physical as well as cognitive frailty [92].

Despite significant associations demonstrated between cognitive and physical frailty, some key aspects remain unresolved including the role of cognitive reserve and the common etiopathogenesis between cognitive and physical impairments. The combination of physical frailty and brain frailty (cognitive impairment) needs to be more clearly understood. Furthermore, in the context of HE, several issues should be addressed including the link between HE and cognitive frailty, underlying pathophysiology in the brain between HE with and without frailty, as well as the interplay between HE, cognitive decline, and aging. Another question that remains to be answered is how to integrate HE, physical frailty, cognitive frailty, and sarcopenia.

Recommendations and Future Research

Sarcopenia and frailty (physical and cognitive) are growing areas of research that are emerging in hepatology. With the aging population, the prevalence of sarcopenia and frailty is likely to rise in both the general population and patients with cirrhosis and HE, suggesting an interplay between chronic liver disease, HE, malnutrition, sarcopenia, and frailty (Fig. 17.1). The international hepatology community therefore needs to establish a consensus on a measurement tool to be used in the liver disease population. Specifically, a consensus for diagnostic criteria for sarcopenia, including sarcopenic obesity, and frailty (physical and cognitive) is urgently needed in cirrhotic patient with HE. In fact, sarcopenia, frailty, and nutritional status should be incorporated into routine assessments of patients with cirrhosis. Also, combining tests and scales may be used to predict outcomes. Recently, a composite score was developed combining the *Montreal Cognitive Assessment* (MoCA) and the *Clinical Frailty Scale* (CFS) to predict HE admissions [93]. CFS is a practical ≤1 min nine-category global frailty scale ranging from "very fit" to "severely frail" that has demonstrated excellent prognostic utility [94, 95]. Keeping with the definition of HE as a brain dysfunction caused by liver insufficiency, screening for cognitive impairment is likely to be a fundamental part of any baseline assessment. MoCA is recognized as a more sensitive measure of mild cognitive impairment than the Mini-Mental State Examination (MMSE) [96, 97] and is an easy to administer paper-pencil test with standardized norms. The MoCa-CFS was revealed as an independent predictor of HE admission and predicted impaired health-related quality of life and all-cause

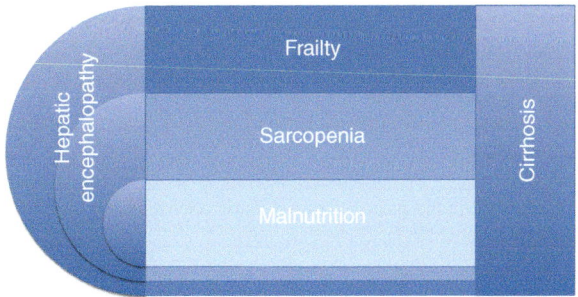

Fig. 17.1 Interplay between hepatic encephalopathy and complications of cirrhosis

admissions within 6 months [93]. Indeed, combining different tools, as exemplified by MoCA-CFS, could lead to better diagnosis of HE.

Furthermore, pathophysiological mechanisms of sarcopenia and frailty in the context of cirrhosis and HE should be further elucidated. This will allow to better elaborate targeted interventions to prevent or stabilize sarcopenia and frailty in patients with HE. Muscle mass optimization by exercise training and nutrition along with the use of technology should be an integral part of cirrhotic patients' management. This can be achieved only by a concerted effort of clinicians; health professionals including dietitians, nurses, physical therapists, psychologists, as well as patients and researchers.

References

1. Montagnese S, Russo FP, Amodio P, Burra P, Gasbarrini A, Loguercio C, et al. Hepatic encephalopathy 2018: a clinical practice guideline by the Italian Association for the Study of the Liver (AISF). Dig Liver Dis. 2019;51(2):190–205.
2. Tapper EB, Parikh ND, Waljee AK, Volk M, Carlozzi NE, Lok AS-F. Diagnosis of minimal hepatic encephalopathy: a systematic review of point-of-care diagnostic tests. Am J Gastroenterol. 2018;113(4):529–38.
3. Ridola L, Nardelli S, Gioia S, Riggio O. Quality of life in patients with minimal hepatic encephalopathy. World J Gastroenterol. 2018;24(48):5446–53.
4. Hartmann IJ, Groeneweg M, Quero JC, Beijeman SJ, de Man RA, Hop WC, et al. The prognostic significance of subclinical hepatic encephalopathy. Am J Gastroenterol. 2000;95(8):2029–34.
5. Allampati S, Duarte-Rojo A, Thacker LR, Patidar KR, White MB, Klair JS, et al. Diagnosis of minimal hepatic encephalopathy using stroop EncephalApp: a multicenter US-based, Norm-Based Study. Am J Gastroenterol. 2016;111(1):78–86.
6. Stewart CA, Malinchoc M, Kim WR, Kamath PS. Hepatic encephalopathy as a predictor of survival in patients with end-stage liver disease. Liver Transpl. 2007;13(10):1366–71.
7. Patidar KR, Thacker LR, Wade JB, Sterling RK, Sanyal AJ, Siddiqui MS, et al. Covert hepatic encephalopathy is independently associated with poor survival and increased risk of hospitalization. Am J Gastroenterol. 2014;109(11):1757–63.
8. Neff G, Iii WZ. Systematic review of the economic burden of overt hepatic encephalopathy and pharmacoeconomic impact of rifaximin. PharmacoEconomics. 2018;36(7):809–22.
9. Smith BW, Adams LA. Non-alcoholic fatty liver disease. Crit Rev Clin Lab Sci. 2011;48(3):97–113.
10. Butterworth RF. Altered glial-neuronal crosstalk: cornerstone in the pathogenesis of hepatic encephalopathy. Neurochem Int. 2010;57(4):383–8.
11. Bosoi CR, Parent-Robitaille C, Anderson K, Tremblay M, Rose CF. AST-120 (spherical carbon adsorbent) lowers ammonia levels and attenuates brain edema in bile-duct ligated rats. Hepatology. 2011;53(6):1995–2002.
12. Rovira A, Alonso J, Córdoba J. MR imaging findings in hepatic encephalopathy. AJNR Am J Neuroradiol. 2008;29(9):1612–21.
13. Bosoi CR, Yang X, Huynh J, Parent-Robitaille C, Jiang W, Tremblay M, et al. Systemic oxidative stress is implicated in the pathogenesis of brain edema in rats with chronic liver failure. Free Radic Biol Med. 2012;52(7):1228–35.
14. Bosoi CR, Rose CF. Identifying the direct effects of ammonia on the brain. Metab Brain Dis. 2009;24(1):95–102.

15. Butterworth RF. Pathophysiology of hepatic encephalopathy: a new look at ammonia. Metab Brain Dis. 2002;17(4):221–7.
16. Rose CF. Increase brain lactate in hepatic encephalopathy: cause or consequence? Neurochem Int. 2010;57(4):389–94.
17. Wright G, Noiret L, Damink SW, Jalan R. Interorgan ammonia metabolism in liver failure: the basis of current and future therapies. Liver Int. 2011;31(2):163–75.
18. Gluud LL, Vilstrup H, Morgan MY. Non-absorbable disaccharides versus placebo/no intervention and lactulose versus lactitol for the prevention and treatment of hepatic encephalopathy in people with cirrhosis. Cochrane Database Syst Rev. 2016;(5):CD003044.
19. van Leeuwen PA, van Berlo CL, Soeters PB. New mode of action for lactulose. Lancet. 1988;1(8575–6):55–6.
20. Teperman LW, Peyregne VP. Considerations on the impact of hepatic encephalopathy treatments in the pretransplant setting. Transplantation. 2010;89(7):771–8.
21. Tarao K, Ikeda T, Hayashi K, Sakurai A, Okada T, Ito T, et al. Successful use of vancomycin hydrochloride in the treatment of lactulose resistant chronic hepatic encephalopathy. Gut. 1990;31(6):702–6.
22. Mas A, Rodés J, Sunyer L, Rodrigo L, Planas R, Vargas V, et al. Comparison of rifaximin and lactitol in the treatment of acute hepatic encephalopathy: results of a randomized, double-blind, double-dummy, controlled clinical trial. J Hepatol. 2003;38(1):51–8.
23. Pedretti G, Calzetti C, Missale G, Fiaccadori F. Rifaximin versus neomycin on hyperammonemia in chronic portal systemic encephalopathy of cirrhotics. A double-blind, randomized trial. Ital J Gastroenterol. 1991;23(4):175–8.
24. Bass NM, Mullen KD, Sanyal A, Poordad F, Neff G, Leevy CB, et al. Rifaximin treatment in hepatic encephalopathy. N Engl J Med. 2010;362(12):1071–81.
25. Kawaguchi T, Suzuki F, Imamura M, Murashima N, Yanase M, Mine T, et al. Rifaximin-altered gut microbiota components associated with liver/neuropsychological functions in patients with hepatic encephalopathy: an exploratory data analysis of phase II/III clinical trials. Hepatol Res. 2019;49(4):404–18.
26. Malaguarnera M, Greco F, Barone G, Gargante MP, Malaguarnera M, Toscano MA. Bifidobacterium longum with fructo-oligosaccharide (FOS) treatment in minimal hepatic encephalopathy: a randomized, double-blind, placebo-controlled study. Dig Dis Sci. 2007;52(11):3259–65.
27. Bajaj JS, Saeian K, Christensen KM, Hafeezullah M, Varma RR, Franco J, et al. Probiotic yogurt for the treatment of minimal hepatic encephalopathy. Am J Gastroenterol. 2008;103(7):1707–15.
28. Dalal R, McGee RG, Riordan SM, Webster AC. Probiotics for people with hepatic encephalopathy. Cochrane Database Syst Rev. 2017;(2):CD008716.
29. Enns GM, Berry SA, Berry GT, Rhead WJ, Brusilow SW, Hamosh A. Survival after treatment with phenylacetate and benzoate for urea-cycle disorders. N Engl J Med. 2007;356(22):2282–92.
30. Sushma S, Dasarathy S, Tandon RK, Jain S, Gupta S, Bhist MS. Sodium benzoate in the treatment of acute hepatic encephalopathy: a double-blind randomized trial. Hepatology. 1992;16(1):138–44.
31. Weiss N, Tripon S, Lodey M, Guiller E, Junot H, Monneret D, et al. Treating hepatic encephalopathy in cirrhotic patients admitted to ICU with sodium phenylbutyrate: a preliminary study. Fundam Clin Pharmacol. 2018;32(2):209–15.
32. Rockey DC, Vierling JM, Mantry P, Ghabril M, Brown RS, Alexeeva O, et al. Randomized, double-blind, controlled study of glycerol phenylbutyrate in hepatic encephalopathy. Hepatology. 2014;59(3):1073–83.
33. Butterworth RF, Kircheis G, Hilger N, McPhail MJW. Efficacy of l-ornithine l-aspartate for the treatment of hepatic encephalopathy and hyperammonemia in cirrhosis: systematic review and meta-analysis of randomized controlled trials. J Clin Exp Hepatol. 2018;8(3):301–13.

34. Butterworth RF, McPhail MJW. L-Ornithine L-Aspartate (LOLA) for hepatic encephalopathy in cirrhosis: results of randomized controlled trials and meta-analyses. Drugs. 2019;79(Suppl 1):31–7.
35. Jalan R, Wright G, Davies NA, Hodges SJ. L-Ornithine phenylacetate (OP): a novel treatment for hyperammonemia and hepatic encephalopathy. Med Hypotheses. 2007;69(5):1064–9.
36. Stravitz RT, Gottfried M, Durkalski V, Fontana RJ, Hanje AJ, Koch D, et al. Safety, tolerability, and pharmacokinetics of l-ornithine phenylacetate in patients with acute liver injury/failure and hyperammonemia. Hepatology. 2018;67(3):1003–13.
37. Ventura-Cots M, Arranz JA, Simón-Talero M, Torrens M, Blanco A, Riudor E, et al. Safety of ornithine phenylacetate in cirrhotic decompensated patients: an open-label, dose-escalating, single-cohort study. J Clin Gastroenterol. 2013;47(10):881–7.
38. Ventura-Cots M, Concepción M, Arranz JA, Simón-Talero M, Torrens M, Blanco-Grau A, et al. Impact of ornithine phenylacetate (OCR-002) in lowering plasma ammonia after upper gastrointestinal bleeding in cirrhotic patients. Ther Adv Gastroenterol. 2016;9(6):823–35.
39. Yamato M, Muto Y, Yoshida T, Kato M, Moriwaki H. Clearance rate of plasma branched-chain amino acids correlates significantly with blood ammonia level in patients with liver cirrhosis. Int Hepatol Commun. 1995;3(2):91–6.
40. Wahren J, Felig P, Hagenfeldt L. Effect of protein ingestion on splanchnic and leg metabolism in normal man and in patients with diabetes mellitus. J Clin Invest. 1976;57(4):987–99.
41. Marchesini G, Dioguardi FS, Bianchi GP, Zoli M, Bellati G, Roffi L, et al. Long-term oral branched-chain amino acid treatment in chronic hepatic encephalopathy. A randomized double-blind casein-controlled trial. The Italian Multicenter Study Group. J Hepatol. 1990;11(1):92–101.
42. Gluud LL, Dam G, Les I, Marchesini G, Borre M, Aagaard NK, et al. Branched-chain amino acids for people with hepatic encephalopathy. Cochrane Database Syst Rev. 2017;(5):CD001939.
43. Malaguarnera M, Pistone G, Astuto M, Vecchio I, Raffaele R, Lo Giudice E, et al. Effects of L-acetylcarnitine on cirrhotic patients with hepatic coma: randomized double-blind, placebo-controlled trial. Dig Dis Sci. 2006;51(12):2242–7.
44. Martí-Carvajal AJ, Gluud C, Arevalo-Rodriguez I, Martí-Amarista CE. Acetyl-L-carnitine for patients with hepatic encephalopathy. Cochrane Database Syst Rev. 2019;(1):CD011451.
45. Gentile S, Guarino G, Romano M, Alagia IA, Fierro M, Annunziata S, et al. A randomized controlled trial of acarbose in hepatic encephalopathy. Clin Gastroenterol Hepatol. 2005;3(2):184–91.
46. Agostoni V, Lee SH, Forster V, Kabbaj M, Bosoi CR, Tremblay M, et al. Liposome-supported peritoneal dialysis for the treatment of hyperammonemia-associated encephalopathy. Adv Funct Mater. 2016;26(46):8382–9.
47. Kurtz CB, Millet YA, Puurunen MK, Perreault M, Charbonneau MR, Isabella VM, et al. An engineered E. coli Nissle improves hyperammonemia and survival in mice and shows dose-dependent exposure in healthy humans. Sci Transl Med. 2019;11(475):eaau7975.
48. Chen Y, Yang F, Lu H, Wang B, Chen Y, Lei D, et al. Characterization of fecal microbial communities in patients with liver cirrhosis. Hepatology. 2011;54(2):562–72.
49. Bajaj JS, Heuman DM, Hylemon PB, Sanyal AJ, White MB, Monteith P, et al. Altered profile of human gut microbiome is associated with cirrhosis and its complications. J Hepatol. 2014;60(5):940–7.
50. Bajaj JS, Kassam Z, Fagan A, Gavis EA, Liu E, Cox IJ, et al. Fecal microbiota transplant from a rational stool donor improves hepatic encephalopathy: a randomized clinical trial. Hepatology. 2017;66(6):1727–38.
51. Adam R, Hoti E. Liver transplantation: the current situation. Semin Liver Dis. 2009;29(1):3–18.
52. Sotil EU, Gottstein J, Ayala E, Randolph C, Blei AT. Impact of preoperative overt hepatic encephalopathy on neurocognitive function after liver transplantation. Liver Transpl. 2009;15(2):184–92.

53. Atluri DK, Asgeri M, Mullen KD. Reversibility of hepatic encephalopathy after liver transplantation. Metab Brain Dis. 2010;25(1):111–3.
54. Weiss N, Thabut D. Neurological complications occurring after liver transplantation: role of risk factors, hepatic encephalopathy, and acute (on chronic) brain injury. Liver Transpl. 2019;25(3):469–87.
55. Bemeur C. Neurological complications post-liver transplantation: impact of nutritional status. Metab Brain Dis. 2013;28(2):293–300.
56. Cruz-Jentoft AJ, Bahat G, Bauer J, Boirie Y, Bruyère O, Cederholm T, et al. Sarcopenia: revised European consensus on definition and diagnosis. Age Ageing. 2019;48(1):16–31.
57. Merli M, Giusto M, Lucidi C, Giannelli V, Pentassuglio I, Di Gregorio V, et al. Muscle depletion increases the risk of overt and minimal hepatic encephalopathy: results of a prospective study. Metab Brain Dis. 2013;28(2):281–4.
58. Selberg O, Böttcher J, Tusch G, Pichlmayr R, Henkel E, Müller MJ. Identification of high- and low-risk patients before liver transplantation: a prospective cohort study of nutritional and metabolic parameters in 150 patients. Hepatology. 1997;25(3):652–7.
59. Hartman C, Eliakim R, Shamir R. Nutritional status and nutritional therapy in inflammatory bowel diseases. World J Gastroenterol. 2009;15(21):2570–8.
60. Montano-Loza AJ, Duarte-Rojo A, Meza-Junco J, Baracos VE, Sawyer MB, Pang JXQ, et al. Inclusion of sarcopenia within MELD (MELD-sarcopenia) and the prediction of mortality in patients with cirrhosis. Clin Transl Gastroenterol. 2015;6(7):e102.
61. Chang K-V, Chen J-D, Wu W-T, Huang K-C, Lin H-Y, Han D-S. Is sarcopenia associated with hepatic encephalopathy in liver cirrhosis? A systematic review and meta-analysis. J Formos Med Assoc. 2019;118(4):833–42.
62. Tapper EB, Jiang ZG, Patwardhan VR. Refining the ammonia hypothesis: a physiology-driven approach to the treatment of hepatic encephalopathy. Mayo Clin Proc. 2015;90(5):646–58.
63. Kumar A, Davuluri G, Silva RNE, Engelen MPKJ, Ten Have GAM, Prayson R, et al. Ammonia lowering reverses sarcopenia of cirrhosis by restoring skeletal muscle proteostasis. Hepatology. 2017;65(6):2045–58.
64. Hanai T, Shirakı M, Watanabe S, Kochi T, Imai K, Suetsugu A, et al. Sarcopenia predicts minimal hepatic encephalopathy in patients with liver cirrhosis. Hepatol Res. 2017;47(13):1359–67.
65. Dasarathy S, Mookerjee RP, Rackayova V, Rangroo Thrane V, Vairappan B, Ott P, et al. Ammonia toxicity: from head to toe? Metab Brain Dis. 2017;32(2):529–38.
66. Kant S, Davuluri G, Alchirazi KA, Welch N, Heit C, Kumar A, et al. Ethanol sensitizes skeletal muscle to ammonia-induced molecular perturbations. J Biol Chem. 2019;294(18):7231–44.
67. Bhanji RA, Moctezuma-Velazquez C, Duarte-Rojo A, Ebadi M, Ghosh S, Rose C, et al. Myosteatosis and sarcopenia are associated with hepatic encephalopathy in patients with cirrhosis. Hepatol Int. 2018;12(4):377–86.
68. Thandassery RB, Montano-Loza AJ. Role of nutrition and muscle in cirrhosis. Curr Treat Options Gastroenterol. 2016;14(2):257–73.
69. Zenith L, Meena N, Ramadi A, Yavari M, Harvey A, Carbonneau M, et al. Eight weeks of exercise training increases aerobic capacity and muscle mass and reduces fatigue in patients with cirrhosis. Clin Gastroenterol Hepatol. 2014;12(11):1920–1926.e2.
70. Román E, García-Galcerán C, Torrades T, Herrera S, Marín A, Doñate M, et al. Effects of an exercise programme on functional capacity, body composition and risk of falls in patients with cirrhosis: a randomized clinical trial. PLoS One. 2016;11(3):e0151652.
71. Kruger C, McNeely ML, Bailey RJ, Yavari M, Abraldes JG, Carbonneau M, et al. Home exercise training improves exercise capacity in cirrhosis patients: role of exercise adherence. Sci Rep. 2018;8(1):99.
72. Amodio P, Bemeur C, Butterworth R, Cordoba J, Kato A, Montagnese S, et al. The nutritional management of hepatic encephalopathy in patients with cirrhosis: international society for hepatic encephalopathy and nitrogen metabolism consensus. Hepatology. 2013;58(1):325–36.

73. Aamann L, Tandon P, Bémeur C. Role of exercise in the management of hepatic encephalopathy: experience from animal and human studies. J Clin Exp Hepatol. 2019;9(1):131–6.
74. Bémeur C, Butterworth RF. Nutrition in the management of cirrhosis and its neurological complications. J Clin Exp Hepatol. [Internet]. 2013 [cited 2013 Jun 24]. Available from: http://www.sciencedirect.com/science/article/pii/S0973688313005550.
75. Fried LP, Tangen CM, Walston J, Newman AB, Hirsch C, Gottdiener J, et al. Frailty in older adults: evidence for a phenotype. J Gerontol A Biol Sci Med Sci. 2001;56(3):M146–56.
76. Landi F, Calvani R, Cesari M, Tosato M, Martone AM, Bernabei R, et al. Sarcopenia as the biological substrate of physical frailty. Clin Geriatr Med. 2015;31(3):367–74.
77. Lai JC, Feng S, Terrault NA, Lizaola B, Hayssen H, Covinsky K. Frailty predicts waitlist mortality in liver transplant candidates. Am J Transplant. 2014;14(8):1870–9.
78. Carey EJ, Steidley DE, Aqel BA, Byrne TJ, Mekeel KL, Rakela J, et al. Six-minute walk distance predicts mortality in liver transplant candidates. Liver Transpl. 2010;16(12):1373–8.
79. Alvares-da-Silva MR, Reverbel da Silveira T. Comparison between handgrip strength, subjective global assessment, and prognostic nutritional index in assessing malnutrition and predicting clinical outcome in cirrhotic outpatients. Nutrition. 2005;21(2):113–7.
80. Tapper EB, Konerman M, Murphy S, Sonnenday CJ. Hepatic encephalopathy impacts the predictive value of the Fried Frailty Index. Am J Transplant. 2018;18(10):2566–70.
81. Lai JC, Dodge JL, Sen S, Covinsky K, Feng S. Functional decline in patients with cirrhosis awaiting liver transplantation: results from the functional assessment in liver transplantation (FrAILT) study. Hepatology. 2016;63(2):574–80.
82. Englesbe MJ, Patel SP, He K, Lynch RJ, Schaubel DE, Harbaugh C, et al. Sarcopenia and mortality after liver transplantation. J Am Coll Surg. 2010;211(2):271–8.
83. Laube R, Wang H, Park L, Heyman JK, Vidot H, Majumdar A, et al. Frailty in advanced liver disease. Liver Int. 2018;38(12):2117–28.
84. Trivedi HD, Tapper EB. Interventions to improve physical function and prevent adverse events in cirrhosis. Gastroenterol Rep (Oxf). 2018;6(1):13–20.
85. Boyle PA, Buchman AS, Wilson RS, Leurgans SE, Bennett DA. Physical frailty is associated with incident mild cognitive impairment in community-based older persons. J Am Geriatr Soc. 2010;58(2):248–55.
86. Rosado-Artalejo C, Carnicero JA, Losa-Reyna J, Guadalupe-Grau A, Castillo-Gallego C, Gutierrez-Avila G, et al. Cognitive performance across 3 frailty phenotypes: Toledo study for healthy aging. J Am Med Dir Assoc. 2017;18(9):785–90.
87. Morley JE, Morris JC, Berg-Weger M, Borson S, Carpenter BD, Del Campo N, et al. Brain health: the importance of recognizing cognitive impairment: an IAGG consensus conference. J Am Med Dir Assoc. 2015;16(9):731–9.
88. Calzà L, Beltrami D, Gagliardi G, Ghidoni E, Marcello N, Rossini-Favretti R, et al. Should we screen for cognitive decline and dementia? Maturitas. 2015;82(1):28–35.
89. Kelaiditi E, Cesari M, Canevelli M, van Kan GA, Ousset P-J, Gillette-Guyonnet S, et al. Cognitive frailty: rational and definition from an (I.A.N.A./I.A.G.G.) international consensus group. J Nutr Health Aging. 2013;17(9):726–34.
90. Davis BC, Bajaj JS. Effects of alcohol on the brain in cirrhosis: beyond hepatic encephalopathy. Alcohol Clin Exp Res. 2018;42(4):660–7.
91. Ahluwalia V, Wade JB, Moeller FG, White MB, Unser AB, Gavis EA, et al. The etiology of cirrhosis is a strong determinant of brain reserve: a multimodal magnetic resonance imaging study. Liver Transpl. 2015;21(9):1123–32.
92. Solfrizzi V, Scafato E, Seripa D, Lozupone M, Imbimbo BP, D'Amato A, et al. Reversible cognitive frailty, dementia, and all-cause mortality. The Italian Longitudinal Study on Aging. J Am Med Dir Assoc. 2017;18(1):89.e1–8.

93. Ney M, Tangri N, Dobbs B, Bajaj J, Rolfson D, Ma M, et al. Predicting hepatic encephalopathy-related hospitalizations using a composite assessment of cognitive impairment and frailty in 355 patients with cirrhosis. Am J Gastroenterol. 2018;113(10):1506–15.
94. Bagshaw SM, Stelfox HT, McDermid RC, Rolfson DB, Tsuyuki RT, Baig N, et al. Association between frailty and short- and long-term outcomes among critically ill patients: a multicentre prospective cohort study. CMAJ. 2014;186(2):E95–102.
95. Sujino Y, Tanno J, Nakano S, Funada S, Hosoi Y, Senbonmatsu T, et al. Impact of hypoalbuminemia, frailty, and body mass index on early prognosis in older patients (≥85 years) with ST-elevation myocardial infarction. J Cardiol. 2015;66(3):263–8.
96. Nasreddine ZS, Phillips NA, Bédirian V, Charbonneau S, Whitehead V, Collin I, et al. The Montreal Cognitive Assessment, MoCA: a brief screening tool for mild cognitive impairment. J Am Geriatr Soc. 2005;53(4):695–9.
97. Pendlebury ST, Cuthbertson FC, Welch SJV, Mehta Z, Rothwell PM. Underestimation of cognitive impairment by Mini-Mental State Examination versus the Montreal Cognitive Assessment in patients with transient ischemic attack and stroke: a population-based study. Stroke. 2010;41(6):1290–3.

Chapter 18
A Research Wish List to Understand, Diagnose, and Manage Frailty and Sarcopenia

Michael A. Dunn

Muscle and the Liver-Brain-Gut Axis

There has been a rapid progress in our understanding of the key connections mediated by substrates, cytokines, and other signaling messengers among the liver, the brain, and the gut, a constellation described as the gut-liver-brain axis [1]. Appreciation of the functions of this axis in response to impaired ammonia metabolism in advanced liver disease, for example, illustrates the impact of interorgan shifts in handling this key substrate on the development of hepatic encephalopathy.

Muscle, as the obligate location where extrahepatic ammonia disposition takes place in advanced cirrhosis, is best understood as the fourth member of this axis. Until now, however, we have mainly thought more about muscle as an end target in these pathologic relationships rather than as a key culprit promoting injury and pathologic signaling.

Are muscle disturbances an independent driver of liver injury in addition to being a consequence? Bhanji et al. reviewed evidence supporting the proposal that sarcopenia could be a contributing cause of nonalcoholic fatty liver disease [2]. They noted that sarcopenia promotes insulin resistance independent of obesity because muscle is the primary tissue responsible for insulin-mediated glucose disposal. In addition, sarcopenia is associated with nonalcoholic fatty liver disease independent of obesity, insulin resistance, or the metabolic syndrome.

As an endocrine organ, muscle produces cytokines such as myostatin, interleukin-6, and irisin. Myostatin impairs muscle protein synthesis and promotes proteolysis. Myostatin also increases adipose tissue mass and leads to decreased adiponectin.

M. A. Dunn (✉)
Center for Liver Diseases, Thomas E. Starzl Transplantation Institute, Pittsburgh, PA, USA

Pittsburgh Liver Research Center, University of Pittsburgh, Pittsburgh, PA, USA
e-mail: dunnma@upmc.edu

© Springer Nature Switzerland AG 2020
P. Tandon, A. J. Montano-Loza (eds.), *Frailty and Sarcopenia in Cirrhosis*,
https://doi.org/10.1007/978-3-030-26226-6_18

Both interleukin-6 and irisin are thought to be protective in fatty liver disease. Could muscle loss result in their deficient production and consequently promote disease progression?

Alcohol, the premier multi-organ toxin, regularly injures both the liver and muscle. The mechanisms involved in alcoholic muscle injury have been recently reviewed [3]. However, whether alcohol-induced muscle loss can potentiate alcoholic liver injury in a similar manner to that proposed above for the impact of sarcopenia on nonalcoholic fatty liver disease is an open question that merits study.

Our understanding of the relationships between perturbations of the gut microbiome, known as dysbiosis, and the progression of cirrhosis complications is rapidly expanding [4]. Microbial products entering the circulation through a permeable gut barrier have cytokine-like deleterious effects. In parallel with these advances, there has also been robust progress in defining the impacts of gut microbial dysbiosis on sarcopenia [5]. Both gut-liver and gut-muscle communications involve similar messengers, so that it now seems opportune to consider effects of common gut-derived signals on the liver and muscle. Defining the components of gut-liver-muscle cross talk could provide new insight for their significance in liver disease.

Adrenergic Signaling and Muscle in Liver Disease

The adrenergic nervous system is highly complex and involves a multitude of important effects on circulation and metabolic processes. In advanced liver disease, we have learned, often by trial and error, how to protect patients from variceal bleeding with nonselective beta blocker treatment while limiting its adverse impacts on patients with impaired cardiac function, ascites, abnormal renal circulation, and increased gut permeability [6]. Evidence that we are only beginning to appreciate the full scope of adrenergic effects in hepatology is emerging from data on the impact of adrenergic signaling in muscle.

Agricultural use of beta agonists in meat production is widespread because of their ability to increase lean muscle mass in cattle, swine, and poultry. Concerning muscle performance, competition athletes frequently engaged in doping with beta agonists for performance enhancement before their prohibition and mandated testing was enforced by the World Anti-Doping Agency. Interestingly, an exception allowing their use by Olympic athletes with exercise-induced asthma had the result that competitors with permission to use the beta agonist salmeterol won twice the expected number of Olympic medals as those who did not [7]. If beta adrenergic stimulation is a trophic requirement for muscle performance and health, could we learn whether nonselective beta blockade in sarcopenic cirrhotic patients affects muscle mass or performance?

The liver is richly innervated with adrenergic and cholinergic afferent and efferent fibers that generate traffic with the brainstem and cerebral cortex. The signaling exerts important known effects on energy intake, glucose utilization, and lipid metabolism [8]. Virtually nothing is known about how structural or inflammatory liver diseases might affect these pathways and consequently impact key substrate flows to muscle. Subjective severe fatigue is commonplace in cirrhosis, and as noted below, cirrhotic patients often grossly overestimate their levels of physical activity. Could aberrant autonomic central nervous system inputs from a cirrhotic organ be part of the explanation for these highly prevalent brain and volitional drivers of cirrhotic frailty and sarcopenia?

Metabolic Priorities

Excess ammonia delivered to muscle is the key multipotent metabolic driver of frailty and sarcopenia in cirrhotic patients. As shown in Fig. 18.1, the obligate need for muscle to process and export excess ammonia as glutamine depletes critical substrates for muscle protein synthesis and mitochondrial function. Ammonia-mediated myostatin release also impairs protein synthesis, and ammonia independently stimulates autophagy and impairs muscle contractility.

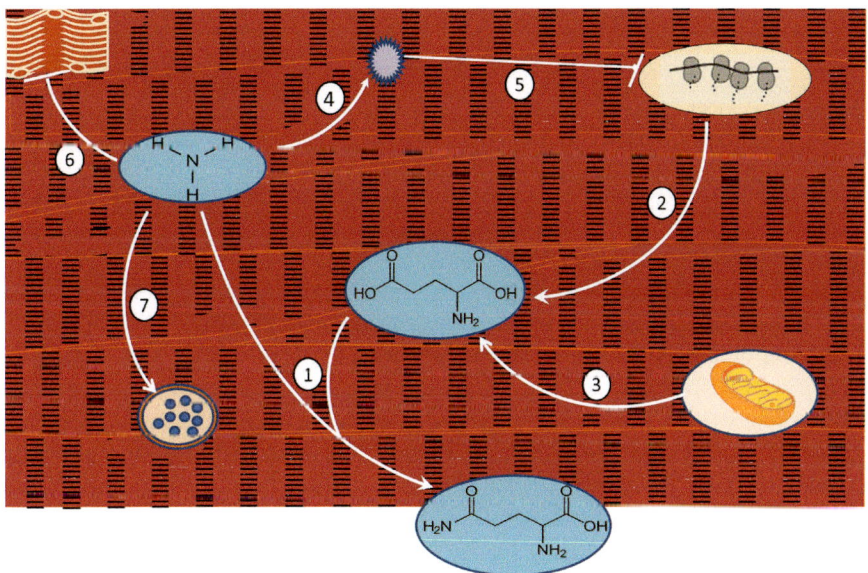

Fig. 18.1 Ammonia, the key metabolic driver of cirrhotic muscle wasting (1). Excess ammonia delivered to muscle combines with glutamic acid to form glutamine. Glutamine delivered to the gut becomes the primary ammonia excretion path in cirrhosis. (2) The increased need for glutamic acid depletes the amino acid pool needed for protein synthesis. (3) Glutamic acid formation from alpha-ketoglutarate depletes that important citric acid cycle intermediate, impairing mitochondrial energy generation. (4, 5) Ammonia triggers formation and release of myostatin, a cytokine that blocks muscle protein synthesis by mTOR inhibition. (6) Ammonia directly inhibits muscle contractility. (7) Ammonia stimulates muscle lysosomal autophagy

Dasarathy and Hatzgolou reviewed the concept of proteostasis in muscle, or maintenance of muscle mass, as the balance between muscle protein synthesis and proteolysis [9]. They describe a hyperammonemic stress response in cirrhosis with both stimulation of myostatin release and phosphorylation of the eukaryotic translation initiation factor 2 (eIF2) alpha subunit; both events inhibit muscle protein synthesis. Davuluri et al. showed that administration of L-leucine in rats and cirrhotic patients could restore muscle protein synthesis and promote proteostasis [10].

While the mechanisms of ammonia-mediated myotoxicity in cirrhosis are now better defined, we lack evidence for safe and effective practical interventions to fully reverse the problem.

At present, our ability to achieve a goal of fully suppressing ammonia excess to the normal range within the muscle and brain using our available medications—lactulose and rifaximin—is limited at best in most cirrhotic patients. If adding a tailored leucine-enriched amino acid mixture to our current treatment regimen could reliably normalize or minimize ammonia excess, would that intervention help to stabilize muscle mass, muscle strength, or muscle protein? Most of the preliminary reports of successful treatment of the problem reported elsewhere in this book have used a combination of nutritional support along with a physical activity regimen. Is there a minimum level of daily physical activity needed to show benefit for a tailored metabolic therapy?

Measuring Frailty and Sarcopenia

Methods to measure frailty and sarcopenia are illustrated in Fig. 18.2 and discussed in depth elsewhere in this volume. The skeletal muscle index, an anatomic measurement of sarcopenia based on segmental analysis of muscle on CT scans at the L3 vertebral level, has now been reported in a multicenter cohort of North American liver transplant candidates with sarcopenia cutoff values of muscle area normalized to patient height of 50 cm^2/m^2 in men and 39 cm^2/m^2 in women [11]. Handgrip, along with performance of chair stands and balance, is a component of the Liver Frailty Index (LFI), a composite frailty measurement with robust predictive accuracy for liver transplant outcomes [12]. Personal activity monitoring, as shown with a Fitbit in Fig. 18.2, has been evaluated in liver transplant candidates in comparison with self-reported activity estimates [13].

Objective activity measurements have strong potential for improving cirrhosis care and monitoring the effectiveness of physical activity interventions.

Anatomic sarcopenia measurements using CT scanning are normally performed when an imaging study with its attendant low-dose radiation exposure is clinically indicated; repetitive scans depend on clinical need. DEXA and bio-impedance methods are subject to variation in body water content, common in cirrhosis, and have not been considered a gold standard for that reason. Very recently a method

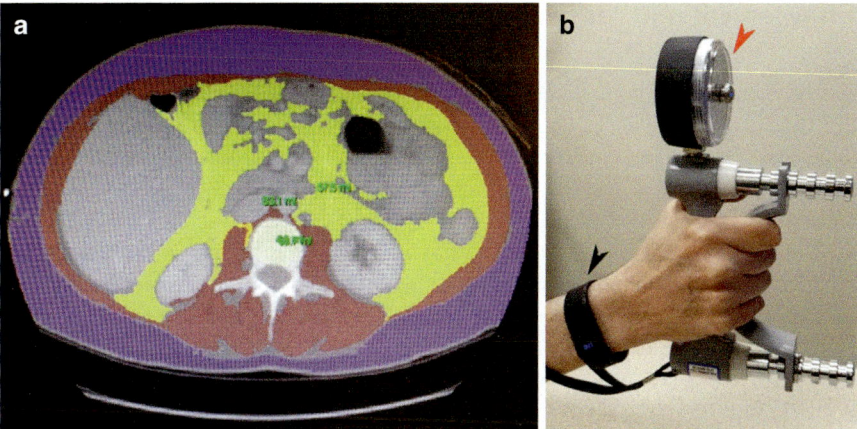

Fig. 18.2 Measuring sarcopenia, physical activity, and frailty. (**a**) A CT cross section at vertebral level L3 with muscle highlighted in red, used for calculation of the skeletal muscle index, SMI, as cm^2 of muscle area divided by patient height in m^2. Gender-specific SMI cutoffs, 50 cm^2/m^2 in men and 39 cm^2/m^2 in women, are used to standardize sarcopenia measurement in liver transplant candidates [11]. (**b**) Black arrow. A wearable personal activity monitor. Web-based transmission delivers step count, heart rate, calories expended, and activity intensity to a user's smartphone and their electronic medical record. (**b**) Red arrow. A dynamometer for measuring grip strength, a component of the Liver Frailty Index [12]

relying on administration of D3-creatine, which distributes rapidly and completely to the muscle compartment, was reported that may prove valuable for the precise, repetitive total muscle mass measurements needed to further study anatomic sarcopenia in cirrhotic patients [14].

Of the functional measurements of frailty reviewed elsewhere in this volume, the LFI has the advantage of ease of performance and robust association with transplant-related outcomes. Its three elements take strength, balance, and performance of chair stands, a task requiring coordination, into account. Gait speed, while slightly less accurate when compared with the LFI for predictive value, also depends on integration of strength, stability, and coordination. As a global index of mobility, it is understood by the general geriatric community and, as a patient reinforcement tool, matches what many patients actually do in home-based walking programs. The 6-minute walk distance also has merit for its strong association with transplant outcomes, and it offers better measurement of sustained activity capacity than provided by other tests [15].

Important research questions that merit exploration for these measurements in general cirrhosis care and transplant hepatology include what their optimal frequency should be over time, how to assess the clinical meaning of changes over time, whether they have prognostic value independent of other measurements, and how they can best be used to engage patients in self-motivation.

Engagement and Motivation

As noted earlier, cirrhotic patients who experience easy fatigue and low energy tend to overestimate their level of activity, with likely deleterious effects on their maintenance of physical capacity to withstand stress such as that of transplantation. Liver transplant candidates who assess themselves as highly or moderately active are among the most sedentary patients ever studied when daily activity is objectively measured [13]. As the proportion of patients with advanced cirrhosis attributed to nonalcoholic steatohepatitis continues to increase, we can only expect inactivity, a cardinal feature of the metabolic syndrome, to intensify rather than improve. In overcoming such a formidable barrier to wellness, it appears important to energetically seek out, assess, and treat depression and substance disorders, to engage supportive family and caregivers, and to consider every available behavioral support option.

Berzigotti et al. reported a promising initiative that capitalized on positive group dynamics and a recreational intervention framework, the SportDiet study, in which 50 of an initial cohort of 60 obese cirrhotic patients with portal hypertension completed a 16-week intensive lifestyle intervention experience with substantial improvements in body mass index and portal pressure gradient [16].

Cirrhosis care is highly dependent on careful compliance with often-demanding treatment programs in a patient population that tends to have limited physical or psychological capacity for full engagement. With respect to research opportunity, there is a great untapped potential for comparative effectiveness study of best practices for tailored care delivery in this demanding population.

Timing Is Everything: Is Change Sustainable?

One of the most important knowledge gaps in cirrhosis care is our limited understanding of the temporal profile associated with potential interventions. We can estimate with reasonable accuracy the time course of likely survival to transplant based on MELD-Na trajectory or progression of CNI-induced renal failure. We lack information on whether recovery of physical performance after completing an exercise program is sustainable, what can be predicted with accuracy about functional recovery after liver transplantation [17], and how an improvement in LFI might be associated with sustained improvement of a quality of life metric. Interest and publications on frailty and sarcopenia in liver disease have attracted a growing interest over the 7 years since its inception. It will be important when possible to determine the sustainability of the improved outcomes that we seek.

References

1. Patel VC, White H, Støy S, et al. Clinical science workshop: targeting the gut-liver-brain axis. Metab Brain Dis. 2016;31:1327–37.
2. Bhanji RA, Narayanan P, Allen AM, et al. Sarcopenia in hiding: the risk and consequence of underestimating muscle dysfunction in NASH. Hepatology. 2017;66:2055–65.
3. Simon L, Jolley SE, Molina PE. Alcoholic myopathy: pathophysiologic mechanisms and clinical implications. Alcohol Res. 2017;38:207–17.
4. Acharya C, Bajaj JS. The microbiome in cirrhosis and its complications. Clin Gastroenterol Hepatol. 2019;17:307–21.
5. Ticinesi A, Lauretani F, Milani C, et al. Aging gut microbiota at the cross-road between nutrition, physical frailty, and sarcopenia: is there a gut–muscle axis? Nutrients. 2017;9:1303.
6. Reiberger T, Mandorfer M. Beta adrenergic blockade and decompensated cirrhosis. J Hepatol. 2017;66:849–59.
7. Jacobson GA, Fawcett JP. Beta2-agonist doping control and optical isomer challenges. Sports Med. 2016;46:1787–95.
8. Kandilis AN, Papadopoulou IP, Koskinas J, et al. Liver innervation and hepatic function: new insights. J Surg Res. 2015;194:511–9.
9. Dasarathy S, Hatzgolou M. Hyperammonemia and proteostasis in cirrhosis. Curr Opin Clin Nutr Metab Care. 2018;21:30–6.
10. Davuluri G, Krowkowski D, Guan BJ, et al. Metabolic adaptation of skeletal muscle to hyperammonemia drives the beneficial effects of L-leucine in cirrhosis. J Hepatol. 2016;65:929–37.
11. Carey EJ, Lai JC, Wang CW, et al. A multicenter study to define sarcopenia in patients with end-stage liver disease. Liver Transpl. 2017;23:625–33.
12. Lai JC, Covinsky KE, Dodge JL, et al. Development of a novel frailty index to predict mortality in patients with end-stage liver disease. Hepatology. 2017;66:564–74.
13. Dunn MA, Josbeno DA, Schmotzer AR, et al. The gap between clinically assessed physical performance and objective physical activity in liver transplant candidates. Liver Transpl. 2016;22:1324–32.
14. Cawthon PM, Orwoll ES, Peters KE, et al. Strong relation between muscle mass determined by D3-creatine dilution, physical performance and incidence of falls and mobility limitations in a prospective cohort of older men. J Gerontol A Biol Sci Med Sci. 2019;74(6):844–52.
15. Carey EJ, Steidley DE, Aqel BA, et al. Six-minute walk distance predicts mortality in liver transplant candidates. Liver Transpl. 2010;16:1373–8.
16. Berzigotti A, Albillos A, Villanueva C, et al. Effects of an intensive lifestyle intervention program on portal hypertension in patients with cirrhosis and obesity: the SportDiet study. Hepatology. 2017;65:1293–305.
17. Lai JC, Segev DL, McCulloch CE, et al. Physical frailty after liver transplantation. Am J Transplant. 2018;18:1986–94.

Index

© Springer Nature Switzerland AG 2020
P. Tandon, A. J. Montano-Loza (eds.), *Frailty and Sarcopenia in Cirrhosis*,
https://doi.org/10.1007/978-3-030-26226-6

Printed by Printforce, the Netherlands